Gunzburg et al. (Eds.) **The Use of Bone Substitutes in Spine Surgery**

Springer
Berlin
Heidelberg
New York
Barcelona
Hong Kong
London
Milan
Paris
Tokyo

R. Gunzburg · M. Szpalski · N. Passuti · M. Aebi
(Editors)

The Use of Bone Substitutes in Spine Surgery

A State of the Art Review

With 61 Figures and 18 Tables

Springer

Dr. Robert Gunzburg
Eeuwfeestkliniek
Harmoniestraat 68
2018 Antwerp
Belgium

Dr. Norbert Passuti
Clinique Chirurgicale Orthopédique
Hôtel Dieu
1, Place Alexis Ricordeau
44093 Nantes Cedex 1
France

Dr. Marek Szpalski
Centre Hospitalier Molière
Longchamps
Rue Marconi 142
1180 Brussels
Belgium

Dr. Max Aebi
McGill University/
Royal Victoria Hospital
Division of Orthopaedic Surgery
Montreal, Quebec
Canada

ISBN 3-540-42687-6 Springer-Verlag Berlin Heidelberg NewYork

Also published as Volume 10, Supplement 2, October 2001
of the European Spine Journal
ISSN 0940-6719

Die Deutsche Bibliothek – CIP-Einheitsaufnahme
The use of bone substitutes in spine surgery: a state of the art review /
ed.: Robert Gunzburg ... – Berlin; Heidelberg; New York; Barcelona;
Hongkong; London; Mailand; Paris; Tokio: Springer, 2002
ISBN 3-540-42687-6

Springer-Verlag Berlin Heidelberg New York
a member of BertelsmannSpringer Science+Business Media GmbH
http://www.springer.de

Cover design: e STUDIO CALAMAR, Pau/Girona
Typesetting, printing and bookbinding: ROTABENE, Rothenburg o. d. T.

Printed on acid-free paper SPIN 10883662 24/3111 5 4 3 2 1

Contents

Robert Gunzburg
Marek Szpalski
Norbert Passuti
Max Aebi

Biomaterials: the new frontiers in spine surgery

Recent developments in surgical techniques have led to an increased demand for bone stock. Fusion enhancement, bone void filling in tumor surgery and trauma are only a few examples. Autologous bone can be considered as the most successful bone graft material, and constitutes the accepted "gold standard", as it combines all the properties required from a bone graft: osteoinductivity, osteoconductivity and osteogenic potential. However, it is linked to a nonnegligible morbidity, and the quantity available for harvesting is limited and may be insufficient. Over the years, many solutions have been proposed, from the use of plaster of Paris to homologous frozen bone (allografts), dried heterologous bone (xenografts) or even corals. Growth of demand combined with the limitations of the "gold standard" has led to wide use of processed allografts. While those materials are always osteoconductive, their possible (but still disputed) osteoinductive properties depend on the processing technique. Those substances carry a minimal, but possible, risk of infectious disease transmission, and the recent discoveries about the almost indestructible properties of prions have to increase our level of caution.

Osteoinductive materials such as demineralized bone matrix (DBM) have been used, and the research on bone morphogenic proteins (BMP) may open the door to fascinating possibilities. It may be that the use of BMP will enable the achievement of better bone healing and/or fusion than using the "gold standard".

Many artificial biodegradable bone substitutes, mostly based on calcium phosphate ceramics, are now commercially available. While their biological safety may be certain, their true value as isolated graft material is still under scrutiny. A lot of work is currently being performed on the use of bone marrow aspirate and BMP in combination with these synthetic cancellous bone substitutes, which may render the need for autografts obsolete in the near future.

The ultimate aim is one of an unlimited supply of material that is both osteoconducting and osteoinducting, with a modulus of elasticity comparable to that of living human bone.

However, despite all the research accomplished, many questions remain about the specific mechanisms involved in spine fusion, and the study of gene expression should help us to better understand the biological processes leading to a solid bone fusion.

In this supplement we present a 'state of the art in bone substitution for the spine'. The general principles of bone biology and bone healing are outlined, as are recent advances in understanding and influencing bone formation. A variety of substitutes are described and compared.

Obviously, such new bone substitutes only represent an adjuvant to surgery and will remain secondary to a proper surgical indication and a sound surgical technique.

R. Gunzburg (✉)
Eeuwfeestkliniek, Harmoniestraat 68, 2018 Antwerp, Belgium
e-mail: r.gunzburg@worldonline.be

M. Szpalski
21 avenue Coghen, Brussels, Belgium

N. Passuti
Clinique Chirurgicale Orthopédique, Nantes, France

M. Aebi
Division of Orthopaedic Surgery, McGill University,
Royal Victoria Hospital, Montreal, Quebec, Canada

D. W. Sommerfeldt
C. T. Rubin

Biology of bone and how it orchestrates the form and function of the skeleton

D.W. Sommerfeldt (✉) · C.T. Rubin
Center for Biotechnology,
State University of New York,
Stony Brook, New York, USA
e-mail: Clinton.Rubin@sunysb.edu,
Tel.: +1-631-632-8521,
Fax: +1-631-632-8577

D.W. Sommerfeldt · C.T. Rubin
Musculo-Skeletal Research Laboratory,
Department of Biomedical Engineering,
State University of New York, Stony
Brook, New York, USA

Abstract The principal role of the skeleton is to provide structural support for the body. While the skeleton also serves as the body's mineral reservoir, the mineralized structure is the very basis of posture, opposes muscular contraction resulting in motion, withstands functional load bearing, and protects internal organs. Although the mass and morphology of the skeleton is defined, to some extent, by genetic determinants, it is the tissue's ability to remodel – the local resorption and formation of bone – which is responsible for achieving this intricate balance between competing responsibilities. The aim of this review is to address bone's form–function relationship, beginning with extensive research in the musculoskeletal disciplines, and focusing on several recent cellular and molecular discoveries which help understand the complex interdependence of bone cells, growth factors, physical stimuli, metabolic demands, and structural responsibilities. With a clinical and spine-oriented audience in mind, the principles of bone cell and molecular biology and physiology are presented, and an attempt has been made to incorporate epidemiologic data and therapeutic implications. Bone research remains interdisciplinary by nature, and a deeper understanding of bone biology will ultimately lead to advances in the treatment of diseases and injuries to bone itself.

Keywords Bone · Skeleton · Orthopedic · Growth Factors · Morphology · Osteoblasts · Osteoclasts · Osteocytes · Remodeling

Introduction

The skeleton's principal role as a structure has predisposed bone to the unfortunate reputation of being an inert and static material. Given bone tissue's ability to adapt its mass and morphology to functional demands, its ability to repair itself without leaving a scar, and its capacity to rapidly mobilize mineral stores on metabolic demand, it is in fact the ultimate "smart" material [43] and a dynamic example of "form follows function" in biological systems [45]. Considering the ever-growing number of patients who suffer from devastating disorders of the skeleton and the ever-increasing opportunities inherent in the post-genomics era to treat diseases and injuries to bone [44], it is critical for both the physician and the scientist to more fully understand the biology of bone and how its ability to form and resorb tissue ultimately orchestrates the structural and metabolic successes of the skeleton.

Cells

Three distinctly different cell types can be found within bone: the matrix-producing osteoblast, the tissue-resorbing osteoclast, and the osteocyte, which accounts for 90% of all cells in the adult skeleton. Osteocytes can be viewed as highly specialized and fully differentiated osteoblasts;

similarly, osteoblasts have recently been described as sophisticated fibroblasts [19]. Fibroblasts, osteoblasts, osteocytes, and adipocytes derive from pluripotent mesenchymal stem cells [3], whereas osteoclasts are of hematopoietic descent and their precursors are located in the monocytic fraction of the bone marrow [22].

Osteoblasts

Functionally, osteoblasts are the cells within bone that lay down the extracellular matrix and regulate its mineralization. Morphologically, these cells are cuboidal in shape and located at the bone surface together with their precursors, where they form a tight layer of cells. Osteoblasts are highly anchorage dependent and rely on extensive cell–matrix and cell–cell contacts via a variety of transmembranous proteins (integrins, connexins, cadherins) and specific receptors (for cytokines, hormones, growth factors) to maintain cellular function and responsiveness to metabolic and mechanical stimuli [21,29].

The lifespan of an osteoblast ranges between 3 days in young rabbits up to 8 weeks in humans, during which time it lays down 0.5–1.5 μm osteoid per day [27,36]. Eventually, some osteoblasts may become "trapped" in their own calcified matrix, changing their phenotype and developing into osteocytes. These cells continue to thrive, but considerably reduce their cell organelles and the production of matrix proteins. They remain connected with other similar cells but also with bone-lining cells (inactive osteoblasts) at the bone's surface, creating an extensive network of intercellular communication. There is accumulating evidence for a functional role of these cellular connections in sensing the need for and directing the site of new bone formation [15,33].

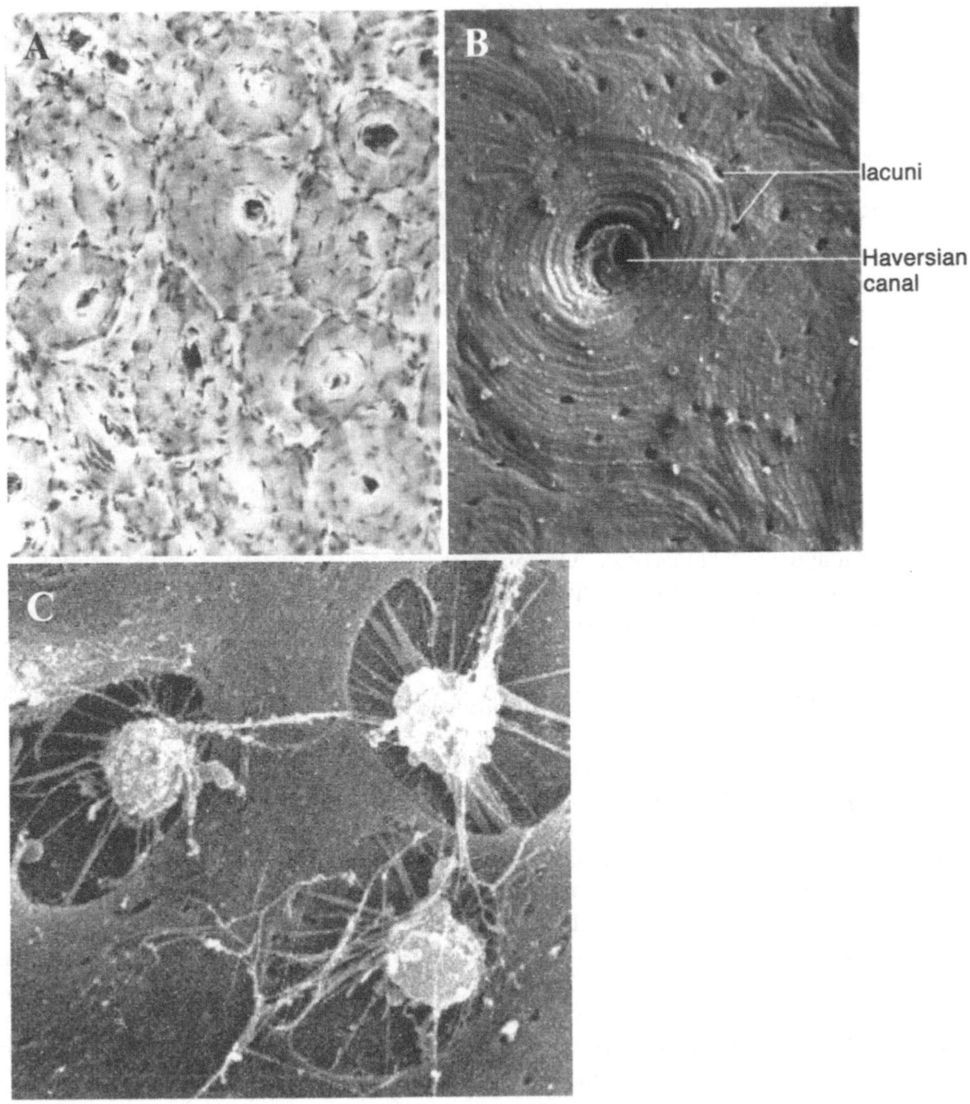

Fig. 1A–C Ultrastructure of bone. **A** Light microscope image of a ground section of compact bone. Osteons or Haversian systems can be seen. The central dark circle is the Haversian canal, which contains a nutrient artery in vivo. It is surrounded by concentric lamellae of calcified bone matrix. The dark spots visible within the compacta are the lacuni in which osteocytes become entrapped. ×350. **B** Scanning electron micrograph (SEM) of a Haversian system. ×800. **C** SEM at higher magnification reveals individual osteocytes with cellular processes reaching out towards the lacunar wall and interconnecting cells in an intricate network. ×1600. (Reproduced with permission from the Dept. of Functional Anatomy of the University of Glasgow, http://www.anatomy.gla.ac.uk/fab/)

Osteoclasts

The main feature of osteoclasts is their ability to resorb fully mineralized bone at sites called Howship's lacunae. Both macrophages and osteoclasts are derived from hematopoietic stem cells and, similar to macrophages, osteoclasts are highly migratory, multinucleated, and polarized cells which carry an arsenal of lysosomal enzymes [46]. They have to be highly specialized to fulfill their task and possess several unique ultrastructural characteristics, such as pleomorphic mitochondria, vacuoles, and lysosomes [47]. Probably the most intriguing feature is the apical membrane, which is able to form a tight seal with the calcified matrix. A resorption bay is formed underneath the cell into which the lytic enzymes are secreted. In addition, proton pumps lower the pH in this subosteoclastic space to values between 2 and 4, activating the secreted enzymes such as tartrate-resistant acid phosphatase [7]. An activated osteoclast is able to resorb 200,000 μm^3/day, an amount of bone formed by seven to ten generations of osteoblasts with an average lifespan of 15–20 days [1].

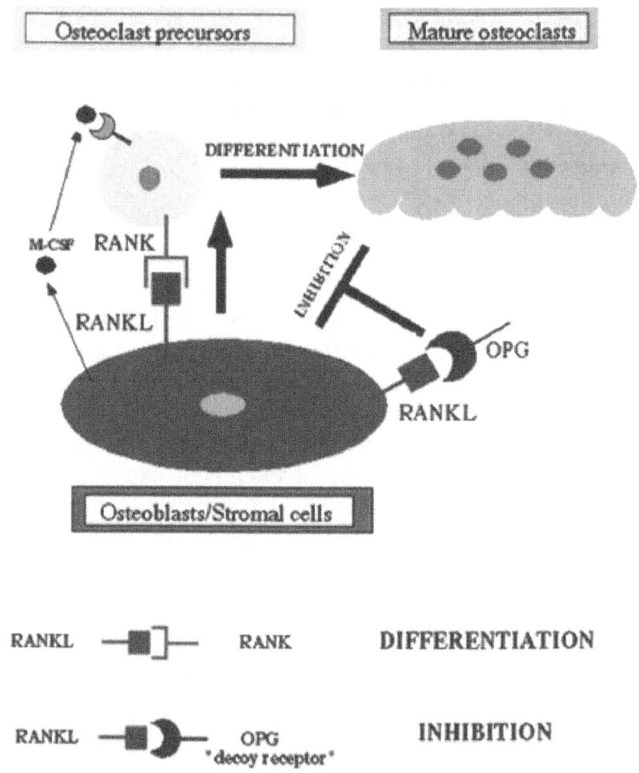

Fig. 2 Schematic of osteoblast–osteoclast interaction via RANK/RANK-L and the soluble protein osteoprotegerin (*OPG*). RANK-L, a transmembranous receptor on the surface of mature osteoblasts, interacts with the transmembranous RANK receptor on osteoblast precursor cells. This interaction induces proliferation and differentiation of osteoclasts in the presence of the permissive factor macrophage colony-stimulating factor (M-CSF) and can be inhibited by OPG. (Reproduced with permission from [4])

Osteocytes

Derived from osteoblasts yet distinctly different in morphology and function, osteocytes are the most abundant cells in bone. They are smaller in size than osteoblasts, contain less cell organelles such as ribosomes and endoplasmatic reticula, and have an increased nucleus to cytoplasm ratio. There is a higher number of filopodia, or cytoplasmatic extensions, which serve to interconnect the osteocytes and to connect them with the bone-lining cells, creating a veritable three-dimensional syncitium (Fig. 1), the function of which is beginning to emerge [12]. Considering that it is osteocytes that are the principal cell in adult bone and that neither osteoclasts nor osteoblasts are evident in any significant numbers in a skeleton with low turnover, it appears that this osteocyte construct may actually orchestrate the spatial and temporal recruitment of the cells that form and resorb bone [9].

Interaction of bone-forming and bone-resorbing cells

Although it was suggested for many years that crosstalk between osteoblasts and osteoclasts must exist to coordinate processes of bone formation and resorption, it was not until 1997 that a molecular basis for this paradigm was discovered in the form of osteoprotegerin (OPG) and, shortly after, its cognate ligand OPG-L, a transmembranous receptor expressed on osteoblasts and immune cells. Both of these molecules can bind to RANK (receptor/activator of NF-κB), a transmembranous receptor expressed on osteoclast precursor cells. Interaction between OPG-L and RANK initiates a signaling and gene expression cascade resulting in the promotion of osteoclast formation from the precursor pool. In this setting, OPG, which is secreted by osteoblasts, but also expressed in many other tissues, acts as a soluble competitive binding partner for RANK-L, which inhibits osteoclast formation and, consequentially, bone resorption [24] (Fig. 2). This crosstalk mechanism also appears to be an endpoint for the action of several calciotropic hormones and cytokines such as 1,25-$(OH)_2D_3$, parathyroid hormone (PTH), estrogen, prostaglandin E_2 (PGE_2), interleukins, and tumor necrosis factor (TNF)-α. As a result of these findings, and a mere 3 years after its discovery, OPG has already entered clinical trials as a promising therapeutic agent for osteoporosis [4,23].

Extracellular matrix

Calcified bone contains about 25% organic matrix, including cells (2–5%), 5% water, and 70% inorganic mineral (hydroxylapatite). Osteoid, the freshly synthesized matrix prior to its mineralization, consists primarily (approx. 94%) of collagen. Other proteins, some of them unique to bone, such as osteocalcin, are embedded in the extracellular matrix and may have important signaling functions (bone morphogeneic proteins, growth factors, cytokines, adhesion molecules) or play a role during the mineralization process (osteopontin, osteonectin, matrix-gla protein). The use of knockout mice lacking the ability to synthesize these proteins has shed light on the individual functions of some of these proteins. Osteocalcin-deficient mice, for example, display increased bone formation [18], whereas mice lacking osteonectin are osteopenic due to reduced bone remodeling [14].

Most of the non-collagenous proteins in bone consist of proteoglycans, the function of which was regarded until recently as structural. Recent findings, however, using transgenic mouse models show that at least some of these molecules such as perlecan and biglycan, in addition to their role in defining the spatial organization of the extracellular matrix (ECM), can also have unique functions at a biochemical level. In the case of perlecan, for example, synthesis of proteoglycan is essential for survival of these animals, possibly due to roles in facilitating cellular signaling and/or interactions with growth factors during development [2].

Ten to 15 days after the organic matrix has been laid down, it begins to mineralize. During this period, the mineral content suddenly increases to 70% of its final amount, whereas deposition of the final 30% takes several months. While the actual process of mineralization remains poorly understood, several investigators believe that the initiators of this process are small, round, extracellular, lipid bilaminar organelles which bud from hypertrophic chondrocytes, or osteoblasts. These matrix vesicles contain phosphatases, phospholipids, and calcium ions. At a point of supersaturation, mineral crystalization begins and as the matrix vesicles disintegrate, the mineral is exposed to the matrix where the process of mineralization proceeds in a self-perpetuating manner. During this process, collagen fibrils, fibronectin, and glycoproteins such as osteonectin and osteopontin determine the orientation and organization of the bone mineral crystal [11]. Other glycoproteins such as matrix-gla protein and glycosaminoglycans appear to play a role in the inhibition of excessive mineralization [50].

Bone mineral is generically referred to as hydroxyapatite [$Ca_{10}(PO_4)_6(OH)_2$], a plate-like crystal 20–80 nm in length and 2–5 nm thick. Because it is four times smaller than naturally occurring apatites and less perfect in structure, it is more reactive and soluble and facilitates chemical turnover [48]. In other words, a more "perfect" crystal would be difficult to resorb, and thus repair of the matrix would be hindered. Typically, the degree of mineralization of bone, or bone mineral density (BMD), is estimated in the clinic via dual-energy X-ray absorptiometry (DXA) or quantitative computed tomography (qCT) and is the principal diagnostic tool for osteoporosis [38].

Development

The vertebrate skeleton is the product of complex, coordinated, and synergistic interaction between three distinctly different cell lines. Cells derived from the neural crest are responsible for the development of the branchial arches and, ultimately, the craniofacial skeleton; sclerotome cells, a subdivision of the somites and of mesodermal origin, give rise to the axial skeleton; and the lateral plate mesoderm is the starting point for limb bud formation and long bone development [6].

Two mechanisms of bone formation can be observed during morphogenesis. One option involves mesenchymal cells differentiating directly into osteoblasts, which then proceed to form bone. This membranous or intramembranous bone formation is found during skull development, but also in maxilla and mandibula morphogenesis. If differentiation of mesenchymal cells proceeds via chondrocytes, which then form cartilaginous templates or so-called anlagen of the future bones, the process is termed endochondral ossification. The cartilage anlagen develop by interstitial and appositional growth and are at some point replaced by invading osteoblasts, which replace the hypertrophic cartilage and allow ossification of the structure [35].

The axial skeleton begins to develop in humans at 4 weeks postgestation, when cells from the paraxial mesoderm condense to form somites and subsequently sclerotomes. After differentiating into chondrocytes and migrating ventral, dorsal, and lateral to the neural tube, the cartilage anlagen for the vertebral body, neural arches, and ribs or transverse processes, respectively, are formed (Fig. 3).

A key aspect during development of the vertebral column is to create a flexible enclosure to allow continuous growth of the neural components, which develop slower and later. During the precartilaginous stage (week 4–6), the vertebral anlage is formed by the sclerotomal mesenchyme surrounding the notochord. Each sclerotome has two components, of which the cranial loose cells fuse with the next segment, whereas the caudal dense cells form the fibrous ring of the intervertebral disk and surround the notochord, which eventually forms the nucleus pulposus. The caudalmost cells then fuse with the cranial cells from the next segment and so on. During the cartilaginous stage, the mesenchymal anlagen are replaced by cartilage (week 7) and finally, during the bony stage of vertebral development (week 7 to year 25), by three primary ossification centers from within the cartilaginous vertebrae. The two dorsal ones form the two vertebral arches, which do not fuse until age 3–5 years, whereas the central and more ventral ossification center forms the vertebral body. Vertebral development is not completed until puberty, as the secondary ossification centers on the vertebral body and facets are formed.

This lengthy process of spine development is under tight and complex genetic control and regulation. A mas-

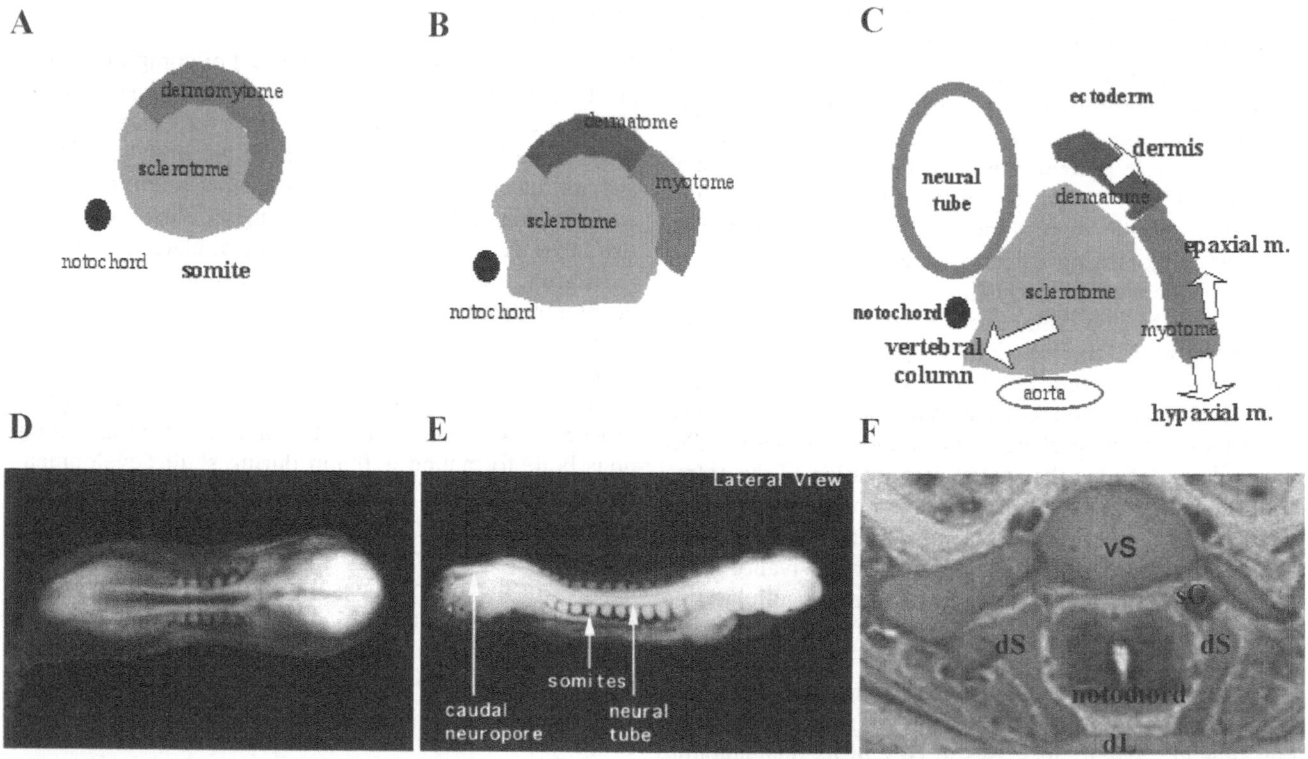

Fig. 3A–F Development of the verterbral column. **A** Somitogenesis begins during week 4 with condensation in the paraxial mesoderm. **B** Cells within the somites further differentiate, and the cells surrounding the notochord then proceed to form the sclerotome. **C** Sclerotome cells then differentiate into chondrocytes that form the anlagen of vertebral bodies. **D,E** Somite formation is clearly visible in a human embryo at day 22.5. (Courtesy of Prof. Kohei Shiota, Congenital Anomaly Research Center, Kyoto University Faculty of Medicine). **F** Section through the cartilaginous anlage of vertebral body Th1 in a human embryo at day 55. The ventral sclerotome (*vS*) forming the vertebral body and the two dorsal sclerotomes (*dS*) forming the vertebral arches, which will fuse after birth, are clearly visible. *dL*, dorsal lamina; *sG*, spinal ganglion. (Courtesy of Dr. Mark Hill, Cell Biology Lab, School of Anatomy, University of New South Wales, Sydney)

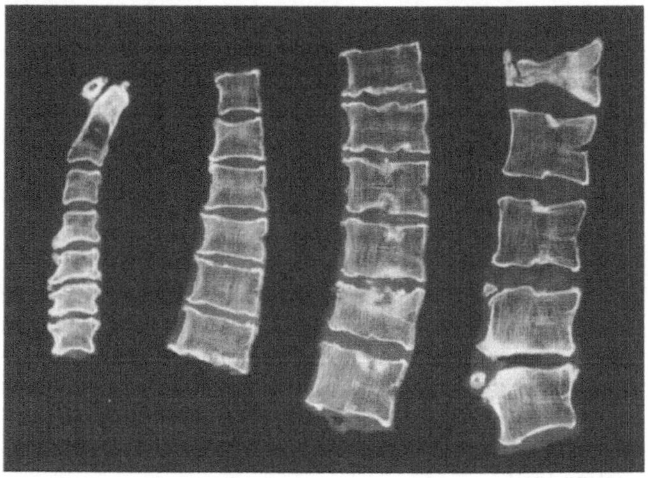

Fig. 4 Contact radiography of a cervical, thoracic, and lumbar human spine. The trabecular architecture within the vertebral body and the orientation of trabeculi preferably in the direction of axial loading are shown. Note the multiple degenerative changes such as C1/C2 fusion with the formation of osteophytes, or the osteoporotic compression fracture of L1. (Courtesy of Dr. M. Amling, Dept. of Trauma and Reconstructive Surgery, University of Hamburg, Germany)

ter gene for development of the vertebral column is the secreted cytokine sonic hedgehog, for example. Mice carrying inactivated alleles of this gene do not form a spine and lack the posterior parts of their ribs [10]. Sonic hedgehog and a number of highly conserved homeobox transcription factors, which have been under intense investigation for the last 4–5 years, are equally important during limb formation, where they control dorsal–ventral, proximal–distal, and posterior–anterior patterning [25].

Architecture

Morphology

Bones are exceptionally well suited for the structural demands placed on them. At the gross morphological level, as hollow tubes they provide great strength and durability against axial compression forces while at the same time minimizing weight to efficiently accomplish this task. The ultimate tensile strength of bone approaches that of cast iron, and its capacity to absorb and release energy is twice that of oak, yet the weight of bone is only one third that of steel [31]. On the next level, the morphology of cortical and cancellous bone is strategically arranged to accommodate input of stresses and strains during weight-bearing. The trabecular cascades of the proximal femur, for example, readily distribute the forces and moments to the cortical shell of the diaphysis. The vertebral body distributes axial compressive forces throughout a tightly woven network of trabecular bone, thus minimizing fracture risk even under extreme conditions (Fig. 4).

Microscopically, bone is made up of two distinct phenotypes: woven and lamellar. As mentioned earlier, woven bone is characteristic of embryonic and fetal development, but it is also found in the healthy adult skeleton at ligament and tendon insertions and under pathologic conditions, such as osteogenic tumor and metastasis formation or in the temporary callus of a healing fracture, where it is usually resorbed and replaced by lamellar bone within a few weeks of deposition. Architecturally, it has an irregular, disorganized pattern of collagen fiber orientation and osteocyte distribution. Mechanical stimulation can cause rapid production of woven bone, which ultimately remodels into dense, lamellar bone [39], indicating that the woven bone response is a strategic means of rapidly responding to changes in functional activity.

Lamellar or mature bone is found in both cortical and trabecular bone. The structural subunits, the lamellae, run parallel to the trabeculae or, as is the case in cortical bone, are arranged in osteons, which are composed of up to 20 concentric lamellar plates forming a cylinder with a diameter of 200–300 μm. A central capillary runs through the osteon, and up to seven concentric rings of osteocytes are incorporated into its wall. A distinction is made between primary osteons, which form de novo, e.g., during woven bone consolidation, and secondary osteons or Haversian systems, which form via resorption of preexisting bone and account for most of the adult human bone tissue [1].

Modeling and remodeling

Modeling is the processes whereby bone is laid down onto surfaces without necessarily being preceded by resorption. In the case of remodeling, osteoclastic resorption of bone leaves pockets that are then filled by osteoblast activity. A classic example of modeling occurs during longitudinal growth of long bones at the metaphysis and diaphysis. To increase the girth of the diaphysis, bone is laid onto the periosteal and endosteal surfaces. As bone length increases, the wider metaphysis has to be remodeled into a leaner diaphyseal shape by periosteal resorption and endosteal apposition of bone. This process is generally referred to as metaphyseal reshaping [20]. In a similar fashion, the sagittal curvature of a femur adapts during growth to accommodate the increasing length of the bone; this is done on the posterior surface through the highly coupled resorption of the periosteal surface and apposition on the endosteal surface and vice versa on the anterior surface by resorption of the endosteal surface and formation on the periosteal surface. This process results in the central section of the bone "drifting" dorsally, a process known as cortical drift [42].

Remodeling as an etiologic factor in skeletal disorders

In the adult skeleton, remodeling is by far the more active process, reflecting the process of "real-time" tissue replacement during bone turnover and repair. In some places, either as bone-lining cells on a trabeculum or as infilling after an osteoclastic cutting cone in cortical bone, osteoblasts lay down new bone; in others, osteoclasts resorb the mineralized matrix. This cyclic sequence is also called the activation–resorption–reversal–formation (ARRF) sequence and takes about 3–6 months to be completed in humans. Remodeling is not only required to replace dead or damaged tissue, it also gives bone the capacity to adapt to changes in loading and to respond to nutritional and/or metabolic changes [5,37].

Ultimately, the pathologies inherent in bone diseases are reflected by this physiologic remodeling sequence, either by influencing bone formation (induction of osteoblast activity or inhibition of osteoclast activity) or resorption (induction of osteoclast activity or inhibition of osteoblast activity). According to this paradigm, osteoporosis is generally viewed as the inability of osteoblasts to fully repair the resorptive defects during normal osteoclast resorption, since mean wall thickness and porosity in cortical bone are generally elevated and trabecular spacing in cancellous bone is increased [13].

The spine consists primarily (75%) of trabecular bone, and the intertrochanteric region of the femur has a cancellous bone content of 50%. Despite the relatively small net amount of cancellous bone (only 15% of the total bone in the body), remodeling events within these parts of the skeleton therefore largely determine whether osteoporotic fractures occur. Bone mass peaks at about 35 years of age. Since a decline in bone mass with age is evident within the entire population, failure of the skeletal structures mentioned above is the result of a host of additional systemic and local factors. These can include perimenopausal decline in estrogen production, heritable, nutritional, and environmental factors, and the absence or reduction of mechanical stimuli, which alone or in combination tend to further aggravate the resorptive component of the bone remodeling equation [34].

Systemic regulation of bone remodeling

Perhaps the principal responsibility of systemic peptide or steroid hormones is to regulate mineral homeostasis rather than locally control skeletal morphology. Nevertheless, PTH, for example, as the main regulator of serum calcium, has significant effects on bone remodeling. By indirectly stimulating osteoclast activity via an increase in OPG-L on the osteoblast membrane and/or inhibition of OPG secretion, PTH is able to release calcium and phosphate into the bloodstream while at the same time inducing net bone resorption [30].

Osteoprotegerin and its ligand also seem to be involved in the action of vitamin D or calcitriol (1,25-$(OH)_2D_3$), as its active metabolite is generally referred to. While adequate levels of it are necessary to provide calcium for bone formation via intestinal reabsorption, supraphysiologic levels induce bone resorption by stimulation of osteoclast differentiation. An increase in OPG-L gene expression in osteoblasts seems to be the mechanism of this effect on bone resorption [32].

As an example of induction of bone formation via the same effector pathway, estrogen, or more correctly 17β-estradiol, protects bone by increasing OPG levels in osteoblasts, thus inhibiting osteoclast differentiation and activation and promoting osteoclast apoptosis. Using the same effector mechanism, namely OPG/OPG-L interaction, many cytokines and calciotropic hormones therefore seem to exert what are sometimes dual effects on bone formation and/or resorption [24].

In addition to these hormonal systemic regulatory mechanisms, exciting data have recently been presented postulating a central control mechanism for bone mass control via the hypothalamus. In this model, leptin not only regulates body mass, but also – and at much lower serum concentrations – has an inhibitory effect on bone mass. This effect is apparently not mediated via a direct effect on bone cells and is also independent of endocrine organs such as the pituitary gland, the parathyroid, or adrenal glands, but rather suggests an additional control of bone mass solely by the central nervous system [17].

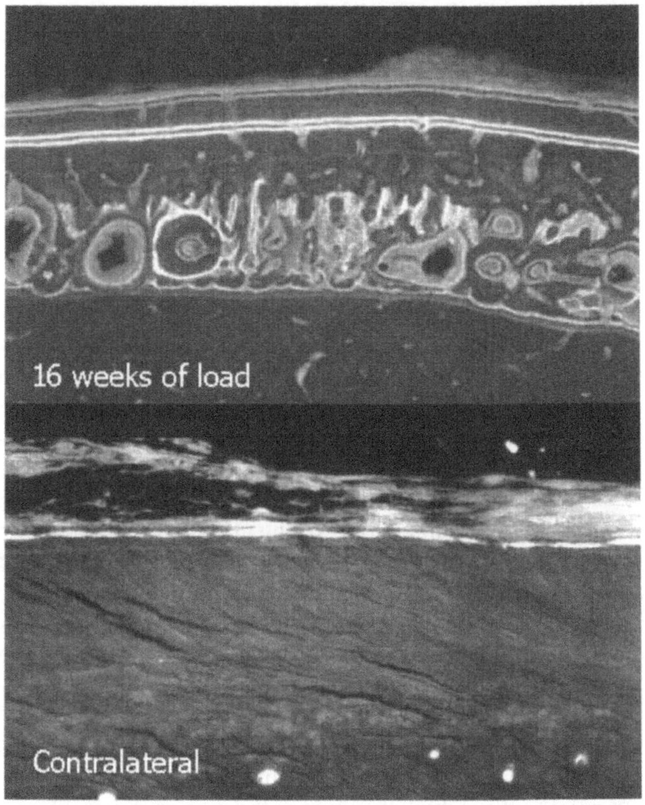

Fig. 5 A fluorescent photomicrograph of the periosteal surface of a turkey ulna diaphysis following 16 weeks of a mechanical regimen sufficient to cause a peak of 2000 microstrain. Remnants of the original woven response can be seen serving as interstitial elements of primary and secondarily remodeled bone. In essence, the woven bone response has served as a strategic stage in the achievement of a structurally appropriate increase in bone mass. Mechanical stimuli are certainly strong, site-specific growth factors. (Reproduced with permission from [28])

Structural adaptation in bone

A great deal of bone's structural success is derived from its ability to constantly redefine its mass and morphology to accommodate subtle changes in mechanical and metabolic demands. It is therefore reasonable to speculate about the signals that regulate the modeling and remodeling processes. Regardless of the genetic predetermination of the shape and structure (i.e., cancellous vs. cortical) of each individual bone in the skeleton, a bone's shape, anatomy, and mechanical properties, such as mechanical strength, stiffness, and toughness, are adapted to mechanical stimuli happens throughout the lifetime of an individual. The "form follows function" concept as it pertains to mechanical adaptation in bone was first proposed in 1892; it is one of the oldest in modern medicine and is widely referred to as Wolff's law [49]. A century later, the parameters in the functional environment that bone is actually responding to still remain unclear. For example, several research teams are strong advocates of the theory that strain magnitude is the key regulatory factor in bone adaptation. However, it is important to emphasize that axial loading accounts for only a small percentage of the total strain measured at the bone surface, with well over 80% of measured strain caused by bending moments. Much smaller strains would certainly be achieved (or much less bone material required) if all strains were a product of axial loads. As it is, though, at most only one small area of the bone is subject to high strains, yet the remodeling of bone correlates only weakly with this area most likely to be subject to microcracks or other forms of damage or extreme signals. Equally surprisingly, it does not appear to be the aim of long bone curvature or cross-sectional geometries to minimize bending moments, but in some cases these morphologic features even accentuate the strain signals [40].

Perhaps contrary to a "static material"-based interpretation of Wolff's concept, it appears that the ultimate goal of bone adaptation is not to minimize strain. Instead, skeletal morphology and functional load-bearing apparently conspire to strive toward a certain type of strain. Peak strain magnitudes measured in a wide range of adult species are remarkably similar, ranging from 2000 to 3500 microstrain (where the yield strain of bone is approximately 7000 microstrain, and the ultimate strain is 25,000 microstrain). This generic peak strain environment has been termed "dynamic strain similarity" and is one argument for the concept of bone working toward achieving a favorable strain environment rather than to reduce it as far as possible [41] (Fig. 5).

Although the cellular and molecular mechanisms have yet to be fully established, there is increasing evidence for the concept of a mechanosensory cell system, such as the osteocyte syncytium, that is able to communicate information to bone-forming and/or bone-resorbing cells. The interspecies similarity in strain magnitudes further suggests the existence of a generic cellular mechanism that strives toward a common structural and beneficial goal.

There are many examples of this structure–function relationship, including the 35% increase in cortical thickness on the humerus of the playing arm of professional tennis players [26] or the striking bone resorption that results from immobilization or space flight; it is thus clear that bone can quickly identify changes in its functional milieu and respond to these changes structurally [16, 26].

Attempts to identify the parameters that bone is sensitive to in terms of an adaptive response have shown that parameters such as strain distribution, gradients, cycle number, and rate critically influence bone mass, turnover, and remodeling. Nevertheless, no single parameter has been shown to reliably predict bone adaptation under all naturally observed or experimentally created conditions [8]. Perhaps we should be more hesitant to presume that skeletal morphology is merely a product of dominant strain parameters with the structural goal of minimizing strain. Instead, incorporating the biological principles that guide the homeostasis of a living tissue, the cellular advantages for a tissue exposed to a dynamic functional milieu such as increased perfusion and nutrition have to be considered in concert with the advantages of an effective structural material.

Whatever the signal transduction pathway of transforming physical information to something the cell population can perceive and respond to, it is clear that the capacity of bone tissue to adapt to the functional demands placed on it is critical to the skeleton's structural success. Indeed, as we attempt to evaluate the cellular mechanisms responsible for the positive control of bone mass, the osteogenic potential of physical stimuli cannot be ignored.

Conclusion

By providing a brief overview of the anatomical, structural, and physiological aspects of bone's form–function relationship, it is hoped that this manuscript has provided at least an appreciation of the great complexity of bone tissue. An exhaustive review of bone biology and its ability to orchestrate the mass and morphology of the skeleton is obviously not possible, not only because of space constraints, but because there is so much about this "smart material" that we still do not understand. In reviewing the means by which bone integrates the fundamental tasks of providing skeletal structure while managing the metabolic responsibilities of an organ under endocrine, and possibly central, control, it is hoped that, at the same time, the physician and scientist will have gained some insight into the challenges – and opportunities – which musculoskeletal science is faced with. Through transgenic approaches, the contributions of individual proteins within bone to its structural and functional integrity can and will continue to be determined. Similarly, cell–cell and cell–matrix interactions within bone are being elucidated on a molecular level using signal transduction studies. The advent of the molecular tools capable of genome-wide gene expression analyses, the search for single nucleotide polymorphisms (SNP), and proteomics will certainly lead to discoveries identifying the responsible genes and proteins for many diseases affecting the bone phenotype. Advances in new biocompatible materials, both osteoconductive and osteoinductive, will also aid in the treatment of bone disorders, while new diagnostic modalities will aid in identifying those at risk of disease perhaps before symptoms are evident.

Other problems, e.g., questions concerning mechanotransduction, a mechanosensory system, and the details of regulation of bone adaptation, are still less clear, even though considerable progress has been made in identifying some of the responsible parameters of bone's functional milieu and the means by which bone can respond to it in terms of modeling and remodeling. An improved understanding of how bone perceives and responds to mechanical signals will certainly aid in accelerating the healing of fractures, augmenting osseointegration into implants, and ensuring that diseases such as osteoporosis can be adequately addressed.

The basic biology of bone is obviously also of concern to the clinician and spine surgeon. Even in a field of medicine where hands-on experience cannot be overestimated, new treatment modalities for diseases and problems of the musculoskeletal system are certain to be derived from the above-mentioned studies. For example, local gene delivery systems to achieve spinal fusion between hypermobile segments in spondylolisthesis are conceivable; tissue engineering approaches to replace and augment bone, cartilage, and muscle are receiving a great deal of attention; and many of the drugs to treat arthritis, osteoporosis, and other diseases of the musculoskeletal system will be based on SNP and complex gene interactions. These are undoubtedly exciting times for everyone working in the bone field, and the interdisciplinary nature of the research that has brought us tremendous insight into bone's complexity on a structural and functional level will serve us well in the future.

Acknowledgments This work was kindly supported by grants from the German Research Foundation (DFG So 427/1–1 to D.W.S.), the National Institutes of Health (AR39278, AR41011, AR41040, and AR43498), and the National Aeronautics and Space Administration (DAG-53950).

References

1. Albright J, Skinner H (1987) Bone: structural organization and remodeling dynamics. In: Albright J, Brand R (eds) The scientific basis of orthopaedics, 2nd edn. Appleton and Lange, East Norwalk, pp 161–198
2. Aszodi A, Bateman JF, Gustafsson E, Boot-Handford R, Fassler R (2000) Mammalian skeletogenesis and extracellular matrix: what can we learn from knockout mice? [In process citation]. Cell Struct Funct 25:73–84
3. Aubin JE (1998) Bone stem cells. J Cell Biochem Suppl 30–31:73–82
4. Aubin JE, Bonnelye E (2000) Osteoprotegerin and its ligand: a new paradigm for regulation of osteoclastogenesis and bone resorption. Medscape Womens Health 5:5
5. Bain SD, Rubin CT (1990) Metabolic modulation of disuse osteopenia: endocrine-dependent site specificity of bone remodeling. J Bone Miner Res 5:1069–1075
6. Beddington RS, Robertson EJ (1999) Axis development and early asymmetry in mammals. Cell 96:195–209
7. Blair HC, Teitelbaum SL, Ghiselli R, Gluck S (1989) Osteoclastic bone resorption by a polarized vacuolar proton pump. Science 245:855–857
8. Brown TD, Pedersen DR, Gray ML, Brand RA, Rubin CT (1990) Toward an identification of mechanical parameters initiating periosteal remodeling: a combined experimental and analytic approach. J Biomech 23:893–905
9. Burger EH, Klein-Nulend J (1999) Mechanotransduction in bone–role of the lacuno-canalicular network. FASEB J 13 Suppl:S101–S112
10. Chiang C, Litingtung Y, Lee E, Young KE, Corden JL, Westphal H, Beachy PA (1996) Cyclopia and defective axial patterning in mice lacking Sonic hedgehog gene function. Nature 383:407–413
11. Christoffersen J, Landis WJ (1991) A contribution with review to the description of mineralization of bone and other calcified tissues in vivo. Anat Rec 230:435–450
12. Curtis TA, Ashrafi SH, Weber DF (1985) Canalicular communication in the cortices of human long bones. Anat Rec 212:336–344
13. Darby AJ, Meunier PJ (1981) Mean wall thickness and formation periods of trabecular bone packets in idiopathic osteoporosis. Calcif Tissue Int 33:199–204
14. Delany AM, Amling M, Priemel M, Howe C, Baron R, Canalis E (2000) Osteopenia and decreased bone formation in osteonectin-deficient mice [published erratum appears in J Clin Invest 105(9):1325]. J Clin Invest 105:915–923
15. Donahue HJ, McLeod KJ, Rubin CT, Andersen J, Grine EA, Hertzberg EL, Brink PR (1995) Cell-to-cell communication in osteoblastic networks: cell line-dependent hormonal regulation of gap junction function. J Bone Miner Res 10:881–889
16. Donaldson CL, Hulley SB, Vogel JM, Hattner RS, Bayers JH, McMillan DE (1970) Effect of prolonged bed rest on bone mineral. Metabolism 19:1071–1084
17. Ducy P, Amling M, Takeda S, Priemel M, Schilling AF, Beil FT, Shen J, Vinson C, Rueger JM, Karsenty G (2000) Leptin inhibits bone formation through a hypothalamic relay: a central control of bone mass. Cell 100:197–207
18. Ducy P, Desbois C, Boyce B, Pinero G, Story B, Dunstan C, Smith E, Bonadio J, Goldstein S, Gundberg C, Bradley A, Karsenty G (1996) Increased bone formation in osteocalcin-deficient mice. Nature 382:448–452
19. Ducy P, Schinke T, Karsenty G (2000) The osteoblast: a sophisticated fibroblast under central surveillance. Science 289:1501–1504
20. Enlow D (1963) Principles of bone remodeling. Thomas, Springfield
21. Ferrari SL, Traianedes K, Thorne M, Lafage-Proust MH, Genever P, Cecchini MG, Behar V, Bisello A, Chorev M, Rosenblatt M, Suva LJ (2000) A role for N-cadherin in the development of the differentiated osteoblastic phenotype. J Bone Miner Res 15:198–208
22. Fujikawa Y, Quinn JM, Sabokbar A, McGee JO, Athanasou NA (1996) The human osteoclast precursor circulates in the monocyte fraction. Endocrinology 137:4058–4060
23. Hofbauer LC, Heufelder AE (2000) Clinical review 114: hot topic. The role of receptor activator of nuclear factor-kappaB ligand and osteoprotegerin in the pathogenesis and treatment of metabolic bone diseases. J Clin Endocrinol Metab 85:2355–2363
24. Hofbauer LC, Khosla S, Dunstan CR, Lacey DL, Boyle WJ, Riggs BL (2000) The roles of osteoprotegerin and osteoprotegerin ligand in the paracrine regulation of bone resorption. J Bone Miner Res 15:2–12
25. Izpisua-Belmonte JC, Duboule D (1992) Homeobox genes and pattern formation in the vertebrate limb. Dev Biol 152:26–36
26. Jones HH, Priest JD, Hayes WC, Tichenor CC, Nagel DA (1977) Humeral hypertrophy in response to exercise. J Bone Joint Surg [Am] 59:204–208
27. Jowsey J (1977) Metabolic diseases of bone. Saunders, Philadelphia
28. Lanyon LE, Rubin CT (1984) Static vs dynamic loads as an influence on bone remodelling. J Biomech 17:897–905
29. Lecanda F, Towler DA, Ziambaras K, Cheng SL, Koval M, Steinberg TH, Civitelli R (1998) Gap junctional communication modulates gene expression in osteoblastic cells. Mol Biol Cell 9:2249–2258
30. Lee SK, Lorenzo JA (1999) Parathyroid hormone stimulates TRANCE and inhibits osteoprotegerin messenger ribonucleic acid expression in murine bone marrow cultures: correlation with osteoclast-like cell formation. Endocrinology 140:3552–3561
31. Martin R, Burr D (1989) Structure, function, and adaptation of compact bone. Raven, New York, pp 1–275

32. Morony S, Capparelli C, Lee R, Shimamoto G, Boone T, Lacey DL, Dunstan CR (1999) A chimeric form of osteoprotegerin inhibits hypercalcemia and bone resorption induced by IL-1beta, TNF-alpha, PTH, PTHrP, and 1, 25(OH)2D3. J Bone Miner Res 14: 1478–1485
33. Mosley JR (2000) Osteoporosis and bone functional adaptation: mechanobiological regulation of bone architecture in growing and adult bone, a review. J Rehabil Res Dev 37:189–199
34. Mundy GR (1987) Bone resorption and turnover in health and disease. Bone 8 Suppl 1:S9–16
35. Olsen BJ (1999) Bone morphogenesis and embryonic development. In: Favus MJ (ed) Primer on the metabolic bone diseases and disorders of mineral metabolism, 4th edn. Lippincott, Williams and Wilkins, Philadelphia, pp 11–14
36. Owen M (1972) Cellular dynamics of bone. In: Bourne G (ed) The biochemistry and physiology of bone, 2nd edn. Academic, New York, pp 271
37. Qin YX, Rubin CT, McLeod KJ (1998) Nonlinear dependence of loading intensity and cycle number in the maintenance of bone mass and morphology. J Orthop Res 16:482–489
38. Rizzoli R, Slosman D, Bonjour JP (1995) The role of dual energy X-ray absorptiometry of lumbar spine and proximal femur in the diagnosis and follow-up of osteoporosis. Am J Med 98:33S–36S
39. Rubin CT, Gross TS, McLeod KJ, Bain SD (1995) Morphologic stages in lamellar bone formation stimulated by a potent mechanical stimulus. J Bone Miner Res 10:488–495
40. Rubin CT, Lanyon LE (1982) Limb mechanics as a function of speed and gait: a study of functional strains in the radius and tibia of horse and dog. J Exp Biol 101:187–211
41. Rubin CT, Lanyon LE (1984) Dynamic strain similarity in vertebrates; an alternative to allometric limb bone scaling. J Theor Biol 107:321–327
42. Ruff CB, Hayes WC (1982) Subperiosteal expansion and cortical remodeling of the human femur and tibia with aging. Science 217:945–948
43. Sabolinski ML, Alvarez O, Auletta M, Mulder G, Parenteau NL (1996) Cultured skin as a 'smart material' for healing wounds: experience in venous ulcers. Biomaterials 17:311–320
44. Service RF (2000) Tissue engineers build new bone [news]. Science 289:1498–1500
45. Sullivan LH (1947) The tall office building artistically considered. In: Athey I (ed) Kindergarten chats (revised 1918) and other writings. Dover, Mineola, NY, pp 202–213
46. Teitelbaum SL (2000) Bone resorption by osteoclasts. Science 289:1504–1508
47. Walker DG (1972) Enzymatic and electron microscopic analysis of isolated osteoclasts. Calcif Tissue Res 9:296–309
48. Weiner S, Traub W (1992) Bone structure: from angstroms to microns. FASEB J 6:879–885
49. Wolff J (1892) Das Gesetz der Transformation des Knochens. Hirschwald, Berlin
50. Yagami K, Suh JY, Enomoto-Iwamoto M, Koyama E, Abrams WR, Shapiro IM, Pacifici M, Iwamoto M (1999) Matrix GLA protein is a developmental regulator of chondrocyte mineralization and, when constitutively expressed, blocks endochondral and intramembranous ossification in the limb. J Cell Biol 147:1097–1108

T. Albrektsson
C. Johansson

Osteoinduction, osteoconduction and osseointegration

Abstract Osteoinduction is the process by which osteogenesis is induced. It is a phenomenon regularly seen in any type of bone healing process. Osteoinduction implies the recruitment of immature cells and the stimulation of these cells to develop into preosteoblasts. In a bone healing situation such as a fracture, the majority of bone healing is dependent on osteoinduction. Osteoconduction means that bone grows on a surface. This phenomenon is regularly seen in the case of bone implants. Implant materials of low biocompatibility such as copper, silver and bone cement shows little or no osteoconduction. Osseointegration is the stable anchorage of an implant achieved by direct bone-to-implant contact. In craniofacial implantology, this mode of anchorage is the only one for which high success rates have been reported. Osseointegration is possible in other parts of the body, but its importance for the anchorage of major arthroplasties is under debate. Ingrowth of bone in a porous-coated prosthesis may or may not represent osseointegration.

Keywords Osteoinduction · Osteoconduction · Osseointegration

T. Albrektsson (✉) · C. Johansson
Department of Biomaterials/
Handicap Research, P.O. Box 412,
SE 405 30 Gothenburg, Sweden
e-mail: tomas.albrektsson@hkf.gu.se

Introduction

The terms osteoinduction, osteoconduction and osseointegration are frequently, but not always correctly, used terms in many orthopaedic papers. To give but one example of incorrect terminology, arthroplasties are commonly claimed to be osseointegrated based only on radiographic evidence, despite the fact that the resolution of radiography alone is too poor to determine whether an implant is osseointegrated or not. The aim of this paper is to first briefly explain and define these terms and then to look at them in some detail. Osteoinduction, osteoconduction and osseointegration are now the subject of much discussion, e.g. in connection with bone morphogenic proteins (BMP), bone growth factors and direct bone anchorage, respectively. Suggested definitions of the terms osteoinduction, osteoconduction and osseointegration read as follows:

Osteoinduction. This term means that primitive, undifferentiated and pluripotent cells are somehow stimulated to develop into the bone-forming cell lineage. One proposed definition is the process by which osteogenesis is induced [43].

Osteoconduction. This term means that bone grows on a surface. An osteoconductive surface is one that permits bone growth on its surface or down into pores, channels or pipes. Wilson-Hench [43] has suggested that osteoconduction is the process by which bone is directed so as to conform to a material's surface. However, Glantz [18] has pointed out that this way of looking at bone conduction is somewhat restricted, since the original definition bears little or no relation to biomaterials.

Osseointegration. This was first described by Brånemark and co-workers [12]. The term was first defined in a paper by Albrektsson et al. [4] as direct contact (at the light microscope level) between living bone and implant. Osseointegration is also histologically defined in *Dorland's Illustrated Medical Dictionary* as the direct anchorage of an implant by the formation of bony tissue around the implant without the growth of fibrous tissue at the bone–implant interface. Since the histological definitions have some shortcomings, mainly that they have a limited clinical application, another more biomechanically oriented definition of osseointegration has been suggested: "A process whereby clinically asymptomatic rigid fixation of alloplastic materials is achieved, and maintained, in bone during functional loading" [46]. The rigid fixation of an implant in orthopaedic praxis can be determined using radio-stereophotogrammetic (RSA) techniques and, at least in craniofacial implantology, resonance frequency analysis (RFA) [28].

Osteoinduction and its importance for bone healing

In addition to the differentiated bone cells, i.e. osteoblasts, osteoclasts and osteocytes, bone and adjacent tissues contain a number of less differentiated cells. These undifferentiated cells are of utmost importance for proper bone healing or anchorage of an implant, since they can be recruited to form osteoprogenitor cells [45] and, with time, develop into differentiated bone cells (Fig. 1). With the correct stimulus (the inductive agent), an undifferentiated mesenchymal cell can be transformed into a preosteoblast, a process which constitutes bone induction. The classical papers describing bone induction at various host sites were published a long time ago [20, 25, 40]. These authors used gall bladder epithelium, alcohol extracts of bone and transplants to muscles or the anterior chamber of the eye, respectively, to demonstrate heterotopic bone formation. The safest way to demonstrate whether a particular agent is osteoinductive or not is still to inject it into a heterotopic bed such as a muscle pouch and to analyse any potential bone formation (Fig. 2). Inductive agents naturally function in bone surroundings too, but it is difficult to differentiate between bone induction and bone conduction in an orthotopic site.

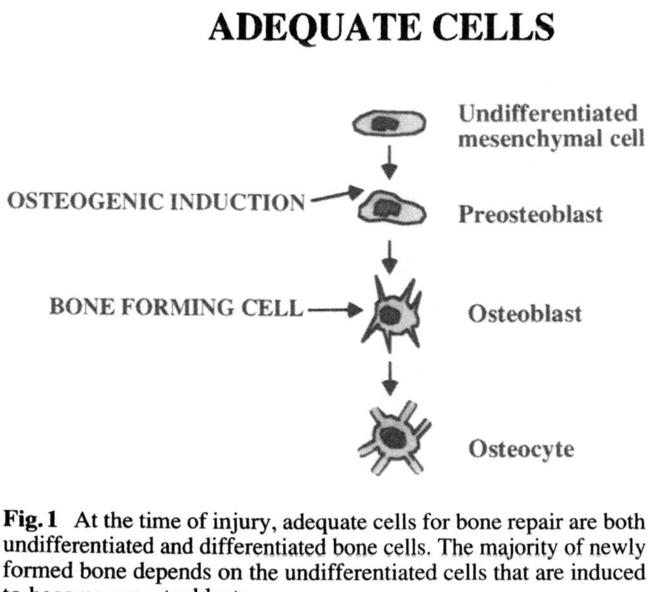

Fig. 1 At the time of injury, adequate cells for bone repair are both undifferentiated and differentiated bone cells. The majority of newly formed bone depends on the undifferentiated cells that are induced to become preosteoblasts

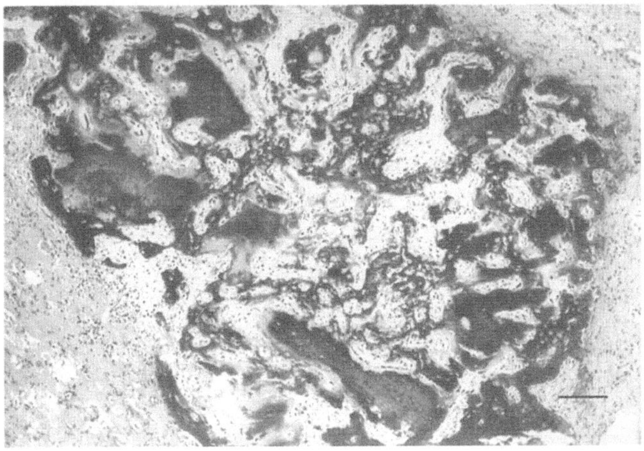

Fig. 2 The best way to demonstrate whether a specific agent is osteoinductive is to inject it into a soft tissue pouch, where bone formation does not occur under normal conditions. BMP-7 induced bone formation 19 days after injection into a subcutaneous site in a rat. Toluidine blue. *Bar*, 100 μm

More modern research into osteoinduction dates back to Urist's experiment in the mid-1960s [39]. Demineralised bone was used as an osteoinductive agent. Later, Urist et al. [41] isolated a soluble glycoprotein called BMP as the inductive agent. The BMP belong to the transforming growth factor (TGF)-β-family of growth factors. There are at least 15 different BMP [34], of which BMP-2 and BMP-7 seem to be particularly interesting. To date, a great number of research projects involving various types of BMP are being conducted (for reviews, see [24, 34]). BMP are naturally released in response to trauma or at bone remodelling and are the only known inducive agents [26]. However, physical stimuli such as stress or types of electrical signals otherwise applied have been regarded as, directly or indirectly, influencing bone induction [10, 13, 14, 44].

Osteoinduction, i.e. the recruitment of immature cells and the stimulation of these cells to develop into preosteoblasts, is a basic biological mechanism that occurs regularly, e.g. in fracture healing and implant incorporation. Even if pre-existing osteoblasts (i.e. before the injury) may help to form new bone, it is generally agreed that such pre-existing cells only contribute a minor portion of the new bone needed in a fracture-healing situation [16, 17]. According to Frost [16, 17] (Fig. 3), the inevitable bone, marrow and soft tissue injury triggers the subsequent repair by sensitising different types of surviving cells. Si-

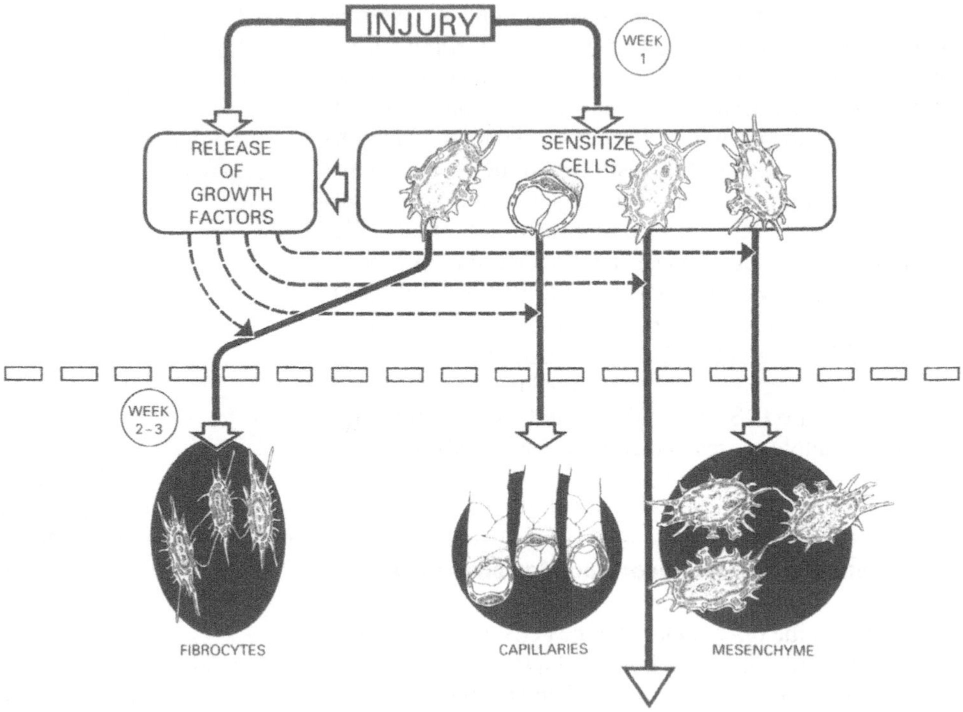

Fig. 3 According to Frost's theory, injury triggers off a healing response by the release of growth factors and sensitising of cells. This is a primitive healing response with stimulation of many different types of cells

multaneously, the injury releases local, biochemical and biophysical messengers that help cells to respond and that guide them to respond in the proper manner. Some of these messengers guide the differentiation and organisation of cells, while others provide mitogens. This initial part of the healing response thus includes osteoinduction, a process that starts immediately after the injury and is very active during the first week thereafter, even though the action of the newly recruited preosteoblasts is not obvious until several weeks later, in the callus stage.

Osteoconduction and its importance for bone healing

Bone growth on an implant surface depends on the action of differentiated bone cells. These cells may originate either in pre-existing preosteoblasts/osteoblasts that are activated by trauma or in cells recruited from primitive mesenchymal cells by osteoinduction [16, 17]. In the practical situation, therefore, osteoconduction (Fig. 4) depends to a fairly large extent on previous osteoinduction. The debate concerning whether or not a particular biomaterial acts as an osteoinductor may be slightly academic, since the injury at placement is sufficient to recruit previously undifferentiated bone cells.

Various types of bone growth factors are necessary for bone formation. Furthermore, bone growth, including bone conduction, does not occur without a proper blood supply. Albrektsson [1] studied bone conduction and remodelling in vivo and came to the conclusion that so-called full vascularisation was necessary for bone formation. It is there-

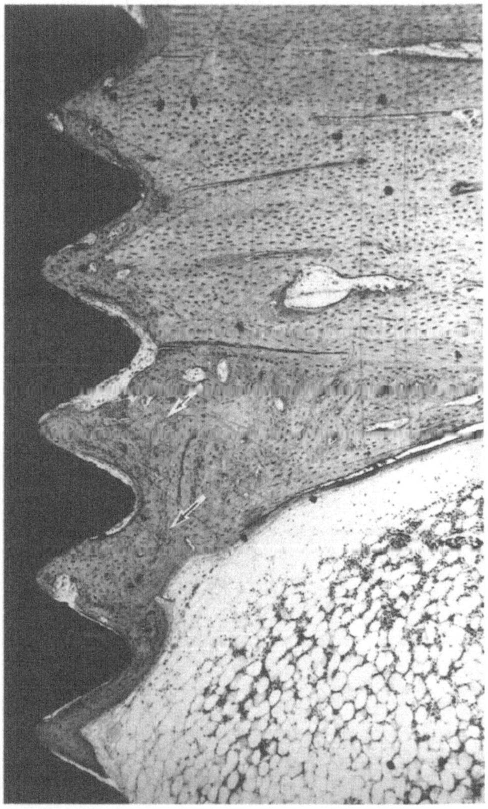

Fig. 4 In biomaterials science, osteoconduction means growth of bone on the surface of a foreign material, as seen in the lower part of this titanium screw implant (*arrows*). Distance between thread peaks, 600 µm

fore not surprising that the principal action of many growth factors is both mitogenic and angiogenic [37]. Growth factors that regulate bone tissue in one way or another include insulin-like growth factor (IGF I, II), fibroblast growth factor (FGF), TGF-β and platelet-derived growth factor (PDGF). The IGF are also called somatomedins. The growth factors are small proteins that serve as signalling agents for cells [37] (see the paper by Lind, this volume, for a more detailed discussion of various growth factors).

However, in the case of implants, bone conduction is not only dependent on conditions for bone repair, but also on the biomaterial used and its reactions. Bone conduction is not possible on certain materials such as copper and silver [3]. However, bone conduction is seen with biomaterials not regarded as ideal from the point of view of biocompatibility, such as stainless steel [22] and obviously materials of high biocompatibility such as commercially pure (c.p.) titanium. Bone conduction on implants may be quantified. There is a significant difference in the amount of bone that grows on seemingly similar materials such as c.p. titanium and titanium 6-aluminum 4-vanadium [23]. However, the clinical implications of this difference remain unknown.

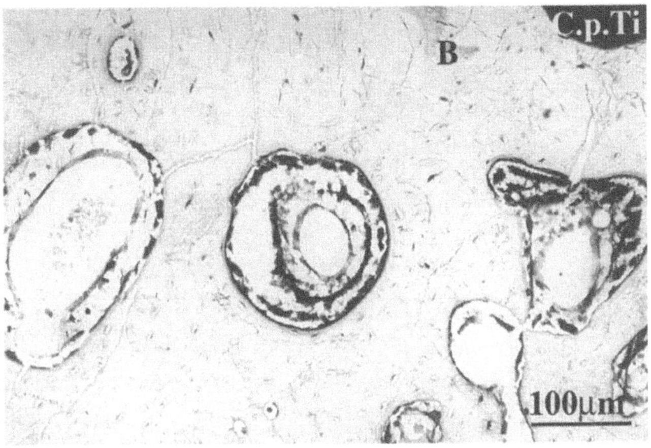

Fig. 5 Simultaneous bone formation and resorption at the interface between bone (*B*) and a commercially pure titanium (*c.p. Ti*) implant. There are three cavities arranged in a horizontal line in the middle of the figure. In the left cavity, red dominates, i.e. positive staining for acid phosphatase meaning active bone resorption. In the middle cavity, blue dominates, i.e. positive staining for alkaline phosphatase, meaning active bone formation. In the right cavity, there is red and blue staining, i.e. both bone formation and resorption. *Bar*, 100 µm

Osseointegration of implants

Brånemark, who introduced this term, suggested the spelling "osseointegration" instead of "osteointegration", and the original spelling is preferred in this paper. Osseointegration is not an isolated phenomenon, but instead depends on previous osteoinduction and osteoconduction. Thus materials that are too toxic to allow osteoconduction will not be osseointegrated either. However, many materials show at least some bone attachment, which has inspired bone pathologists to regard osseointegration as a simple foreign body reaction [15], whereas more clinically oriented scientists have rejected such a view. Osseointegrated implants have undergone a real breakthrough in oral and craniofacial implantology, yielding excellent functional results, in contrast to alternatively anchored implants, which have generally shown very poor success rates [6, 12, 35, 36]. Even if initial osseointegration is dependent on bone induction and conduction, the term implies that the bone anchorage is maintained over time. Cylindrical implant designs (without threads), rough plasma-sprayed surfaces and overloading represent factors that may lead to secondary failure of osseointegration [2, 4].

The ultrastructure of the bone–titanium interface in osseointegration demonstrates an amorphous layer from 20–40 to 500 nm thick. Some investigators [5] have described collagen and calcified tissue in this zone, whereas others [32] have failed to verify these findings. This zone is too narrow to be seen at the light microscope level of resolution. At the light microscope level, direct bone contact, osteogenesis and bone resorption occur simultaneously [31] (Fig. 5). From a purely biomechanical viewpoint, Skalak and Zhao [33] have demonstrated that when a hole slightly smaller than the implant diameter is prepared for implant placement, force-fitting stress increases installation torque and initial stability can be induced at a similar magnitude as seen with roughened implants.

Oral implants retrieved from patients despite remaining stability have shown that there does not seem to be 100% bone attachment. Implants retrieved after clinical function for up to 17 years showed an average of 70–80% bone contact with an absolute minimum of 60% [7]. Functioning osseointegrated implants demonstrate interfacial bone density similar to that of the bone in which the implant was implanted [38]. Even if long-term functioning osseointegrated implants show what seems to be similar bone tissue reactions, osseointegration might be able to be achieved more rapidly than otherwise observed. Such potentially accelerated osseointegration has been indicated by results from experiments with hydroxyapatite coating [19], using intermediary roughened implants [42], after hyperbaric oxygen treatment [30] or by using anodised c.p. titanium with artificially enhanced oxide layers [9]. Acceleration of osseointegration may depend on the removal of negative tissue conditions or optimisation of the biomaterial rather than on an actual increase in the rate of bone response.

Much less attention has been paid to the possibility of establishing osseointegration in orthopaedic surgery than in oral and craniofacial surgery. The original notion that polymerised bone cement may be histologically osseointegrated has not been confirmed in more recent investigations [29]. Histological sections to reveal true bone-to-im-

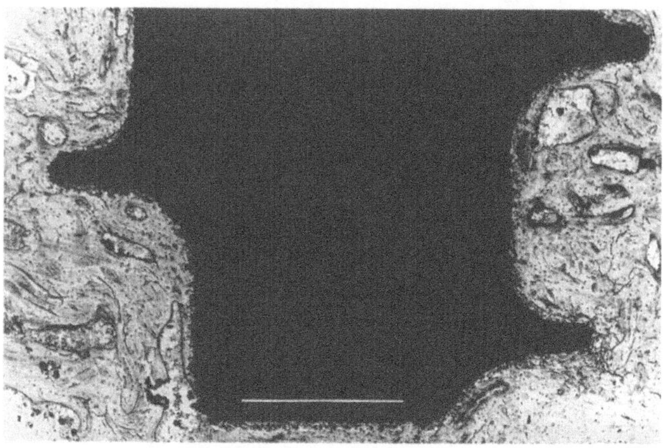

Fig. 6 Hydroxyapatite-coated vertebral screw in a goat. Osseointegration is evident. *Bar*, 1000 μm (Courtesy of Dr. B. Sandén, Uppsala University)

plant contact need to be quite thin (of the order of 10–20 μm) to really reveal osseointegration. Thicker sections have a shadow effect [21] that make it impossible to state whether or not true direct bone contact has been achieved. Apart from poor resolution, this is the reason why common radiographs are of little value in the diagnosis of osseointegration. The question is whether it is really possible to establish osseointegration of conventional orthopaedic arthroplasties with the combined use of less biocompatible materials, interfacial heat due to curing bone cement, drilling or reaming without a cooling agent and too rapid loading. It is known that interfacial implant movement of more than 150 μm will inevitably lead to soft tissue formation instead of bone, for instance [11]. Even if one- or two-point bone contact can be demonstrated, this need not represent actual osseointegration of the entire implant.

Screw-type implants inserted using a modified minimally traumatising technique have been convincingly osseointegrated, e.g. in hip arthroplasties [8] and interphalangeal implants [27] or vertebral screws (Fig. 6). However, whether or not osseointegration will become as important a type of anchorage in orthopaedics as in oral and craniofacial implantology will depend on the reported long-term clinical results of this type of anchorage.

Conclusion

Osteoinduction, osteoconduction and osseointegration are interrelated, but not identical phenomena. Osteoinduction is part of normal bone healing and is responsible for the majority of newly formed bone, e.g. after a fracture or the insertion of an implant. The implant itself may be osteoinductive, but this is not a prerequisite for bone induction. Osteoconduction is a term now usually used in conjunction with implants. Osteoconduction and osseointegration both depend not only on biological factors, but also on the response to a foreign material. The osteoconductive response may be rather short lived, but successful osseointegration maintains its bone anchorage over a long period.

References

1. Albrektsson T (1980) The healing of autologous bone grafts after varying degrees of surgical trauma. J Bone Joint Surg [Br] 32:403–410
2. Albrektsson T (1993) On long-term maintenance of the osseointegrated response. Aust Prosthodont J 7 [Suppl]: 15–24
3. Albrektsson T (1995) Principles of osseointegration. In: Hobkirk JA, Watson K (eds) Dental and maxillofacial implantology. Mosby-Wolfe, London, pp 9–19
4. Albrektsson T, Brånemark PI, Hansson HA, Lindström J (1981) Osseointegrated titanium implants. Requirements for ensuring a long-lasting, direct bone anchorage in man. Acta Orthop Scand 52:155–170
5. Albrektsson T, Brånemark PI, Hansson HA, Ivarsson B, Jönsson U (1982) Ultrastructural analysis of the interface zone of titanium and gold implants. Adv Biomaterials 4:167–177
6. Albrektsson T, Brånemark PI, Hansson HA, Kasemo B, Larsson K, Lundström I, McQueen D, Skalak R (1983) The interface zone of inorganic implants in vivo: titanium implants in bone. Ann Biomed Eng 11:1–27
7. Albrektsson T, Eriksson AR, Friberg B, Lekholm U, Lindahl L, Nevins M, Oikarinen V, Roos J, Sennerby L, Åstrand P (1993) Histologic investigations on 33 retrieved Nobelpharma implants. Clinical Implants 12:1–9
8. Albrektsson T, Carlsson LV, Jacobsson M, Macdonald W (1998) The Gothenburg osseointegrated hip arthroplasty: experience with a novel type of hip design. Clin Orth Rel Res 352:81–94
9. Albrektsson T, Johansson C, Lundgren AK, Sul YT, Gottlow J (2000) Experimental studies on oxidized implants. A histomorphometrical and biomechanical analysis. Appl Osseointegration Res 1:21–24
10. Bassett CAL (1968) Biological significance of piezo-electricity. Calcif Tissue Res 1:252–261
11. Brunski JB (1988) The influence of force, motion and related quantities on the response of bone to implants. In: Fitzgerald AF (ed) Non-cemented total hip arthroplasty. Raven, New York, pp 7–19
12. Brånemark PI, Hansson BO, Adell R, Breine U, Lindström J, Hallén O, Öhman A (1977) Osseointegrated titanium implants in the treatment of the edentulous jaw. Scand J Plast Reconstr Surg 11 [Suppl 16]:1–175
13. Buch F (1985) On electrical stimulation of bone tissue. PhD thesis, Dept of Biomaterials/Handicap Research, University of Gothenburg, Sweden, pp 1–139
14. Dealler SF (1981) Electrical phenomena associated with bones and fractures and the therapeutic use of electricity in fracture healing. J Med Eng Tech 5: 73–82

15. Donath K, Laass M, Günzl HJ (1992) The histopathology of different foreign-body reactions in oral soft tissue and bone tissue. Virchows Archiv [A] 420:131–137
16. Frost HM (1989) The biology of fracture healing. An overview for clinicians, part I. Clin Orthop Rel Res 248: 283–293
17. Frost HM (1989) The biology of fracture healing. An overview for clinicans, part II. Clin Orthop Rel Res 248: 294–309
18. Glantz PO (1987) Comment. In: Williams DF (ed) Progress in biomedical engineering, vol 4. Definitions in biomaterials. Elsevier, Amsterdam, p 24
19. Gottlander M (1994) On hard-tissue reactions to hydroxyapatite-coated titanium implants. PhD thesis, Dept of Biomaterials/Handicap Research, University of Göteborg, Sweden, pp 1–192
20. Huggins CB (1931) The formation of bone under the influence of epithelium of the urinary tract. Arch Surg 22:377–386
21. Johansson CB(1991) On tissue reactions to metal implants. PhD thesis, Dept of Biomaterials/Handicap Research, University of Göteborg, Sweden, pp 1–203
22. Johansson C, Albrektsson T, Roos A (1992) A biomechanical and histomorphometric comparison between different types of bone implants evaluated in a rabbit model. Eur J Exp Musculoskel Research 1:51–61
23. Johansson C, Han CH, Wennerberg A, Albrektsson T (1998) A quantitative comparison of machined commercially pure titanium and titanium-aluminum-vanadium implants in rabbit bone. Int J Oral Maxillofac Implants 13:315–321
24. Korhonen LK, Väänänen K (1992) Bone inductive molecules and enhancement of repair and regeneration. In: Hall BK (ed) Fracture repair and regeneration, vol 5. CRC, Boca Raton, pp 209–232
25. Levander G (1938) A study of bone regeneration. Surg Gynec Obstet 67:705–714
26. Lind M (1996) Growth factors: possible new clinical tools. Acta Orthop Scand 67:407–417
27. Lundborg G, Brånemark PI (2000) Osseointegrated proximal interphalangeal joint prostheses with a replaceable flexible joint spacer – long term results. Scand J Plast Reconstr Surg 34:345–353
28. Meredith N (1997) On the clinical measurement of implant stability and osseointegration. PhD thesis, Dept of Biomaterials/Handicap Research, University of Göteborg, Sweden, pp 1–200
29. Morberg P (1991) On bone tissue reactions to acrylic cement. PhD thesis, Dept of Biomaterials/Handicap Research, University of Göteborg, Sweden, pp 1–139
30. Nilsson LP, Granström G, Albrektsson T (1987) The effect of hyperbaric oxygen treatment of bone regeneration. An experimental study in the rabbit. Int J Oral Maxillofac Implants 3:43–48
31. Röser K, Johansson C, Donath K, Albrektsson T (2000) A new approach to demonstate cellular activity in bone formation adjacent to implants. J Biomed Mater Res 51:280–291
32. Sennerby L, Ericson LE, Thomsen P, Lekholm U, Åstrand P (1991) Structure of the bone titanium interface in retrieved clinical oral implants. Clin Oral Impl Res 2:103–111
33. Skalak R, Zhao Y (2000) Interaction of force-fitting and surface roughness of implants. Clin Implant Dent Rel Res 2:219–224
34. Solheim E (1998) Growth factors in bone. Int Orthop (SICOT) 22:410–416
35. Tjellström A, Lindström J, Hallén O, Albrektsson T, Brånemark PI (1981) Osseointegrated titanium implants in the temporal bone. A clinical study on bone-anchored hearing aids. Am J Otol 2:303–310
36. Tjellström A, Lindström J, Nylén O, Albrektsson T, Brånemark P-I, Birgersson B, Nero H, Sylvén C (1981) The bone-anchored auricular epithesis. Laryngoscope 91:811–815
37. Trippel SE, Coutts RD, Einhorn TA, Mundy GR, Rosenfeld RG (1996) Growth factors as therapeutic agents. J Bone Joint Surg [Am] 78:1272–1286
38. Tsuboi N, Sennerby L, Johansson C, Albrektsson T, Tsuboi Y, Iizika T (1996) Histomorphometric analysis of bone-titanium interface in human retrieved implants. In: Ueda M (ed) Proceedings of the third international congress on tissue integration in oral and maxillofacial reconstruction. Quintessence, Tokyo, pp 84–85
39. Urist MR (1965) Bone: formation by autoinduction. Science 150:893–899
40. Urist MR, McLean FC (1952) Osteogenic potency and new bone formation by induction in transplants to the anterior chamber of the eye. J Bone Joint Surg [Am] 34:443–452
41. Urist MR, Mikulski A, Lietze A (1979) Solubilized bone morphogenetic protein. Proc Natl Acad Sci USA 76: 1828–1832
42. Wennerberg A (1996) On surface roughness and implant incorporation. PhD thesis, Dept of Biomaterials/ Handicap Research, University of Göteborg, Sweden, pp 1–212
43. Wilson-Hench J (1987) Osteoinduction. In: Williams DF (ed) Progress in biomedical engineering, vol 4. Definitions in biomaterials. Elsevier, Amsterdam, p 29
44. Yasuda I (1953) Fundamental aspects of fracture treatment. J Kyoto Med Soc 4:395–404
45. Young RW (1963) Nucleic acids, protein synthesis and bone. Clin Orthop Rel Res 26:147–156
46. Zarb G, Albrektsson T (1991) Osseointegration – a requiem for the periodontal ligament? – An editorial. Int J Periodont Rest Dentistry 11:88–91

Martin Lind
Cody Bünger

Factors stimulating bone formation

M. Lind (✉) · C. Bünger
Orthopaedic Research Laboratory,
Nørrebrogade 44 blg 1A,
University Hospital of Aarhus,
8000 Aarhus C, Denmark
e-mail: martinlind@dadlnet.dk,
Tel.: +45-89-494134,
Fax: +45-89-494150

Abstract The aim of this review is to describe major approaches for stimulating bone healing and to review other factors affecting bone healing. Spinal bone fusion after surgery is a demanding process requiring optimal conditions for clinical success. Bone formation and healing can be enhanced through various methods. Experimental studies have revealed an array of stimulative measures. These include biochemical stimulation by use of hormones and growth factors, physical stimulation through mechanical and electromagnetic measures, and bone grafting by use of bone tissue or bone substitutes. Newer biological techniques such as stem cell transplantation and gene therapy can also be used to stimulate bone healing. Apart from bone transplantation, clinical experience with the many stimulation modalities is limited. Possible areas for clinical use of these novel methods are discussed.

Keywords Bone healing · Bone graft · Growth factors · Stimulation · Stem cells · Gene therapy

Introduction

Osseous spinal fusion remains a cornerstone of surgical treatment of severe spinal disorders. However, the success rate is still debated and difficult to assess in the presence of metal implant material. A general failure rate of 5–30% is reported in lumbar spinal fusion [58]. Fusion capacity is influenced by numerous factors: individual biological factors, the bone graft material, and biomechanical and external factors. Predictive factors for good osseous fusion are uniformly associated with good functional outcome, for which psychosocial factors, the presence of neurodeficit, and the primary diagnosis also seem to have major importance.

The individual biological factors governing spinal fusion are related to bone homeostasis and thereby to age. Little is known about individual variations in spinal fusion capacity, although it is generally accepted that young patients heal well. Recent studies have shown that all osteotropic growth factors known to be sequentially involved in the spinal fusion process [6] are present in iliac crest bone autografts of all age groups but with higher variation in older people [3, 16]. Other growth factors that regulate vascular ingrowth have not been addressed and might be equally important. Osteotropic growth factors such as TGF β, BMP2, and BMP7 have been shown experimentally to induce/provide sufficient bone formation for both intracorporal and posterolateral spinal fusion at the level of bone autografts in sheep, rabbits, and baboons [9, 22], but the clinical effectiveness has yet to be determined in controlled studies and negative and positive results have been reported [7, 38, 39]. At present, the cost effectiveness of osteotropic growth factors for humans seems very high compared to combined femoral ring allograft and autograft for anterior interbody fusion or to morselized human allograft in posterolateral fusion.

Bone autograft harvesting is associated with high donor site morbidity (15–20%), even in long-term follow-up. Limited amounts of material are available in osteoporotic patients and for multilevel procedures. Bone cement, structural bone allograft, and metal spacers are viable alternatives to bone autograft in anterior reconstruction. In many less invasive procedures such as cervical and lumbar fusion with cages, bone harvest is time-consuming, and alternative solutions with biologically active substances have found increasing popularity in these procedures [44].

The development of so-called biological cages for intercorporal fusion seems near. The primary goal is sufficient peripheral biomechanical stability. Then an osteogenic potential to bridge bone from one endplate to the other is required for long-term stability. Whether osteogenic growth factors are able to produce bone fusion alone or in combination with new carriers inside stress-shielding cages in older humans is an important question. In posterolateral fusion, additional support of the fusion process by supplementary growth factors or other osteoinductive principles would improve fusion and clinical outcome. However, the clinical effect of exogenic growth factors in the metabolic active fusion bed in humans is mostly unknown and needs further research.

The aim of this review is to present the current knowledge of stimulated bone healing and the basic biological mechanisms involved.

Principles for enhancing bone healing and bone formation

Three basic principles apply to the enhancement of bone healing and bone formation (Table 1). When investigating experimental enhancement, the following principles must be considered:

- Bone induction is new bone formation from determined osteogenic precursor cells
- Bone conduction is enhanced bone formation due to a favorable structural environment where bone is formed
- Bone genesis is stimulated by modulations of natural biochemical processes that initiate and maintain bone formation during a healing response

Bone induction can be obtained by two approaches: cell-mediated and growth factor-mediated. In the first, bone precursor cells can be harvested from bone marrow and placed in, for example, bone defects requiring bone induction to heal sufficiently. Bone precursor cells can also be cultured from crude bone marrow, and by this method large numbers of bone precursor cells can be obtained for bone induction. During osteoinduction, osteogenic precursor cells can proliferate in both osseous and nonosseous biological environments and differentiate to form mature osteoblasts, forming bone matrix that subsequently mineralizes to mature bone tissue.

Table 1 Basic principles for enhancement of bone healing and bone formation and their mechanisms

Osteoinduction	Osteogenesis	Osteoconduction
Bone precursor cells	Growth factors	Porous coatings
TGF-β superfamily	Ca/P ceramics	Ca/P ceramics
Bone autograft	Bone autograft	Bone allograft

In growth factor-mediated bone induction, a special family of growth factors called bone morphogenetic proteins (BMP) have the unique property of stimulating mesenchymal stem cells to differentiate towards chondro- and osteoblastic lineage. Local application of BMP induces extensive bone induction and can be used for bone formation in bone defects and as a substitute for bone grafts. After implantation of autologous bone graft, bone formation is probably accomplished by both cell- and growth factor-mediated bone induction, which occurs with viable precursor cells from the bone marrow stroma and BMP growth factors released from the bone matrix.

In bone conduction, normal bone formation is helped to extend due to a favorable structural environment in which the bone conductive material serves as a scaffold for new bone formation. An example of such an environment is a porous coating with the optimal pore size of 100–400 μm, which is able to favor bone ingrowth into endoprosthetic components. Allogenic bone grafts and other processed bone graft materials probably function mainly as bone conductive materials. Materials such as calcium phosphate ceramics and glass ceramics have osteoconductive properties but have also been suggested to stimulate osteogenesis by releasing nonorganic mineral ions, which activates cellular processes during bone formation and healing [62].

Bone matrix is a storage medium for growth factors that participate in activation and maintenance of cellular processes during bone formation and healing. Some of these growth factors have been shown to accelerate bone formation and bone healing when applied locally to intact and healing bone tissue. However, this principle is pure osteogenesis stimulation. The main topic of this review is to describe principles for stimulated bone healing and formation.

Patient-related factors

Age

Age is a definite determining factor for bone healing. One probable cause for reduced healing potential with increasing age is the reduction in the number of mesenchymal stem cells in bone tissue with increasing age [12]. With bone trauma, this means that stem cell recruitment for the healing response is reduced with increasing age. This limited access to biochemical factors during a healing response contributes to the already weakened healing response in older patients. Some evidence exists that the growth factor levels within bone matrix also decline with age [54, 59].

Osteoporosis

Osteoporosis leads to a decrease in bone volume, especially in areas with trabecular bone tissue. The reduced thickness and number of trabeculae resulting from osteoporosis compromise mechanical properties, especially of metaphyseal bone regions, and lead to increased fracture risk. Until recently, osteoporotic bone was thought to have the same healing potential as nonosteoporotic bone. However, recent studies demonstrated reduced fracture healing in osteoporotic rats [67].

Smoking

Smoking has been demonstrated to inhibit fracture healing and spinal fusion both experimentally and clinically [6, 36]. In experimental studies, nicotine demonstrated negative effects on callus formation, cortical remodeling, and mechanical properties [55]. In a spinal fusion model in rabbits, nicotine stimulation resulted in nonunion in all cases, as opposed to only 44% in the control group [60]. The negative influence of nicotine on the healing process is thought to be due mainly to inhibition of vascularization [56].

Drugs

Systemically administered drugs can potentially modulate bone formation and repair. Several drugs are known that have adverse effects on bone formation. Few anabolic hormones have been demonstrated to stimulate bone healing. Growth hormone has been demonstrated experimentally to enhance fracture healing [5]. No clinical study has demonstrated advantageous effects of growth hormone on fracture healing.

Biphosphonates, which block osteoclastic bone resorption, can increase bone mineral content (BMC) in osteoporotic patients. Some speculation existed as to whether interference with the bone remodeling process affects bone healing. Experimental and clinical studies have tested the effects of biphosphonates during fracture healing. In a randomized controlled study of patients with Colles' fractures, alendronate increased BMC at the fracture site and had no other adverse effects [1]. Similar effects have been found experimentally in rat diaphyseal fractures, with increased BMC and no effect on remodeling and mechanical properties of the fracture [46]. Today, no knowledge exists concerning the effects of bisphosphonates on the healing of bone grafts during spinal fusion.

Cytotoxic drugs used for chemotherapy can naturally exhibit negative effects on bone formation. Experimental studies have shown that even short-term administration of methotrexate reduces trabecular bone volume and the bone formation rate. Fractures in rats also heal more slowly and with weaker mechanical properties after methotrexate treatment [27, 53]. Corticosteroids have well-known adverse effects on bone remodeling, leading to osteoporosis. Also, bone healing is adversely affected by corticosteroids [25]. Nonsteroidal anti-inflammatory drugs (NSAID) are known to inhibit ectopic bone formation [29]. Some experimental data provide evidence that these drugs can inhibit fracture healing [28, 35]. Unfortunately, there is no certainty concerning the effects of NSAID on bone graft healing during spinal fusion or for osseointegration of spinal implants.

Adjuvant factors stimulating bone formation

Bone grafting

Principles

Bone grafts have two main functions: (1) promote bone formation or osteogenesis and (2) provide structural support. Osteogenesis may originate from the bone graft itself or from the host bed. Graft osteogenesis can occur when cells are transplanted, remain viable through diffusion, and produce new bone at the transplantation site. More significant contributions to osteogenesis, however, occur through the processes of osteoinduction and osteoconduction.

Osteoinduction occurs when pleuripotential mesenchymal cells in the host bed are recruited to differentiate into bone-forming cells known as osteoblasts. This process is mediated by BMP, a glycoprotein found in the matrix of bone grafts, and other growth factors [66]. Osteoconduction is the process whereby a bone graft serves as a scaffold or lattice facilitating migration of host cells for osteogenesis. Osteoconduction eventually leads to partial resorption of the graft and replacement by new host bone. This process is known as creeping substitution. Incorporation of bone grafts through osteoconduction, osteoinduction, and osteogenesis occurs in sequential phases similar to those of fracture healing. The length of time required for a bone graft to incorporate depends on a number of factors including the type of graft utilized and its structure.

Types of bone grafts

Three main types of bone grafts are used in clinical practice: autografts, allografts, and bone graft substitutes.

Autografts. Autogenous bone grafts (ABG) have been proven as the most reliable method of stimulating bone healing. Sources for these grafts include but are not limited to the patient's iliac crest, proximal femur or tibia, femoral head, and a resected rib. ABG incorporate more quickly than allografts by their greater capacity for osteoconduction and osteoinduction. Another advantage is that they may retain the capability of graft osteogenesis through viable osteoblasts in the graft. Autograft application is the gold standard for obtaining spinal fusion during all kinds of spinal surgery.

Allografts. Because of the aforementioned disadvantages, alternatives to ABG have been researched extensively. Allografting (transplanting bone from one patient to another) has become a popular substitute. Allografts have mainly osteoconductive properties. Allograft chips are often used to supplement bone autograft when large amounts of bone graft material are needed during spine fusion.

Bone graft substitutes. To avoid immunologic graft rejection, eliminate disease risk, and have an unlimited supply of graft material, interest in bone graft substitutes has mounted. Bone graft substitutes include ceramics, demineralized bone matrix (DBM), and composite grafts. Most ceramics currently under investigation are synthetic and composed of hydroxyapatite (HA), tricalcium phosphate (TCP), or combinations of the two [15, 31, 48]. Ceramics simply provide an osteoconductive lattice upon which host osteogenesis can occur. They completely lack osteoinductive properties. Experimental animal studies have consistently demonstrated the superior performance of ABG over ceramic implants alone. However, Bucholz [15] found a similar efficacy of calcium phosphate ceramics and autogenous bone for certain clinical applications in humans such as filling defects under tibial plateau fractures, where the graft material would be under compressive forces. DBM is formed through acid extraction of bone, leaving a composite of noncollagenous proteins, bone growth factors, and collagen in continuity. Currently, DBM is available freeze-dried and processed from cortical or corticocancellous bone as a powder, crushed granules, or chips. It is also available as a gel called Grafton (Osteotech, Shrewsbury, N.J., USA), which can be applied intraoperatively with a syringe [52].

Composite grafts incorporate the favorable properties of different materials into a single compound. They include materials providing both an osteoconductive matrix and osteoinductive properties. Composites of TCP and BMP are currently in use, with TCP ceramic providing an osteoconductive matrix and the BMP stimulating bone healing through osteoinduction. Collagraft (Zimmer, Warsaw, Ind., USA) is a commercially available composite consisting of bovine fibrillar collagen and porous calcium phosphate ceramic. The mixture is nonosteoinductive, but adding autogenous bone marrow provides osteoinductive potential [18, 23].

Biochemical stimulation

Biochemical stimulation of bone healing is a new approach to the above mentioned clinical problems and has become increasingly relevant with the discovery more than a decade ago of peptide regulator molecules called growth factors. Growth factors have been found in all tissues and are today known to regulate local cell-to-cell metabolism and mediate the cellular effects of various hormones. Bone matrix is known to be a large reservoir for numerous growth factors that have been suggested as regulators of bone remodeling and initiators of the bone healing process [47]. In vitro studies have documented that bone growth factors exert numerous regulating effects on bone cells [73], while in vivo studies have shown that a small number of growth factors can stimulate bone healing processes in animals [4, 34, 71]. These data are promising for future possibilities in growth factor-stimulated bone formation and bone healing in orthopedic surgery.

Growth factors

Aside from structural proteins, bone matrix also contains small amounts of very potent regulators of bone cell metabolism. These proteins, called bone-derived growth factors, are produced by osteoblasts and incorporated into the extracellular matrix during bone formation, but small amounts can also be trapped systemically from serum and incorporated into the matrix. The growth factors are located within the matrix until remodeling or trauma causes solubilization and release of the proteins [17, 33]. After release, the growth factors are able to regulate osteoblast and osteoclast metabolism during bone remodeling and may initiate and control a healing response after bone trauma. Thus, they are recognized as the main regulators of bone cell metabolism.

Bone morphogenetic proteins

In 1965, Marshall Urist made the discovery that DBM could induce bone formation when placed ectopically in subcutaneous tissue [63]. This ability of DBM was ascribed to a protein which Urist named BMP [64, 65]. These are the only growth factors with a known ability to stimulate differentiation of mesenchymal stem cells in chondro- and osteoblastic directions [19, 64, 70]. Recent studies have demonstrated that BMPs are expressed during the early phases of fracture healing [32, 50]. The novel recombinant BMPs have intact bone-inducing capacity but need special carriers to exert their activity at low doses [24, 45, 57, 68]. Functional carriers for BMP are: collagen matrix, DBM, and various synthetic polysaccharide matrices [72].

The function of the carrier matrix is to immobilize bone-inducing protein at a particular site for a sufficient time to allow bone induction to occur. In vivo studies of BMP have primarily focused on its use in stimulating the healing of bone defects [21, 61, 71]. A novel clinical approach was performed by Cook, who used BMP-7 and collagen as a substitute for autologous bone in spine fusions in dogs [22]. Although the cellular mechanisms for BMP-stimulated bone induction are only vaguely understood, the in vivo bone induction activity of this group of growth factors is unique, and BMP appears very promising for clinical use in any situation requiring stimulation of bone healing.

Transforming growth factor β

Transforming growth factor beta (TGF-β) is a multifunctional cytokine with a broad range of biological activities. These include regulation of growth and differentiation of many cell types. In general, TGF-β has stimulative effects on cells of mesenchymal origin. Applied continuously to a healing osteotomy in rabbits, TGF-β stimulated increased callus formation and increased maximal bending strength of the osteotomy [43]. In vivo studies have demonstrated stimulatory effects of recombinant human (rh)TGF-β1 on bone healing to both unloaded and weight-loaded TCP and HA ceramic-coated implants in dogs [40, 41, 42]. The in vivo data on TGF-β's ability to stimulate bone formation are very promising, and TGF-β and BMP are probably the most realistic candidates as growth factors for stimulating bone healing and bone induction in orthopedic surgical situations.

Clinical experience with growth factors

So far, only limited data exist concerning the effects of growth factors on human bone tissue and in clinical scenarios. Growth factors in the BMP family are currently being tested and under evaluation for clinical use. BMP-2 and BMP-7 (the latter also designated osteogenic protein, or OP-1) have been tested mainly in clinical cases for salvage purposes. One randomized clinical trial was performed using OP-1 in combination with type 1 bovine collagen. The study addressed treatment of pseudarthrosis. Autogenous bone graft was tested against OP-1 in a randomized multicenter study including 150 patients [20]. Patients were followed for 1 year. Results of the study demonstrated equal effects of OP-1 and autograft treatments according to patient-based clinical evaluation. Radiographic evaluation demonstrated a slightly higher degree of healing in the autograft group. This result, however, could be biased because the autograft used has an independent radiodensity, whereas the OP-1 does not. One controlled study of the effects of OP-1 on bone formation in humans was performed by Geesink [26]. Patients with tibial osteotomies for surgical treatment of osteoarthrosis had additional fibular defects that were stimulated with OP-1 in combination with type 1 bovine collagen, collagen alone, empty gap, and DBM. The OP-1 stimulated healing of the defects, whereas collagen alone did not.

In conclusion, research during the last decade has shown increasing evidence that growth factors can be used as in vivo stimulators of bone healing and bone formation and therefore have therapeutic potential in a variety of clinical situations in orthopedic surgery.

Cell-mediated bone healing

Recently, efforts have focused on the possibility of osteogenic cell transplants for enhancing bone healing and formation. Osteogenic stem cells have been identified, characterized, and isolated for culture expansion [30]. These cells, which are retrieved from bone marrow, can be grown and multiplied in vitro. Multiplied osteogenic stem cell suspensions can be used as transplants for local implantation at sites requiring enhanced bone formation. Preclinical studies have demonstrated the in vivo potential for bone regeneration of locally implanted osteogenic stem cells. Healing of critically sized defects in long bone has been demonstrated in rats and dogs by the use of culture-expanded autologous osteogenic stem cells combined with porous ceramic implants [13, 14]. Bone formation and mechanical properties were enhanced in groups whose ceramic implants were loaded with osteogenic cells. Combinations of osteogenic stem cells and growth factors have been shown to stimulate bone healing in critically large defects. A combination of BMP-2 and nonpurified marrow cells demonstrated 100% healing at 6 weeks, whereas BMP-2 alone, marrow cells alone, and autologous bone graft all demonstrated less than 100% healing at 12 weeks [37]. Cell-mediated stimulated bone healing is very interesting clinically because of the easy access to bone marrow and the high degree of safety using autologous tissue. Additional preclinical studies and clinical studies are necessary to define indications and effects of this new treatment modality.

Gene therapy of bone healing

Osteogenic stem cell transplantation has been further developed using principles of gene therapy. Gene therapy for local enhancement of bone healing is accomplished by transfecting bone stem cells with genes encoding for growth factors that stimulate bone healing. The stem cells then function as growth factor factories with overexpression of a single growth factor. Other phenotypic characteristics of the stem cells which favor bone formation are retained. Typically, the growth factor overexpression is maintained for several weeks. Stem cells transfected with growth factors of the BMP family have been the most successful. Recent studies have described successful stimulation of bone formation using adenovirus-mediated direct gene transfer of BMP [2, 49]. In these studies, direct injections of BMP expressing adenovirus or cells transfected with BMP virus were able to induce bone formation in muscle tissue. More clinically related animal studies were performed in a long bone defect model and a spine fusion model. In the former, marrow cells were transfected with BMP-2-expressing adenovirus [39]. The BMP-2-expressing marrow cells were subsequently injected into critically sized defects in rat femur. A substantially higher healing rate was seen in the BMP-2 marrow-treated group than with BMP-2 protein alone or marrow cells alone. In the spine fusion study, DBM was soaked with marrow transfected and subsequently expressing a novel osteoinductive protein called latent membrane protein (LMP)-1 [8]. Fusion rates were 100% in the LMP marrow cell group and 0% in the marrow cell alone group.

The principle of gene therapy is very interesting as a future clinical tool for stimulation of bone formation and healing, and extensive research is being performed to determine potential advantages and indications for this method. However, concern exists about clinical safety issues and the long-term complications of injecting genetically altered cells into humans.

Physical factors

Electrical

Electrical stimulation of bone healing has existed for three decades and is an FDA-approved treatment for nonunion. The theoretical and biological background for why electrical stimuli can accelerate bone repair is not fully understood, but some knowledge is available. Electrical processes are thought to play a significant role in the mechanically mediated stimulation of bone healing and bone modeling. Charged molecules of bone matrix proteins can generate streaming potentials during mechanical deformation. Also, ion flux can be generated in interstitial fluid of bone tissue during mechanical deformation [69]. Such endogenous electromechanical phenomena affect osteoblasts and osteocytes and alter transmembrane ion channel properties, leading to increased metabolic activity.

Three different types of electrical stimulation have been developed for clinical use. Direct current generators use 5–20 mA. The anode is placed cutaneously some distance from the stimulation site [11]. Alternating current generators use a 5 V, 60 kHz signal to develop a 5–10 mA current at skin level. These methods are also called capacitively coupled electrical stimulation. Using a noninvasive approach, electrodes are placed on each side of the extremity being treated. Pulsed electromagnetic fields (PEMF), also called inductive coupling, represent a different concept in which electrical currents are induced magnetically to microenvironments such as cells and extracellular matrix [10, 51]. Presently, electrical stimulation has obtained limited clinical application. For fresh fractures, this effect is so moderate and therefore clinically insignificant. For nonunion, more recent treatment methods combining intramedullary nailing and bone grafting are successful in up to 90% of cases. This has diminished the relative advantages of electrical stimulation for treating nonunion.

Conclusion

Numerous stimulatory modalities for bone healing have proven effective in preclinical experimental settings. However, limited clinical data exist that address what types of stimulation are beneficial to patients. Also, no data exist concerning which pathological conditions respond to stimulation of bone healing. The growth factors from the TGF superfamily, BMP and TGF, have demonstrated potent stimulatory capability for bone healing and bone formation in vivo. The major problem of these growth factors in clinical use is appropriate delivery systems to ensure sufficient biological activity for optimal effects on bone healing and formation. In the future, the use of bone grafting could probably be reduced considerably by employing growth factors in collagenous or other matrices. Animal experiments have demonstrated that BMP can form bone to the same extent as autologous bone for spine fusions in dogs [22]. New techniques such gene therapy and autologous bone stem cell transplantation might help improve stimulation approaches so that bone grafting can be reduced.

The biological state of the bone tissue to be stimulated is important for the possibility of obtaining stimulatory effects. Most studies on stimulation of bone healing were performed in healthy bone with good vascularization. It should be speculated that impaired vascularization and poor bone quality could reduce the stimulatory effects of growth factors and other adjuvant therapies. However, it could also be speculated that exogenous stimulation is especially advantageous when endogenous healing is compromised. Additional studies are needed to answer these questions and to find ways of improving the biological response to stimulation with various qualities of bone and vascularization.

One major problem is to identify patients and conditions in which impaired bone healing response is likely to lead to poor clinical results such as nonfusion after spinal stabilizing procedures. Therefore, new diagnostic tools are needed that test preoperative healing capacity. This would enable surgeons to determine which patients need adjuvant therapies to improve bone healing.

The coming decade will possibly define indications for the new clinical tools for stimulating bone healing in clinical practice. These tools could increase fusion rates after spine surgery and reduce morbidity after autograft harvest.

References

1. Adolphson P, Abbaszadegan H, Boden H, Salemyr M, Henriques T (2000) Clodronate increases mineralization of callus after Colles' fracture: a randomized, double-blind, placebo-controlled, prospective trial in 32 patients. Acta Orthop Scand 71:195–200
2. Alden TD, Pittman DD, Hankins GR, Beres EJ, Engh JA, Das S, Hudson SB, Kerns KM, Kallmes DF, Helm GA (1999) In vivo endochondral bone formation using a bone morphogenetic protein 2 adenoviral vector. Hum Gene Ther 10:2245–2253
3. Andersen T (2000) Localization and quantification in human bone autograft by means of of semi-quantitative image analysis and ELISA-technique. Aarhus University, Denmark
4. Aspenberg P, Lohmander LS (1989) Fibroblast growth factor stimulates bone formation. Bone induction studied in rats. Acta Orthop Scand 60:473–476
5. Bak B, Jorgensen PH, Andreassen TT (1991) The stimulating effect of growth hormone on fracture healing is dependent on onset and duration of administration. Clin Orthop 295–301
6. Boden SD (1998) The biology of posterolateral lumbar spinal fusion. Orthop Clin North Am 29:603–619
7. Boden SD (2000) Biology of lumbar spine fusion and use of bone graft substitutes: present, future, and next generation. Tissue Eng 6:383–399
8. Boden SD, Titus L, Hair G, Liu Y, Viggeswarapu M, Nanes MS, Baranowski C (1998) Lumbar spine fusion by local gene therapy with a cDNA encoding a novel osteoinductive protein (LMP-1). Spine 23:2486–2492
9. Boden SD, Martin GJ, Jr., Morone MA, Ugbo JL, Moskovitz PA (1999) Posterolateral lumbar intertransverse process spine arthrodesis with recombinant human bone morphogenetic protein 2/hydroxyapatite-tricalcium phosphate after laminectomy in the nonhuman primate. Spine 24:1179–1185
10. Borsalino G, Bagnacani M, Bettati E, Fornaciari F, Rocchi R, Uluhogian S, Ceccherelli G, Cadossi R, Traina GC (1988) Electrical stimulation of human femoral intertrochanteric osteotomies. Double-blind study. Clin Orthop 256–263
11. Brighton CT, Shaman P, Heppenstall RB, Esterhai JL Jr, Pollack SR, Friedenberg ZB (1995) Tibial nonunion treated with direct current, capacitive coupling, or bone graft. Clin Orthop 223–234
12. Bruder SP, Fink DJ, Caplan AI (1994) Mesenchymal stem cells in bone development, bone repair, and skeletal regeneration therapy. J Cell Biochem 56: 283–294
13. Bruder SP, Kraus KH, Goldberg VM, Kadiyala S (1998) The effect of implants loaded with autologous mesenchymal stem cells on the healing of canine segmental bone defects. J Bone Joint Surg Am 80:985–996
14. Bruder SP, Kurth AA, Shea M, Hayes WC, Jaiswal N, Kadiyala S (1998) Bone regeneration by implantation of purified, culture-expanded human mesenchymal stem cells. J Orthop Res 16: 155–162
15. Bucholz RW, Carlton A, Holmes RE (1987) Hydroxyapatite and tricalcium phosphate bone graft substitutes. Orthop Clin North Am 18:323–334
16. Bünger M (2000) Predictive factors for bone helaing at lumbar spine fusion. Quantification of osteotropic growth factors in human autograft bone tissue by means of PCR technique. Aarhus University, Denmark
17. Canalis E, McCarthy TL, Centrella M (1988) Growth factors and the regulation of bone remodeling. J Clin Invest 81:277–281
18. Chapman MW, Bucholz R, Cornell C (1997) Treatment of acute fractures with a collagen-calcium phosphate graft material. A randomized clinical trial. J Bone Joint Surg Am 79:495–502
19. Chen P, Carrington JL, Hammonds RGJ, Reddi AH (1991) Stimulation of chondrogenesis in limb bud mesoderm cells by recombinant human bone morphogenetic protein 2B (BMP-2B) and modulation by transforming growth factor beta 1 and beta 2. Exp Cell Res 195:509–515
20. Cook SD (1999) Preclinical and clinical evaluation of osteogenic protein-1 (BMP-7) in bony sites. Orthopedics 22: 669–671
21. Cook SD, Baffes GC, Wolfe MW et al (1993) rhOP-1 heals segmental long-bone defects in non-human primates. [Abstract]. Trans ORS 484
22. Cook SD, Dalton JE, Tan EH, Whitecloud-III TS, Rueger DC (1994) In vivo evaluation of recombinant human osteogenic protein (rhOP-1) implants as a bone graft substitute for spinal fusions. Spine 19:1655–163
23. Cornell CN, Lane JM, Chapman M, Merkow R, Seligson D, Henry S, Gustilo R, Vincent K (1991) Multicenter trial of Collagraft as bone graft substitute. J Orthop Trauma 5:1–8
24. Cox K (1991) Histological and ultrastructural comparison of the in vivo activities rhBMP 2 and 5. [Abstract]. J Bone Min Res 6:S155
25. Duncan H (1972) Osteoporosis in rheumatoid arthritis and corticosteroid induced osteoporosis. Orthop Clin North Am 3:571–583
26. Geesink RG, Hoefnagels NH, Bulstra SK (1999) Osteogenic activity of OP-1 bone morphogenetic protein (BMP-7) in a human fibular defect. J Bone Joint Surg Br 81:710–718
27. Gerster JC, Bossy R, Dudler J (1999) Bone non-union after osteotomy in patients treated with methotrexate. J Rheumatol 26:2695–2697
28. Hogevold HE, Grogaard B, Reikeras O (1992) Effects of short-term treatment with corticosteroids and indomethacin on bone healing. A mechanical study of osteotomies in rats. Acta Orthop Scand 63:607–611
29. Hoikka V, Lindholm TS, Eskola A (1990) Flurbiprofen inhibits heterotopic bone formation in total hip arthroplasty. Arch Orthop Trauma Surg 109:224–226
30. Jaiswal N, Haynesworth SE, Caplan AI, Bruder SP (1997) Osteogenic differentiation of purified, culture-expanded human mesenchymal stem cells in vitro. J Cell Biochem 64:295–312
31. Jarcho M (1981) Calcium phosphate ceramics as hard tissue prosthetics. Clin Orthop 259–278
32. Jin Y, Yang L, White FH (1994) An immunocytochemical study of bone morphogenetic protein in experimental fracture healing of the rabbit mandible. Chin Med Sci J 9:91–95
33. Joyce ME, Jingushi S, Bolander ME (1992) Transforming growth factor in the regulation of fracture repair. Orthop Clin North Am 21:199–209
34. Joyce ME, Roberts AB, Sporn MB, Bolander ME (1990) Transforming growth factor beta and the initiation of chondrogenesis and osteogenesis in the rat femur. J Cell Biol 110:2195–207
35. Keller J, Bunger C, Andreassen TT, Bak B, Lucht U (1987) Bone repair inhibited by indomethacin. Effects on bone metabolism and strength of rabbit osteotomies. Acta Orthop Scand 58: 379–383
36. Kwiatkowski TC, Hanley EN Jr, Ramp WK (1996) Cigarette smoking and its orthopedic consequences. Am J Orthop 25:590–597
37. Lane JM, Yasko AW, Tomin E, Cole BJ, Waller S, Browne M, Turek T, Gross J (1999) Bone marrow and recombinant human bone morphogenetic protein-2 in osseous repair. Clin Orthop 216–227
38. Laursen M, Hoy K, Hansen ES, Gelineck J, Christensen FB, Bünger CE (1999) Recombinant bone morphogenetic protein-7 as an intracorporal bone growth stimulator in unstable thoracolumbar burst fractures in humans: preliminary results. Eur Spine J 8:485–490

39. Lieberman JR, Daluiski A, Stevenson S, Wu L, McAllister P, Lee YP, Kabo JM, Finerman GA, Berk AJ, Witte ON (1999) The effect of regional gene therapy with bone morphogenetic protein-2-producing bone-marrow cells on the repair of segmental femoral defects in rats. J Bone Joint Surg Am 81:905–917
40. Lind M, Overgaard S, Nguyen T, Ongpipattanakul B, Bünger C, Soballe K (1996) Transforming growth factor-beta stimulates bone ongrowth. Hydroxyapatite-coated implants studied in dogs. Acta Orthop Scand 67:611–616
41. Lind M, Overgaard S, Ongpipattanakul B, Nguyen T, Bünger C, S¢balle K (1996) Transforming growth factor-beta stimulates bone ongrowth to weight-loaded tricalcium phosphate coated implants. J Bone Joint Surg Br 78:377–382
42. Lind M, Overgaard S, S¢balle K, Nguyen T, Ongpipattanakul B, Bünger C (1996) Transforming growth factor-beta 1 enhances bone healing to unloaded tricalcium phosphate coated implants: an experimental study in dogs. J Orthop Res 14:343–350
43. Lind M, Schumacker B, Søballe K, Keller J, Bünger C (1993) Transforming growth factor- enhances fracture healing in rabbit tibiae. Acta Orthop Scand 64:553–556
44. Ludwig SC, Kowalski JM, Boden SD (2000) Osteoinductive bone graft substitutes. Eur Spine J [Suppl 1]:S119–25
45. Luyten FP, Cunningham NS, Vukicevic S, Paralkar V, Ripamonti U, Reddi AH (1992) Advances in osteogenin and related bone morphogenetic proteins in bone induction and repair. Acta Orthop Belg 58 [Suppl 1]:263–267
46. Madsen JE, Berg-Larsen T, Kirkeby OJ, Falch JA, Nordsletten L (1998) No adverse effects of clodronate on fracture healing in rats. Acta Orthop Scand 69:532–536
47. Mohan S, Baylink DJ (1991) Bone growth factors. Clin Orthop 263:30–48
48. Moore DC, Chapman MW, Manske D (1987) The evaluation of a biphasic calcium phosphate ceramic for use in grafting long-bone diaphyseal defects. J Orthop Res 5:356–365
49. Musgrave DS, Bosch P, Ghivizzani S, Robbins PD, Evans CH, Huard J (1999) Adenovirus-mediated direct gene therapy with bone morphogenetic protein-2 produces bone. Bone 24:541–547
50. Nakase T, Nomura S, Yoshikawa H, Hashimoto J, Hirota S, Kitamura Y, Oikawa S, Ono K, Takaoka K (1994) Transient and localized expression of bone morphogenetic protein 4 messenger RNA during fracture healing. J Bone Miner Res 9:651–659
51. Ostrum R, Chao EYS, Bassett et al (1994) Bone injury, regeneration, and repair. In: Simon SR (ed) Orthopaedic basic science. American Academy of Orthopaedic Surgeons, pp 277–323
52. Pals SD, Wilkins RM (1992) Giant cell tumor of bone treated by curettage, cementation, and bone grafting. Orthopedics 15:703–708
53. Pelker RR, Friedlaender GE, Panjabi MM, Markham T, Hausman M, Doganis AC, McKay J (1985) Chemotherapy-induced alterations in the biomechanics of rat bone. J Orthop Res 3: 91–95
54. Pfeilschifter J, Diel I, Scheppach B, Bretz A, Krempien R, Erdmann J, Schmid G, Reske N, Bismar H, Seck T et al (1998) Concentration of transforming growth factor beta in human bone tissue: relationship to age, menopause, bone turnover, and bone volume. J Bone Miner Res 13:716–730
55. Raikin SM, Landsman JC, Alexander VA, Froimson MI, Plaxton NA (1998) Effect of nicotine on the rate and strength of long bone fracture healing. Clin Orthop 231–237
56. Riebel GD, Boden SD, Whitesides TE, Hutton WC (1995) The effect of nicotine on incorporation of cancellous bone graft in an animal model. Spine 20:2198–2202
57. Ripamonti U, Ma S, Cunningham NS, Yeates L, Reddi AH (1992) Initiation of bone regeneration in adult baboons by osteogenin, a bone morphogenetic protein. Matrix 12:369–380
58. Roye DP, Farcy JP (1987) Lumbosacral fusion. In: Camins M, O'Leary P (eds) The lumbar spine. Raven, New York
59. Seck T, Scheppach B, Scharla S, Diel I, Blum WF, Bismar H, Schmid G, Krempien B, Ziegler R, Pfeilschifter J (1998) Concentration of insulin-like growth factor (IGF)-I and -II in iliac crest bone matrix from pre- and postmenopausal women: relationship to age, menopause, bone turnover, bone volume, and circulating IGFs. J Clin Endocrinol Metab 83:2331–2337
60. Silcox DH 3rd, Daftari T, Boden SD, Schimandle JH, Hutton WC, Whitesides TE Jr (1995) The effect of nicotine on spinal fusion. Spine 20:1549–1553
61. Stevenson S, Cunningham J, Toth J et al (1992) Osteogenin in conjunction with ceramic induces bone formation in orthopic segmental defects in rats. [Abstract]. Trans ORS 579
62. Teti A, Tarquilio A, Grano M, Colucci S, Laforgia A, Mangini F, Zambonin Zallone A (1991) Effects of calcium-phosphate-based materials on proliferation and alkaline phosphatase activity of newborn rat periosteal cells in vitro. J Dent Res 70:997–1001
63. Urist MR (1965) Bone formation by autoinduction. Science 159:893–899
64. Urist MR, DeLange RJ, Finerman GAM (1983) Bone cell differentiation and growth factors. Science 220:680–686
65. Urist MR, Huo YK, Brownell AG, Hohl WM, Buyske J, Lietze A, Tempst P, Hunkapiller M, DeLange RJ (1984) Purification of bovine bone morphogenetic protein by hydroxy apatite chromatography. Proc Natl Acad Sci USA 81:371–376
66. Urist MR, O'Connor BT, Burwell GR (1994) Bone grafts, derivatives and substitutes. Butterworth, Oxford
67. Walsh WR, Sherman P, Howlett CR, Sonnabend DH, Ehrlich MG (1997) Fracture healing in a rat osteopenia model. Clin Orthop 218–227
68. Wang EA, Rosen V, D'alessandro JS, Bauduy M, Cordes P, Harada T, Israel DI, Hewitt AT, Kerns KM, LaPan P et al (1990) Recombinant human morphogenic protein induces bone formation. Proc Natl Acad Sci USA 87: 2220–2224
69. Wang Q, Zhong S, Ouyang J, Jiang L, Zhang Z, Xie Y, Luo S (1998) Osteogenesis of electrically stimulated bone cells mediated in part by calcium ions. Clin Orthop 259–268
70. Yamaguchi A, Katagiri T, Ikeda T, Wozney JM, Rosen V, Wang EA, Kahn AJ, Suda T, Yoshiki S (1991) Recombinant human bone morphogenetic protein-2 stimulates osteoblastic maturation and inhibits myogenic differentiation in vitro. J Cell Biol 113: 681–687
71. Yasko AW, Cole BJ, Lane JM, Tomin M, Peterson M, Ron E, Turek T, Wang EA (1992) The healing of segmental bone defects induced by rhBMP-2. J Bone Joint Surg Am 74:659–670
72. Yasko AW, Cole BJ, Lane JM et al (1993) Comparison of rh BMP-2 versus cancellous bone to heal segmental bone defects. [Abstract]. Trans ORS 100
73. Zheng MH, Wood DJ, Papadimitriou JM (1992) What's new in the role of cytokines on osteoblast proliferation and differentiation? Pathol Res Pract 188:1104–1121

Joël Delécrin
Cédric Deschamps
Mostafa Romih
Dominique Heymann
Norbert Passuti

Influence of bone environment on ceramic osteointegration in spinal fusion: comparison of bone-poor and bone-rich sites

J. Delécrin (✉) · N. Passuti
Department of Orthopaedic Surgery,
Hôtel Dieu, University Hospital of Nantes,
44093 Nantes, France
e-mail: joel.delecrin@chu-nantes.fr,
Tel.: +33-2-40084860,
Fax: +33-2-40084908

C. Deschamps · M. Romih · D. Heymann
Laboratoire de Physiopathologie
de la Résorption Osseuse,
Faculté de Médecine,
Université de Nantes, Nantes, France

Abstract Quantitative experimental data showed differences in bone quality and ceramic incorporation between bone-rich and bone-poor implantation sites. Bone in-growth was significantly lower for ceramic implanted at a lumbar intertransverse than a laminar site. Bone-marrow enrichment of the lumbar intertransverse site (regarded as bone-poor) greatly facilitated ceramic osteointegration. The vertebral interbody site, despite theoretical richness in osteogenic precursor cells, might be bone-poor at the time of grafting as compared to the reference iliac crest site. These data have important clinical implications concerning the potential benefit of enriching both bone-poor and bone-rich sites.

Keywords Bone substitutes · Spinal fusion · Calcium phosphate ceramics · Osteogenic precursor cells

Introduction

The biological processes of ceramic osteointegration depend partly on the quality of host bone surrounding bone graft material [6]. The ideal recipient site should be conducive to osteoconduction, osteoinduction and osteogenesis [6]. In practice, these general conditions require either extensive contact or a small space between local host bone and bone substitute in the presence of viable osteogenic precursor cells. These conditions relate to surgical preparation of the recipient site, i.e. the quality of local decortication, the technique of bone substitute positioning and the intrinsic state of the implantation site (quantity of host bone surface available, local richness in osteoprogenitor cells, etc.).

Thus, the potential for bone growth into a bone graft substitute may differ depending on whether the material is on the lamina in contact with host bone or positioned laterally close to the transverse process and surrounded mainly by muscle tissue. Moreover, the addition of progenitor cells from a bone-marrow puncture to graft materials, i.e. enrichment of the graft area with osteogenic cells, may improve the outcome of bone substitute osteointegration [2, 8].

In cases of spinal fusion, the clinical validation of these basic concepts is not very apparent. The present study, based on experimental data from the literature and personal work, attempted to quantify the differences between bone-rich and bone-poor implantation sites in terms of bone quality and ceramic incorporation. The main considerations were the differences between laminar and intertransverse sites at the lumbar level, the benefit of enriching the poor intertransverse site with bone-marrow aspirate, and the richness in osteoprogenitor stem cells at the rich vertebral interbody site as compared to the reference iliac crest site.

Laminar versus intertransverse process site

The posterolateral lumbar fusion site can be divided into two areas with respect to the local biological and mechan-

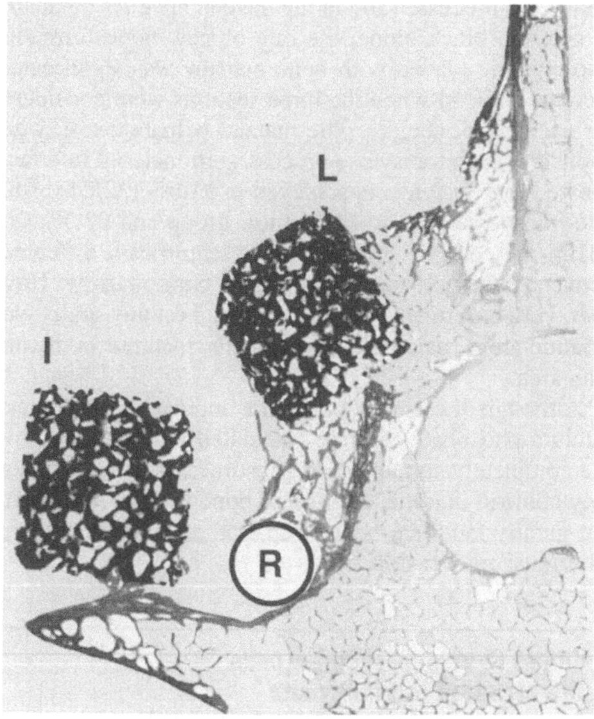

Fig. 1 Juxtaposed microradiographs of ceramic blocks at the laminar (*L*) and intertransverse (*I*) process sites. (*R* indicates location of the rod)

ical environment: a laminar area associated with the facet joint and an area between and including the transverse processes. This distinction is clinically relevant, since the intertransverse site constitutes the poorer bone environment and is often used alone as a surgical site, given the frequency of bilateral laminectomy combined with facetectomy.

In a previous study [4], we evaluated bone growth into calcium phosphate ceramic in a canine model with respect to localization on the lamina or transverse process sites of the lumbar spine. This model represented a clinically relevant setting for the use of pedicular instrumentation and the achievement of posterolateral arthrodesis. The ceramic used was a macroporous biphasic calcium phosphate (40% β-tricalcium and 60% hydroxyapatite) in parallelepipedic block form implanted into both laminar and intertransverse sites, from L2 to L4, on eight dogs. The animals were sacrificed 9 months after surgery.

In the present study, the local environment was taken into account in characterizing each site, i.e. in determining whether bone contact occurred for each side of the square section of the block. Bone in-growth was determined as a function of the local environment by comparing the laminar and intertransverse sites as well as each block side in contact or not with bone within each site.

Analysis within each site confirmed the influence on bone in-growth of close contact between macroporous osteoconductive material and host bone. Ceramic block sides in direct or close contact with the bone of lamina or intertransverse processes exhibited the greatest amount of new bone formation (Fig. 1). These results indicate that a suitable surgical technique requires that ceramic blocks be in contact with host bone.

The comparison of laminar and intertransverse sites showed a significant difference in bone formation. The 9% lower bone growth at the intertransverse site represented nearly one-third of the total amount of bone growth into ceramic at the laminar site (17% vs 26%). This difference, which may have potential clinical relevance, suggests that bone substitutes for posterolateral arthrodesis should be evaluated separately for each site, since good results for the laminar site are not necessarily valid for the intertransverse site. Finally, the intertransverse site appears to be bone-poor, and could benefit from enrichment with osteogenic precursor cells obtained, for example, from an iliac crest puncture.

Addition of bone marrow to a bone-poor intertransverse process site

The osteogenic potential of marrow-derived cells has been largely demonstrated [2, 9]. However, only a few experimental studies have considered the application of bone marrow to the spine as a useful adjunct to enhance rates of bone formation and fusion [1, 3, 5].

In a rabbit posterolateral fusion model grafted with autogenous iliac crest bone, Curylo et al. [3] quantified the effect of bone-marrow enhancement of spinal arthrodesis. The measured mean bone volume determined from computed tomography images was almost 30% greater when bone marrow was added to autogenous iliac crest bone. The fusion rate was achieved in 61% of cases versus 25% in the control group.

Lindholm et al. [5], who added bone marrow obtained by aspiration from the femoral medullar cavity to demineralized bone matrix in a posterior thoracic spinal fusion model in rabbits, found that transplantation of both materials provided more rapid fusion than that of demineralized bone matrix alone.

The association of ceramics with bone marrow has shown osteogenic potential in in vivo situations, e.g. in a rat model in which a combination of bone-marrow cells and calcium phosphate ceramic allowed bone formation in extraosseous sites and also potentiated bone in-growth in osseous sites [8]. It has also been shown in vitro that human marrow-derived cells cultured on macroporous calcium phosphate ceramic express and conserve their osteoblastic phenotype, and that these osteogenic cells are able to form new bone matrix in a ceramic in vitro [10]. Macroporous calcium phosphate ceramics are a main vector associating a mineral volume beneficial to mineralization with a wide specific surface allowing attachment of a large number of cells.

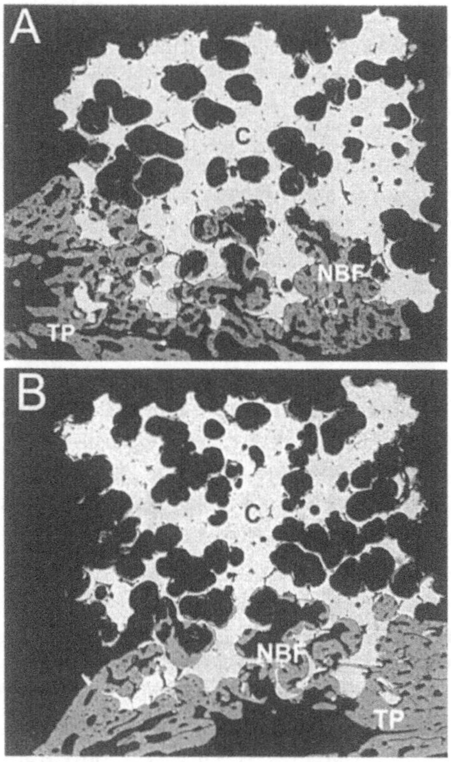

Fig. 2 Scanning electron photomicrographs: transverse sections of calcium phosphate ceramic blocks (*C*) loaded with autologous bone-marrow aspiration (*A*) or grafted alone (*B*) on transverse processes (*TP*). Bone-marrow loading obviously increased new bone formation (*NBF*)

However, Boden et al. [1] found that the use of a ceramic corallin hydroxyapatite with bone marrow did not provide an acceptable bone graft substitute (no solid fusions) in a posterolateral lumbar arthrodesis rabbit model.

In the present study involving a biphasic calcium phosphate ceramic (40% β-tricalcium and 60% hydroxyapatite), the enhancement of bone formation was quantified after addition of bone marrow in an original rabbit intertransverse process lumbar fusion model. Three graft materials were compared: iliac bone grafts (controls) and ceramics, associated or not with a standardized bone-marrow puncture. The originality of this method consisted in performing two independent intertransverse grafts by two independent lateral approaches and stabilizing the spine with posterior instrumentation to minimize movements that might cause non-union. With the transverse process, the graft materials were also secured by a suture.

Ceramic parallelepipedic blocks were randomly loaded with bone-marrow cells. After 6 weeks, the fusion rate was assessed by a manual test and determined for each interface between transverse processes and graft materials. Bone formation was compared on three sections for each specimen using quantitative histomorphometry performed in the coronal plane at the level of the two decorticated transverse processes and in the median area. As compared to ceramic block alone, the rate of new bone formation into ceramic loaded with bone marrow was significantly increased (50%) when the three sections were considered for each block (Fig. 2). The manual palpation test, when applied to each transverse process/graft material interface, showed that fusion was achieved in 91.6% (22/24) of the intertransverse sites in the control group and 92.5% (37/40) in the ceramic group, with no significant difference between blocks loaded or not with bone marrow. However, vertebral fusion was not achieved for any grafts with ceramic alone, as all the blocks were fractured in the median area.

Although these results do not indicate that biphasic calcium phosphate ceramic associated with bone marrow is a completely suitable graft substitute for lumbar fusion, they confirm that the addition of bone marrow to ceramic can greatly facilitate bone formation at a bone-poor (e.g. intertransverse) fusion site.

Richness in osteoprogenitor cells at the vertebral interbody site as compared to the reference iliac crest site

The vertebral interbody site surrounded mainly by spongy bone was presumably bone-rich. The potential richness of this site in osteogenic precursor cells suggests that ceramic material for implantation would not require addition of a bone-marrow puncture from the reference iliac crest site.

The number of alkaline phosphatase-positive colony-forming units was used to estimate the amount of osteoblast progenitor cells contained in bone-marrow aspirates [9] obtained from vertebral interbody and iliac crest sites in the same patient during 25 anterior spinal surgery cases for scoliosis treatment. A syringe containing heparin was used to collect 2–3 ml of sample from the medullary cavity of the iliac crest and the cancellous bone of the vertebral body reached through the interbody space after removal of the disk and subchondral bone. The bone-marrow samples were placed in tissue-culture medium, and the number of alkaline phosphatase-positive colony-forming units was counted after 9 days of culture, using appropriate staining.

No correlation was found between richness in osteoprogenitor bone-marrow cells at the iliac crest and vertebral interbody sites. In most cases, a large difference was observed between the two sites within the same patient. In some cases, the vertebral interbody site was poorer in osteoprogenitor bone-marrow cells.

The number of osteoprogenitor cells from a puncture may vary for different reasons. In histological terms, the number of nucleated cells may increase if local bone marrow is highly cellular and loosely connected, allowing bone-marrow cells in marrow space to flow into the aspiration needle [7]. Apparently, no histological studies have documented differences in cellularity and cancellous bone architecture between iliac crest and vertebral body sites. However, it has been reported that the concentration of bone-marrow-derived cells obtained by puncture depends on the rate of dilution with local blood [7]. The rate at which dilution occurs probably depends at least on the density of the local vessels within cancellous bone. Muschler et al. [7] noted that variation in the dilution rate is due primarily to puncture volume, since contamination by peripheral blood becomes greater as aspiration volume increases. In our study, the dilution effect was partly minimized, as approximately the same volume was collected from both sites.

The differences between the two sites in the same patient could have been due to another cause of blood contamination. As the puncture within the vertebral interbody site was made in spongy bone below the decorticated osseous surface, bleeding may have modified the cell content of the surrounding spongy bone.

In terms of grafting conditions, our results are probably more indicative of cell richness at the interbody site than in the vertebral body itself. Moreover, the vertebral interbody site might be bone-poor at the time of grafting. Therefore, from a clinical point of view, it would seem advisable to perform an iliac crest puncture even when ceramic is implanted in an interbody site, in order to provide a potentially abundant and readily available source of osteoprogenitor cells.

Conclusion

The benefit of adding a bone-marrow puncture from the iliac crest to ceramic is two fold. First, it serves in all cases as a binding medium between ceramic granules, making them easier to handle and place in the graft site. More specifically, it maximises the number of viable osteogenic precursor cells at both bone-rich and bone-poor sites, especially since a site theoretically rich in bone cells could be poor at the time of implantation because of local bleeding.

References

1. Boden SD, Martin GJ, Morone M, Ugbo JL, Titus L, Hutton WC (1999) The use of corallin hydroxyapatite with bone marrow, autogenous bone graft, or osteoinductive bone protein extract for posterolateral lumbar spine fusion. Spine 24:320–327
2. Bruder SP, Fink DJ, Caplan AI (1994) Mesenchymal stem cells in bone development. Bone repair and skeletal regeneration therapy. J Cell Biochem 56:283–294
3. Curylo LJ, Johnstone B, Petersilge CA, Janicki JA, Yoo JU (1999) Augmentation of spinal arthrodesis with autologous bone marrow in a rabbit: posterolateral spine fusion model. Spine 24:434–439
4. Delecrin J, Aguado E, Nguyen JM, Pyre D, Royer J, Passuti N (1997) Influence of local environment on incorporation of ceramic for lumbar fusion. Comparison of laminar and intertransverse sites in a canine model. Spine 22:1683–1689
5. Lindholm TS, Ragni P, Linholm TC (1988) Response of bone marrow stroma cells to demineralized cortical bone matrix in experimental spinal fusion in rabbits. Clin Orthop 230:296–302
6. Marchesi DJ (2000) Spinal fusions: bone and bone substitutes. Eur Spine J 9:372–378
7. Muschler GF, Boehm C, Easley K (1997) Aspiration to obtain osteoblast progenitor cells from human bone marrow: the influence of aspiration volume. J Bone Joint Surg Am 79:1699–1709
8. Ohgushi H, Goldberg VM, Caplan AI (1989) Heterotopic osteogenesis in porous ceramics induced by marrow cells. J Orthop Res 7:568–578
9. Rickard DJ, Kassem M, Hefferan TE, Sakar G, Selsberg TC, Riggs BL (1996) Isolation and characterisation of osteoblast precursor cells from human bone marrow. J Bone Min Res 11:312–324
10. Toquet J, Rohanizadeh R, Guicheux J, Couillaud S, Passuti N, Heymann D (1999) Osteogenic potential in vitro of human bone marrow cells cultured on macroporous biphasic calcium phosphate ceramic. J Biomed Mater Res 44:98–108

M. Bohner

Physical and chemical aspects of calcium phosphates used in spinal surgery

Abstract In 1983, Brown and Chow [10] discovered the first calcium phosphate cement (CPC). This discovery opened a new era in the use of calcium phosphates (CaP) as bone substitute. The first commercial CPC have now been introduced, and porous CaP with totally new properties should follow soon. In this article, the CaP traditionally used in spinal surgery are compared with these new CaP. Particular emphasis is placed on the use of CPC for bone augmentation.

Keywords Calcium phosphate · Cement · Bone · Substitute · Spine

M. Bohner (✉)
Dr. h.c. Robert Mathys Foundation,
Bischmattstr. 12,
2544 Bettlach, Switzerland
e-mail: bohnerm@rms-foundation.ch,
Tel.: +41-32-6441413,
Fax: +41-32-6331176

Introduction

Calcium phosphates (CaP) have been studied as bone repair materials for the last 80 years [1]. CaP only began to be used in spinal surgery more recently, but CaP such as β-tricalcium phosphate (β-TCP), hydroxyapatite (HA), and their composites (biphasic calcium phosphate, BCP) are commonly used as granules or blocks in interbody fusion and scoliosis surgery [29, 41, 43]. Recently, new CaP denominated calcium phosphate cements (CPC) have been introduced [10]. These materials are made of one or several CaP powders and an aqueous solution. When the CaP powders and the aqueous solution are mixed together, a paste is obtained that sets within a few minutes. CPC are usually injectable and have therefore been proposed as a possible alternative to polymethylmetacrylate (PMMA), e.g., to reinforce osteoporotic vertebral bodies [4, 44] and thoracolumbar burst fractures [33] and to restore pedicle screw fixation [36]. CPC can also be used to make granules and blocks out of low-temperature CaP [6]. These CaP are very similar to the CaP present in bone. They possess a very large specific surface area, which makes them biologically much more (re)active than traditional CaP. Despite the increasing use of CPC in medicine, particularly in spinal surgery, there are still very few articles in the medical literature describing CaP other than β-TCP, HA, and BCP [7]. The aim of this article is therefore to describe the differences between these new CaP and the more traditional CaP. Two different categories of CaP should be distinguished: (a) CaP obtained by precipitation from an aqueous solution at or around room temperature (*low-temperature CaP*) and (ii) CaP obtained by a thermal reaction, typically above 1000°C (*high-temperature CaP*). All CPC (e.g., α-BSM, Bone-Source, Norian SRS) belong to the first category, whereas most other CaP products (e.g., chronOS, Endobon, BCP, Pro Osteon, Triosite) belong to the second category. In the first part of this article, low-temperature CaP will be compared with high-temperature CaP; in the second part, CPC will be presented. Particular emphasis is placed on the use of CPC as bone augmentation material in spinal surgery.

Low-temperature calcium phosphates

Low-temperature CaP have a different chemical composition and structure than high-temperature CaP (Table 1), except for stoichiometric hydroxyapatite (Ca:P molar ratio of 1.67), which can precipitate at room temperature and which is stable up to 1300°C. As hydroxyapatite can precipitate over a large range of Ca:P molar ratios (1.50–

Table 1 Main calcium phosphate compounds

Name	Formula	Ca/P	Mineral	Symbol
Monocalcium phosphate monohydrate	$Ca(H_2PO_4)_2{\cdot}H_2O$	0.50	–	MCPM
Dicalcium phosphate	$CaHPO_4$	1.00	Monetite	DCP
Dicalcium phosphate dihydrate	$CaHPO_4{\cdot}2H_2O$	1.00	Brushite	DCPD
Octocalcium phosphate	$Ca_8H_2(PO_4)_6{\cdot}5H_2O$	1.33	–	OCP
Precipitated hydroxyapatite	$Ca_{10-x}(HPO_4)_x(PO_4)_{6-x}(OH)_{2-x}$	1.50–1.67	–	PHA
Tricalcium phosphate	$Ca_9(HPO_4)(PO_4)_5(OH)$	1.50	–	TCP
Amorphous calcium phosphate	$Ca_3(PO_4)_2{\cdot}nH_2O^a$	1.50	–	ACP
Monocalcium phosphate	$Ca(H_2PO_4)_2$	0.50	–	MCP
α-Tricalcium phosphate	α-$Ca_3(PO_4)_2$	1.50	–	α-TCP
β-Tricalcium phosphate	β-$Ca_3(PO_4)_2$	1.50	–	β-TCP
Sintered hydroxyapatite	$Ca_5(PO_4)_3OH$	1.67	Hydroxyapatite	HA
Oxyapatite	$Ca_{10}(PO_4)_6O$	1.67	–	OXA
Tetracalcium phosphate	$Ca_4(PO_4)_2O$	2.00	Hilgenstockite	TetCP
Carbonated apatite	$Ca_{8.8}(HPO_4)_{0.7}(PO_4)_{4.5}(CO_3)_{0.7}(OH)_{1.3}$		Dahlite	CAP

The first six compounds precipitate at room temperature in aqueous systems. The last six compounds are obtained by thermal decomposition or thermal synthesis.
[a] n=3–4.5; 15–20% H_2O.

1.67), a distinction is made between the low-temperature form, referred to here as precipitated hydroxyapatite (PHA), and the high-temperature form, referred to here as hydroxyapatite (HA). PHA is very similar to the mineral part of bone, whereas HA is the hydroxyapatite traditionally used in medicine. Low-temperature CaP are characterized by their large specific surface area (Fig. 1). For example, PHA can have a specific surface area as large as 100 m^2/g, whereas HA has a specific surface area of around 1 m^2/g. This large specific surface area makes low-temperature CaP biologically much more (re)active than high-temperature CaP. Low-temperature CaP have different solubilities than high-temperature CaP (Fig. 2). Differences in the in vivo bioresorption rate can therefore be expected [14].

Among the low-temperature CaP, dicalcium phosphate dihydrate (DCPD; $CaHPO_4{\cdot}2H_2O$) and PHA are particularly interesting. DCPD is the most bioresorbable biocompatible CaP (MCPM is more soluble but is not biocompatible; Fig. 2), whereas PHA is the CaP most similar to the mineral part of bone. DCPD is the CaP that can be most easily synthesized. It has been detected in fracture callus [32], bone [38], and kidney stones [47] and is also sometimes considered to be a precursor of HA in bone [20]. DCPD is biocompatible and osteoconductive. At physiological pH, DCPD is the most soluble low-temper-

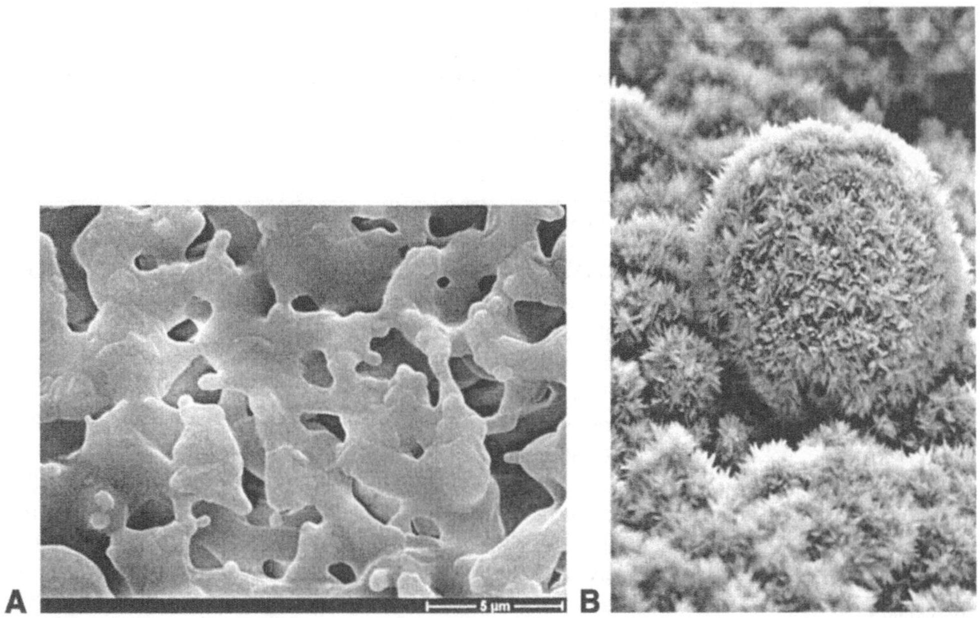

Fig. 1a,b Typical microstructure of **a** a high-temperature calcium phosphate (CaP) (chronOS, Mathys, Switzerland; specific surface area, ≈1 m^2/g) and **b** a low-temperature CaP (CDHA; specific surface area, ≈22 m^2/g). The width of the right photo is 8 µm. (Courtesy of P. Buffat, Swiss Federal Institute of Technology, Lausanne, Switzerland)

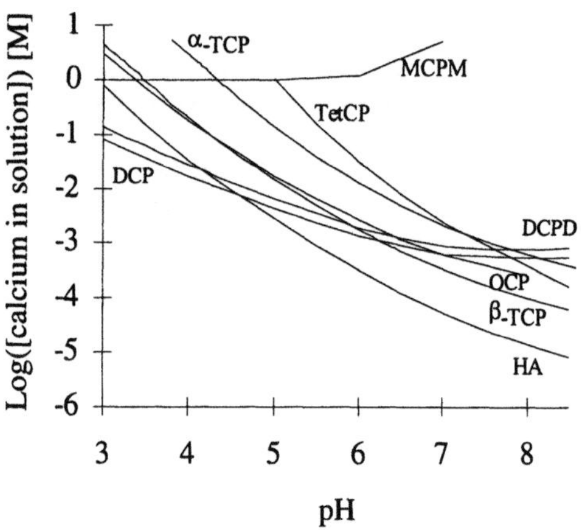

Fig. 2 Solubility isotherms of several calcium phosphates (CaP) in water. The solubility is expressed as the total amount of calcium ions in solution. The solubility data were taken from Vereecke and Lemaître [46]

ature CaP (Fig. 2). It is therefore metastable and can be converted into other low-temperature CaP, such as dicalcium phosphate (DCP; $CaHPO_4$; at pH<6), octocalcium phosphate (OCP; $Ca_8H_2(PO_4)_6 \cdot 5H_2O$; at pH≈6–7), or PHA (at pH>~7). In vivo DCPD is normally rapidly bioresorbed and replaced by new bone [39]. However, DCPD has been observed to transform into PHA, especially in a location poorly irrigated with blood [11]. The addition of small amounts of magnesium, which is an inhibitor of the precipitation of PHA, is believed to prevent the transformation of this magnesium-containing DCPD into PHA [8], hence making DCPD the most bioresorbable biocompatible CaP.

PHA is less soluble than DCPD, but accurate values are lacking due to the fact that PHA can have a Ca:P molar ratio of between 1.50 and 1.67 [9] and sometimes even outside this range [12] (Table 1). The solubility of PHA is believed to increase as the Ca:P molar ratio decreases. Another difficulty in determining the solubility of PHA stems from the fact that PHA can easily incorporate foreign ions such as carbonates, chloride, fluoride, and magnesium ions. These ions may have a very strong influence on the solubility (e.g., fluoride). Finally, the size of the particle crystals is very small in PHA, typically close to 10–20 nm. In this range, the solubility depends on the particle size: the smaller the particle size, the greater the solubility. PHA with a Ca:P molar ratio of 1.50 is often called calcium-deficient hydroxyapatite (CDHA) or tricalcium phosphate (TCP). The latter term has led to it being confused with β-TCP, which has almost the same chemical composition, but a different crystallographic structure. The solubility of TCP is estimated to be close to that of β-TCP [13]. Therefore and contrary to HA, most PHA should be considered as bioresorbable. Apart from brushite CPC, all commercial CPC have PHA (BoneSource, Cementek, α-BSM, Biopex, Mimix) or carbonated PHA (Norian SRS and CRS, Biocement D) as the main end product of the setting reaction. The main difference between the cements after the setting reaction lies in the Ca:P molar ratio, the presence of impurities (e.g., carbonate groups for Norian SRS and Biocement D), the cement porosity, and the crystal size of the PHA. All these parameters influence the bioresorbability of PHA.

With the discovery of CPC [10] and the use of CaP emulsions [6], low-temperature CaP can be produced in almost any shape and porosity. Granules and porous blocks can therefore be made out of CaP other than the traditionally used CaP, i.e., β-TCP, HA, and BCP. These new possibilities are particularly interesting for applications where a fast bioresorption rate or a large specific surface area is required, e.g., tissue engineering or drug delivery. An interesting assumption is that, having a large specific surface area, CaP can adsorb large amounts of endogenous proteins, such as growth factors. Low-temperature CaP might then be indirectly osteoinductive and could therefore be used in applications where fast bone ingrowth is required. To test this hypothesis, intervertebral body fusion cages were filled with an open macroporous CDHA block and implanted in sheep. The 6-month results are expected soon (T. Steffen, private communication). If this assumption proves to be correct, the use of CaP as bone substitute could spread very quickly. Presently,

Table 2 Main apatite calcium phosphate cements (CPC)

Cement name	Company	Components	End product
α-BSM	ETEX	ACP, DCPD [46]	PHA
Biobone	Merck GmbH	–	–
Embarc	Lorenz Surgical	–	–
Norian SRS Norian CRS	Norian (Synthes-Stratec)	α-TCP, $CaCO_3$, MCPM [12]	CAP
Bonesource	Leibinger	TetCP, DCP [10]	PHA
Cementek	Teknimed	α-TCP, TetCP, $Ca(OH)_2$, H_3PO_4	PHA
Mimix	Lorenz Surgical	α-TCP, TetCP, citric acid	PHA
Biocement D	Merck GmbH	α-TCP, DCP, $CaCO_3$, PHA [26]	CAP*
Biopex	Mitsubishi Materials	α-TCP, TetCP, DCPD [28]	PHA
Fracture Grout	Norian (Synthes-Stratec)	TetCP, $CaCO_3$, H_3PO_4 [21]	PHA
chronOS Inject	Mathys Medical	β-TCP, MCPM	DCPD

ACP, amorphous calcium phosphate; CAP, carbonato-apatite; DCP, dicalcium phosphate; DCPD, dicalcium phosphate dihydrate; MCPM, monocalcium phosphate monohydrate; PHA, precipitated hydroxyapatite; TCP, tricalcium phosphate; TetCP, tetracalcium phosphate.

the only commercial products on the market based on low-temperature CaP are CPC (Table 2). CPC have the disadvantage that they bioresorb layer by layer as they do not have any pores large enough to enable bone ingrowth.

High-temperature calcium phosphates

Until the discovery of CPC, it was not possible to synthesize CaP granules or blocks without thermal treatment (typically above 1000°C). All the traditional CaP used in medicine are therefore high-temperature CaP, mostly β-TCP, HA, and β-TCP/HA composites [3]. Due to the low toughness of CaP, the use of high-temperature CaP in spinal surgery has been mainly restricted to non-load-bearing applications. Nevertheless, high-temperature CaP have been used to make cervical cages for interbody fusion [27].

The most soluble high-temperature CaP are tetracalcium phosphate (TetCP; $Ca_4(PO_4)_2O$) and α-tricalcium phosphate (α-TCP; α-$Ca_3(PO_4)_2$). TetCP and α-TCP are about two orders of magnitude more soluble than HA at physiological pH (Fig. 2). TetCP and α-TCP therefore tend to transform into PHA when implanted in vivo. Both compounds are difficult to synthesize, so TetCP and α-TCP have mostly been used as the main constituents of CPC (Table 2). One known commercial α-TCP product is BioBase (BioVision, Germany).

β-TCP has the same composition as α-TCP, but a different crystallographic structure. As a result, β-TCP is one order of magnitude less soluble than α-TCP (Fig. 2). β-TCP can be obtained by thermal treatment above at least 650°C [5], e.g., by heating up CDHA above ~700°C [37]. It has been extensively used as bone substitute, either as granules or as blocks, and is bioresorbable, typically in the range of 1–2 years. Bioresorption occurs via osteoclastic activity [19]. There are a few products on the market, such as chronOS (Mathys, Switzerland), Vitoss (Orthovita, USA), and Biosorb (SBM, France). β-TCP has been successfully used in clinical practice, e.g., for interbody fusion in combination with spinal cages [23] and in scoliosis [29].

HA is the most stable CaP in an aqueous solution (Fig. 1) and is sometimes considered to be the most biocompatible CaP. It is also the CaP with the largest mechanical properties at a given porosity. HA is obtained by sintering stoichiometric PHA (Ca:P molar ratio, 1.67) above ~700°C. At temperatures higher than ~900°C, partial dehydration of HA may take place, eventually resulting in oxyapatite (OXA) [25]. This reaction only takes place in the absence of water vapor [14]. As OXA is difficult to detect, most commercial HA products may contain some OXA. The best-known commercial products are Pro Osteon (Interpore Cross, USA), Endobon (Merck, Germany), and Pyrost (Stryker Howmedica, USA). These products should be considered as non-bioresorbable, as they have a resorption time of decades rather than years.

Biphasic calcium phosphate (BCP) is a composite β-TCP-HA. It is obtained by calcining PHA (with a molar ratio Ca:P<1.67) above ~700°C [5]. BCP has intermediate properties compared with β-TCP and HA. Most commercial products, e.g., Triosite (Zimmer, USA) and BCP (Sofamor Danek, France), contain 60% HA and 40% β-TCP. BCP has been widely used in spinal surgery, e.g., for scoliosis [41, 43].

Calcium phosphate cements

CPC were discovered by Brown and Chow in the 1980s [10]. Since then, many compositions have been proposed [15, 16, 30]. However, despite the large number of formulations, CPC can only have three different end products: apatite (PHA), brushite (DCPD), and amorphous calcium phosphate (ACP). The only study performed with ACP [17] shows that the cement is rapidly converted into PHA. We can therefore classify all CPC formulations into two categories: (a) apatite CPC and (b) brushite CPC. Research effort has largely focused on apatite CPC, despite some interesting features of brushite CPC, mainly its large bioresorption rate. The following aspects of CPC will be considered here: chemistry, mixing, rheological properties, mechanical properties, porosity, heat release, volume change, and bioresorbability.

CPC are made of an aqueous solution and of one or several calcium phosphates. Upon mixing, the calcium phosphate(s) dissolve and precipitate into a less soluble CaP. Two types of setting reaction are possible. First, the setting reaction can occur according to an acid–base reaction, i.e., a relatively acidic CaP reacts with a relatively basic CaP to produce a relatively neutral CaP. A typical example is the cement developed by Brown and Chow [10], in which TetCP (basic) reacts with DCP (neutral) to form PHA (slightly basic):

$$Ca_4(PO_4)_2O + CaHPO_4 \rightarrow Ca_5(PO_4)_3OH \quad (1)$$

Another example is the cement developed by Lemaître [31], in which β-TCP (slightly basic) reacts with MCPM (acidic) to form DCPD (neutral):

$$\beta\text{-}Ca_3(PO_4)_2 + Ca(H_2PO_4)_2 \cdot H_2O + 7H_2O \rightarrow 4CaHPO_4 \cdot 2H_2O \quad (2)$$

The second type of setting reaction occurs when the initial and final CaP have the same Ca:P molar ratio. Typical examples are ACP and α-TCP, which form PHA upon contact with an aqueous solution:

$$3Ca_3(PO_4)_2 \cdot nH_2O \rightarrow Ca_9(PO_4)_5(HPO_4)OH + (3n-1)H_2O \quad (3)$$

$$3\alpha\text{-}Ca_3(PO_4)_2 + H_2O \rightarrow Ca_9(PO_4)_5(HPO_4)OH \quad (4)$$

An important requirement for the clinician is the mixing procedure of the CPC. So far, most CPC are mixed by hand with a mortar and either a pestle or a spatula. To be injected, the cement paste must be transferred into a syringe. Three commercial products are sold with an appropriate mixing device. Norian SRS is sold as a reactant pack containing the powder mixture and the mixing liquid and requires the use of a rather complicated and not always reliable system, i.e., a very large mixing machine and an injection gun. The large pressure obtained with the gun makes it easier to inject the cement, e.g., into a porous and fine structure such as osteoporotic bone. α-BSM is also a two-component system. The powder is in a soft pouch, and the liquid is in a flask. After injecting the liquid into the powder pouch, the cement paste is mixed with the fingers. After 3 min, the paste can be injected. This method is easy and very elegant, but as the setting time of α-BSM is temperature dependent, results may not be always reproducible. Moreover, the pressure that can be applied on the cement is limited. In the product Biopex, the cement is mixed with a spatula in a syringe that can be opened from the front. After mixing, the front part is closed, a needle is inserted into this front part, and the cement paste can be injected by hand.

To be injected in vivo, e.g., in an osteoporotic vertebra, the CPC paste must have two features: (a) injectability and (b) cohesion. Injectability means that the cement paste can be extruded through a long, small needle (e.g., 2 mm diameter and 10 cm length) without demixing. Demixing occurs when the mixing liquid is too fluid compared with the size of the cement powders, resulting in filter pressing: the liquid comes out without the CaP particles. The risk of demixing increases with the applied pressure. A cement paste with an appropriate cohesion sets in a fluid without disintegrating. This can be obtained by maintaining a high viscosity for the CPC paste. Some CPC pastes fulfill these two criteria, e.g., Norian SRS and α-BSM, but other CPC fulfill only one or neither of these requirements. For example, blood must be kept away from the implanting site of BoneSource and Cementek until setting. The loss of cohesion of the cement during mixing may lead to inflammatory reactions [34].

Several approaches can be adopted to improve the injectability and cohesion of a CPC. First, the powder-to-liquid ratio, P/L, can be decreased. The resulting paste is less viscous and can be more easily injected. A similar phenomenon is seen with PMMA cements when the monomer-to-powder ratio is increased. However, a decrease in the powder-to-liquid ratio of the CPC leads to a decrease in the mechanical properties of the CPC, and the cohesion of the CPC may be destroyed. This method is therefore only valid to a certain extent. For example, the manufacturers of Biopex suggest using a P/L ratio of 2.8 or 3.3 g/ml. A second approach is to decrease the particle size of the CPC components. For example, α-BSM, which has a small particle size, is well injectable. However, a small particle size requires a large amount of mixing liquid, which decreases the cohesion of the paste and also leads to greater porosity and lower mechanical properties. A third approach is to modify the interactions between the particles by shifting the isoelectric point by adding so-called surfactants. This approach has recently been used by Friberg et al. [22], but has not been applied in commercial products. An indirect approach is to add CaP particles which act as spacers between other CaP particles. For example, DCP is added to the formulation of Biocement D to improve the injectability of the paste. Finally, a fourth approach is to replace the mixing solution by a viscous polymeric solution [2]. Polysaccharides are particularly interesting due to their compatibility and good rheological properties. Most polysaccharide solutions are thixotropic, i.e., the viscosity of the solution decreases as the shear rate increases. A CPC made using a polymeric solution can therefore be easily injected and has a good cohesion in the absence of shear stresses. Only small amounts (a few weight%) of polysaccharides are normally needed to dramatically increase the viscosity of the mixing liquid. For example, Biopex uses a 5%w sodium chondroitin sulfate solution as mixing liquid. However, only very few polysaccharides are accepted for parenteral use. Moreover, the polymer solution can usually only be sterilized by ultrafiltration.

Another important aspect of cement injectability is the radiopacity. None of the CPC is as radiopaque as PMMA cement. Several research groups have tried to add a radiopacifier to CPC, but the biological outcome of the addition of small radiopaque particles to a bioresorbable CPC is not clear. Nevertheless, radiopacity differences can be expected between different formulations, i.e., the radiopacity should increase as the cement porosity decreases.

Considering their properties, CPC might potentially be used to reinforce osteoporotic vertebral bodies [4, 44] and thoracolumbar burst fractures [33] and to restore pedicle screw fixation [36]. Despite encouraging results, surgeons' expectations have not been met. This is not only due to the lower mechanical properties of CPC compared with PMMA cements, but also, and more importantly, to the greater difficulties encountered in filling the vertebral bodies. Several causes can be suggested: (a) in order to maintain their cohesion, CPC need to be more viscous than PMMA cement, hence rendering CPC less injectable than PMMA cement, and (b) CPC are hydrophilic, whereas PMMA cements are hydrophobic. CPC therefore tend to mix with body fluids and lose their cohesion, whereas PMMA cements tend to stay compact. To prevent these problems, several approaches have been proposed. In one approach, a cavity is created in the vertebral body, e.g., by means of an expandable balloon. The cavity is then filled with the CPC. In another approach, bone marrow is removed from the vertebra using a suction device [44], and the CPC is then injected.

During the setting reaction of the cement, CaP crystals grow and become partly interlocked, hence making the cement mechanically rigid. As CaP are brittle, the compressive strength of a CPC is always much greater than its tensile strength. Most CPC have a tensile strength of

1–10 MPa, whereas the compression strength varies between 10 and 100 MPa. For comparison, the tensile strength of PMMA is 30 MPa [40]. The mechanical properties of a CPC depend on its composition. The main determining factor is the ratio between the amount of cement powder (P) and mixing liquid (L). If this P/L ratio is large, the porosity of the CPC is low. As the mechanical properties decrease exponentially as porosity increases, low porosity always corresponds to large mechanical properties. As a rule of thumb, the tensile strength increases twofold with a 10 vol% decrease in porosity. The mechanical properties reported by CPC manufacturers are never documented, so it is difficult to compare CPC. Several authors have attempted to compare CPC cements. For example, Driessens [18] established compression strengths of 33±5, 8±2, 83±4, and 4±1 MPa and setting times of 8.5±0.5, 17±1,6.5±0.5, and 19±1 min for Norian SRS, Cemetek, Biocement D, and α-BSM, respectively. Biocement D has by far the greatest compressive strength, but this value does not mean that Biocement D is the least breakable implant. In vivo, shear and tensile forces play a very important role. The tensile strength of the CPC therefore also needs to be considered, e.g., using the Mohr circle approach [42]. Finally, it should be kept in mind that the initial mechanical properties of the apatite CPC may vary with implantation time. Animals studies indicate that the mechanical properties of apatite CPC tend to increase continually [35], in contrast to those of brushite CPC, which initially decrease and then increase when bone grows [24].

CPC typically have a porosity of 30–60%vol depending on the cement formulation. The porosity is open, i.e., the pores are perfectly interconnected. The pore size is close to 1 μm. Thus the pores are too small to allow fast bone ingrowth and the CPC bioresorbs layer by layer. This feature is the main drawback of CPC when compared to open macroporous CaP blocks. The porosity of the CPC is due to the excess water used in the CPC composition. Attempts have been made to reduce the amount of water in order to decrease the porosity and hence increase the mechanical properties, but a decrease in porosity also leads to a decrease in the CPC bioresorption rate. Moreover, the amount of water determines the rheological properties of the cement paste: a decrease in the CPC water content leads to a large increase in the viscosity of the cement paste, eventually leading to a nonflowable mixture.

Most CPC release some heat during setting. However, CPC are not as exothermic as PMMA cements or, if they are (e.g., BoneSource, a mixture of TetCP and DCP), the release rate is low enough to allow good dissipation of the heat.

In contrast to PMMA cements, CPC set at an almost constant volume. The final cement porosity can therefore be accurately predicted from the initial composition. The absence of shrinkage enables good contact between bone and CPC during and after setting.

The bioresorption rate of brushite CPC (e.g., chronOS Inject) is higher than that of apatite CPC (e.g., α-BSM), which in turn is higher than that of HA. However, the bioresorption rate of apatite CPC is still very slow, particularly due to the fact that CPC are not macroporous. For example, Young et al. [48] reported a 30% decrease in the amount of Norian SRS after 24 months in a rabbit femur. Some differences in bioresorption rate can be expected depending on the type of apatite CPC. Generally speaking, a longer bioresorption time is expected when the crystal size increases or when the porosity decreases. Norian SRS and α-BSM are therefore expected to bioresorb faster than BoneSource, Biopex, and Cementek.

Conclusion

Traditional CaP (HA, BCP, β-TCP) have commonly been used as granules or blocks to accelerate or improve spinal fusion. The discovery of CPC has opened up new horizons in the use of CaP in spinal surgery. CPC can be injected into osteoporotic bone to reinforce it or can be used to make granules and blocks out of low-temperature CaP. Several CPC are now on the market, while low-temperature CaP granules and blocks are still being tested. However, CPC already need to be improved; in particular, their bioresorption needs to be accelerated and their injectability and mechanical properties improved.

References

1. Albee FH, Morrison HF (1920) Studies in bone growth. Ann Surg 71:32–38
2. Andrianjatovo H, Lemaître J (1995) Effects of polysaccharides on the cement properties in the monocalcium phosphate/β-tricalcium phosphate system. Innov Tech Biol Med 16[1]:140–147
3. Association pour l'étude des greffes et substituts tissulaires en orthopédie (ed) (1999) Les substituts osseux en 1999. Copy 74, Annecy
4. Bai B, Jazrawi LM, Kummer FJ, Spivak JM (1999) The use of an injectable, biodegradable calcium phosphate bone substitute for the prophylactic augmentation of osteoporotic vertebrae and the management of vertebral compression fractures. Spine 24[15]:1521–1526
5. Bénard J (1958) Combinaisons avec le phosphore. In: Bénard J, Bouissières G, Brusset H, Dupuis T, Maillard A, Pascal P, Rinck E, Silber P (eds) Nouveau traité de chimie minérale, vol 4. Masson, Paris, pp 455–488
6. Bohner M (2001) Calcium phosphate emulsions: possible applications. Key Eng Mater 192–195:765–768

7. Bohner M (2000) Calcium orthophosphates in medicine: from ceramics to calcium phosphate cements. Injury 31:S-D37–47
8. Bohner M, Matter S (1999) Brushite hydraulic cement stabilized with a magnesium salt. Patent application PCT/CH99/00595, Switzerland
9. Brown PW, Martin RI (1999) An analysis of hydroxyapatite surface layer formation. J Phys Chem B 103: 1671–1675
10. Brown WE, Chow LC (1985) Dental restorative cement pastes. US Patent no. 4518430
11. Constantz BR, Barr BM, Ison IC, Fulmer MT, Baker J, Mckinney L, Goodman SB, Gunasekaren S, Delaney DC, Ross J, Poser RD (1998) Histological, chemical, and crystallographic analysis of four calcium phosphate cements in different rabbit osseous sites. J Biomed Mater Res (Appl Biomater) 43:451–461
12. Constantz BR, Ison IC, Fulmer MT, Poser RD, Smith ST, VanWagoner M, Ross J, Goldstein SA, Jupiter JB, Rosenthal DI (1995) Skeletal repair by in situ formation of the mineral phase of bone. Science 267:1796–1799
13. Driessens FCM, Verbeeck RMH (1990) Biominerals. CRC Press, Boca Raton
14. Driessens FCM, Verbeeck RMH (1988) Relation between physicochemical solubility and biodegradability of calcium phosphates. In: de Putter C, de Lange GL, de Groot K, Lee AJC (eds) Implant materials in biofunction. Elsevier, Amsterdam, pp 105–111
15. Driessens FCM, Planell JA, Boltong MG, Khairoun I, Ginebra MP (1998) Osteotransductive bone cements. Proc Instn Mech Engrs 212(H):427–435
16. Driessens FCM, Planell JA, Gil FJ (1995) Calcium phosphate bone cements. In: Wise DL, Trantolo DJ, Altobelli DE, Yaszemski MJ, Cresser JD, Schwartz ER (eds) Encyclopedic handbook of biomaterials and bioengineering, part B, vol 2. Dekker, New York, pp 855–877
17. Driessens FCM, DeMayer EAP, Fernandez E, Boltong MG, Berger G, Verbeeck RMH, Ginebra MP, Planell JA (1996) Amorphous calcium phosphate cements and their transformation into calcium deficient hydroxyapatite. Bioceramics 9:231–234
18. Driessens FCM (1999) Chemistry and applied aspects of calcium phosphate bone cements. In: Concepts and clinical applications of ionic cements. Presented at the 15th European Conference on Biomaterials, ESB 99, Arcachon (France), 8–12 September 1999
19. Eggli PS, Müller W, Schenk RK (1988) Porous hydroxyapatite and tricalcium phosphate cylinders with two different pore size ranges implanted in the cancellous bone of rabbits. Clinical Orthop 232:127–138
20. Francis MD, Webb NC (1972) Hydroxyapatite formation from a hydrated calcium monohydrogen phosphate precursor. Calcified Tissue Res 10:82–90
21. Frankenburg EP, Goldstein SA, Bauer TW, Harris SA, Poser RD (1998) Biomechanical and histological evaluation of a calcium phosphate cement. J Bone Joint Surg 80-A[8]:1112–1124
22. Friberg J, Fernandez E, Sarda S, Nilsson M, Ginebra MP, Martinez S, Planell JA (2001) An experimental approach to the study of the rheology behavior of synthetic bone calcium phosphate cements. Key Eng Mater 192–195:777–780
23. Husson JL, Le Huec JC, Polard JL, Trebuchet G, Lesprit E, Bossis JM (1998) Interbody arthodesis of the lumbar vertebrae using retroperitonal videoendoscopy. A preliminary study of 38 cases. Chirurgie 123[5]:491–499
24. Ikenaga M, Hardouin P, Lemaître J, Andrianjatovo H, Flautre B (1998) Biomechanical characterization of a biodegradable calcium phosphate hydraulic cement: a comparison with porous biphasic calcium phosphate ceramics. J Biomed Mater Res 40:139–144
25. Kanazawa T (1989) Inorganic phosphate materials. Materials science monographs, vol 52. Kodansha, Tokyo
26. Khairoun I, Driessens FCM, Boltong MG, Planell JA, Wenz R (1999) Addition of cohesion promotors to calcium phosphate cements. Biomaterials 20: 393–398
27. Kim P, Wakai S, Matsuo S, Moriyama T, Kirino T (1998) Bisegmental cervical interbody fusion using hydroxyapatite implants: surgical results and long-term observation in 70 cases. J Neurosurg 88:21–27
28. Kurashina K, Kurita H, Hirano M, Kotani A, Klein CPAT, de Groot K (1997) In vivo study of calcium phosphate cements: implantation of an α-tricalcium phosphate/dicalcium phosphate dibasic/tetracalcium phosphate monoxide cement paste. Biomaterials 18:539–543
29. Le Huec JC, Lesprit E, Delavigne C, Clement D, Chauveaux D, Le Rebeller A (1997) Tricalcium phosphate ceramics and allografts as bone substitutes for spinal fusion in idiopathis scoliosis: comparative clinical results at four years. Acta Orthop Belg 63[3]:202–211
30. Lemaître J (1995) Injectable calcium phosphate hydraulic cements: new developments and potential applications. Innov Tech Biol Med 16[1]:109–120
31. Lemaître J, Mirtchi AA, Mortier A (1987) Calcium phosphate cements for medical use: state of the art and perspectives of development. Silicates Industriels 9–10:141–146
32. Lenárt G, Bidló G, Pintér J (1972) Some basic problems in the examination of the calcium hydrogen phosphates of bone. Clin Orthop Rel Res 83:263–272
33. Mermelstein LE, McLain RF, Yerby SA (1998) Reinforcement of thoracolumbar burst fractures with calcium phosphate cement. Spine 23[6]:664–671
34. Miyamoto Y, Ishikawa K, Takechi M, Toh T, Yuasa T, Nagayama M, Suzuki K (1999) Histological and compositional evaluations of three types of calcium phosphate cements when implanted in subcutaneous tissue immediately after mixing. J Biomed Mater Res Appl Biomater 48:36–42
35. Miyamoto Y, Ishikawa K, Fukao H, Sawada M, Nagayama M, Kon M, Asaoka K (1995) In vivo setting behaviour of fast-setting calcium phosphate cement. Biomaterials 16:855–860
36. Moore DC, Maitra R S, Farjo LA, Graziano GP, Goldstein SA (1997) Restoration of pedicle screw fixation with an in situ setting calcium phosphate cement. Spine 22[15]:1696–1705
37. Mortier A, Lemaître J, Rouxhet PG (1989) Temperature-programmed characterization of synthetic calcium-deficient phosphate apatites. Thermochim Acta 143:265–282
38. Muenzenberg KJ, Gebhardt M (1973) Brushite, octocalcium phosphate, and carbonate-containing apatite in bone. Clin Orthop Rel Res 90:271–273
39. Munting E, Mirtchi AA, Lemaître J (1993) Bone repair of defects filled with a phosphocalcic hydraulic cement: an in vivo study. J Mater Sci Mater Med 4:337–344
40. Park JB (1995) Orthopedic prosthesis fixation. In: Bronzino JD (ed) The biomedical engineering handbook. CRC Press, Boca Raton, pp 704–724
41. Passuti N, Daculsi G, Rogez JM, Martin S, Bainvel JV (1989) Macroporous calcium phosphate ceramic performance in human spine fusion. Clin Orthop 248:169–176
42. Pittet C, Lemaître J, Chevalley F (2000) Mechanical characterization of brushite cements – a Mohr circles approach. J Biomed Mater Res (Appl Biomater) 53:769–780

43. Ransford AO, Morley T, Edgar MA, Webb P, Passuti N, Chopin D, Morin C, Michel F, Garin C, Pries D (1998) Synthetic porous ceramic compared with autograft in scoliosis surgery. J Bone Joint Surg 80B[1]:13–18
44. Schildhauer TA, Bennett AP, Wright TM, Lane JM, O'Leary PF (1999) Intravertebral body reconstruction with an injectable in situ-setting carbonated apatite: biomechanical evaluation of a minimally invasive technique. J Bone Joint Surg 17:67–72
45. Tofighi A, Mounic S, Chakravarthy P, Rey C, Lee D (2001) Setting reactions involved in injectable cements based on amorphous calcium phosphate. Key Eng Mater 192–195:769–772
46. Vereecke G, Lemaître J (1990) Calculation of the solubility diagrams in the system $Ca(OH)_2$-H_3PO_4-KOH-HNO_3-CO_2-H_2O. J Crystal Growth 104:820–832
47. Werness PG, Bergert JH, Smith LH (1981) Crystalluria. J Crystal Growth 53:166–181
48. Young SW, Holde M, Gunasekaran S, Poser RD, Constantz BR (1998) The correlation of radiographic, MRI, and histological evaluations over two years of a carbonated apatite cement in a rabbit model. In: Andersson GBJ (ed) Transactions of the 44th Annual Meeting of the Orthopaedic Research Society, vol 23, sect 2. Dickerson, Chicago, p 846

H. S. Sandhu
S. N. Khan
D. Y. Suh
S. D. Boden

Demineralized bone matrix, bone morphogenetic proteins, and animal models of spine fusion: an overview

H.S. Sandhu (✉) · S.N. Khan
Spinal Surgical Service,
Hospital for Special Surgery,
Weill Medical College
of Cornell University,
535 East 70th Street,
New York, NY 10021, USA
e-mail: SandhuH@HSS.EDU

D.Y. Suh
Department of Neurological Surgery,
Emory University School of Medicine,
Atlanta, Georgia, USA

S.D. Boden
Department of Orthopaedic Surgery,
Emory University School of Medicine,
Atlanta, Georgia, USA

Abstract Preclinical investigations on the use of bone morphogenetic proteins (BMP) in the spine have yielded promising results. This has led to the preliminary introduction of these growth factors in controlled clinical trials. Initial data made available suggest that these differentiating factors will play a major role in the treatment of spinal disorders in the future. This article reviews key preclinical studies and their results that formed the basis for introduction into clinical trials. Non-primate and non-human primate models of spine fusion with BMP are reviewed objectively, and important issues regarding carrier, dose, and site of implantation are discussed. Finally, exciting new gene therapy research is discussed, with comments made on its applicability for the future.

Keywords Recombinant bone morphogenetic proteins · Non-primate models · Non-human primate models · Delivery vehicles · Gene therapy models

Introduction

The last few decades have seen the remarkable development of spinal fixation devices. In current clinical use, devices are used to attach nearly every component of the spinal anatomy, including lamina, pedicles, spinous processes, facet joints, pars interarticuli and vertebral bodies. Unstable motion segments are often fused using constructs composed of plates, rods, wires and cages. Metals used include stainless steel, titanium and tantalum alloys. Ultimately, however, the success of any spinal fusion is dictated by biologic principles. Only a biologic environment conducive to bone formation and consolidation will allow successful osseous arthrodesis to occur.

Research efforts in the last decade have focused on morphogenetic proteins, opening exciting new avenues in spinal fusion surgery. Several osteoinductive growth factors, referred to as the bone morphogenetic proteins (BMP), have been shown to induce the transformation of undifferentiated mesenchymal cells into chondroblasts and osteoblasts, resulting in the formation of de novo bone [2, 18, 19, 22, 36, 42, 43, 47, 55, 72, 73]. Numerous preclinical animal studies have demonstrated the superiority of BMP implants over traditional autogenous bone grafts for a variety of orthopedic applications [17, 25, 29, 32, 37, 49, 66]. Considerable attention has been focused towards spinal applications for these innovative biologic tools, particularly for augmenting spinal fusion. Indeed, with the advances in molecular biology techniques, these proteins have been used in conjunction with gene therapy principles to deliver the protein at the desired fusion site in rats, leading to speculation as to "percutaneous" fusion in humans! The following sections thus summarize the key preclinical studies involving the BMPs and spinal fusion.

Non-primate models

Demineralized bone matrix

The bone inductive activity of demineralized bone matrix (DBM) has been well established [15, 21, 24, 28, 34, 39, 68, 69, 71]. The primary osteoinductive component of DBM is a series of low-molecular-weight glycoproteins that includes the bone morphogenetic proteins (BMPs). The decalcification of cortical bone exposes these osteoinductive growth factors buried within the mineralized matrix, thereby enhancing the bone formation process [72]. The addition of autologous bone marrow and/or autograft to DBM provides an immediate source of osteogenic precursor cells at the implant site that may provide an additional biochemical contribution to osteogenesis [14, 69, 71]. DBM also appears to support new bone formation through osteoconductive mechanisms [45]. A number of well-controlled studies in a well-established and validated animal model of posterolateral spine fusion have demonstrated the suitability of various forms of DBM as a graft extender and, in some cases, as a graft enhancer and a graft substitute [45, 48]. Moreover, experimental studies have shown that osteoinductive bone protein growth factors combined with DBM produce biomechanically enhanced fusions as compared to autograft alone [4, 5, 6, 65]. DBM has a number of additional advantages that make it an attractive bone graft alternative. It is cost-effective and readily available from tissue banks. The demineralization process destroys the antigenic materials in bone, making DBM less immunogenic than mineralized allograft [30].

DBM products were introduced clinically in 1991, and have since become the most widely used alternative graft product in spinal fusion surgery [57]. Case reports and analyses of several nonrandomized, retrospective clinical series suggest that DBM in combination with autologous marrow or bone demonstrates similar performance characteristics to autograft in posterolateral lumbar spine fusion [41, 61, 67, 70].

Early experimental studies using DBM alone or in combination with autologous bone marrow (BM), autograft, or graft substitutes have reported spinal fusion rates comparable to autograft alone in rats [30], rabbits [38, 39, 50, 51, 52, 53, 54], and dogs [27]. In addition, a number of studies have shown that DBM-autograft or BM composites demonstrate more rapid spinal fusion and appear to achieve radiographic and biomechanical stability earlier than autograft alone [27, 38, 39, 52]. Extrapolating these findings to humans is problematic, however, especially given that the majority of these studies have demonstrated efficacy of DBM in the less challenging anterior or posterior spine rather than the posterolateral spine and/or used animal models of spinal fusion that have not been characterized fully. Moreover, in many of these studies, all groups including the autograft group demonstrated 100% fusion rates, making it difficult to determine the added benefit of DBM over and above autograft [30, 50, 52].

Boden and his colleagues conducted a series of investigations evaluating the efficacy of DBM in a well-characterized and validated animal model of posterolateral lumbar intertransverse process spinal fusion that closely resembles the surgical technique done in humans [4, 5, 6, 45, 48]. These authors have reliably demonstrated an outcome rate of fusion (nonunion rate of 35%) using autologous iliac crest graft that is similar to the rate of pseudoarthroses reported in humans. Moreover, the percentage of fusions that become solid does not change after 4–5 weeks. In these studies, fusion rates using DBM alone or in combinations with a variety of graft materials, including autograft, growth factors, and organic graft substitutes, have been compared to fusion rates using autograft iliac crest graft. Generally accepted measures of fusion based on manual palpation, histology, radiographs and/or biomechanical measures of stability were reported in all of these studies. In general, these studies have shown that certain formulations of DBM, when used alone, are insufficient to promote spinal fusion when placed in the more challenging posterolateral lumbar spinal fusion model in rabbits. When compared to autologous iliac crest bone graft, allogenic rabbit DBM alone resulted in significantly lower rates of fusion [4, 5]. The lower rate of fusion with allogenic DBM alone, as compared to autograft, was even more pronounced when DBM was evaluated in the highly challenging non-human primate model of lumbar posterolateral intertransverse process spinal fusion [5]. In primates, allogenic DBM alone resulted in minimal bone induction with no evidence of fusion at 12 weeks. Similar results were obtained using the gel form of DBM (Grafton) in a rabbit posterolateral lumbar arthrodesis model [48]. In this study, gel-DBM did not increase the fusion rate when added to a standard amount of iliac crest autograft. The addition of gel-DBM to less than the standard amount of autograft did, however, result in fusion rates (70% and 66%) that were comparable to autograft alone (73%). Gel-DBM was most effective in producing fusion rates that mirrored those of autograft when used with autograft in a 3:1 ratio. These authors concluded that, while gel-DBM did not meet criteria as a graft substitute or a graft enhancer (i.e., when added to the usual or a decreased amount of autogenous bone yields a higher rate of successful fusion than autograft alone), gel-DBM did demonstrate properties of a viable graft extender (i.e., when added to autologous bone yields a rate of successful fusion equal to that of autologous bone graft alone).

Other formulations of DBM have shown greater success at inducing spinal fusion when used as stand-alone agents. In a recent study by Martin et al., two new formulations of Grafton DBM (flex-DBM and putty-DBM) were found to be effective as both a graft extender and graft enhancer in the challenging rabbit model of posterolateral spine fusion, as well as demonstrating the capacity to serve as a potential osteoconductive graft substitute [45]. Historical controls allowed comparisons to gel-DBM. In contrast to gel-DBM, which is particle based, the new formulations of Grafton are fiber-containing, and demonstrate improved handling characteristics compared with the gel. Flex-DBM is a flexible sheet of Grafton fibers, whereas putty-DBM is made in a malleable consistency. Previous studies, conducted by Edwards and co-workers in an athymic rat heterotopic implant model, demonstrated that the gel-DGM, flex-DBM and putty-DBM had equivalent osteoinductive capacities [23]. Both the flex- and putty-DBM showed significantly superior fusion rates to gel-DBM and to autograft alone (100%, 83%, 58% and 73%, respectively). When combined with a less than standard amount of autograft (1.5 ml), both composites had significantly superior fusion rates (100%) to autograft alone (33%) and to gel-DBM combined with autograft (70%). Edwards concluded that these two formulations of DBM demonstrated a potential as both a graft extender and graft enhancer, since each performed better than autograft alone when used as stand-alone agents or when combined with autograft. They further postulated that the new formulations of DBM enhance fusion over and above that of gel-DBM combined with autograft, because these fiber-containing formulations may be more osteoconductive than gel-DBM. When flex-, putty- and gel-DBM were devitalized by guanidine extraction, thereby removing the osteoinductive factors, and then compared to devitalized gel-DBM in terms of bone formation, the devitalized flex- and putty-DBM formulations showed significantly more new bone formation than devitalized gel-DBM, suggesting an enhanced ability to serve as an osteoconductive graft substitute. The flex formulation used in these studies was fluffier than the original human flex, and this form has now been produced for human use and is called Grafton Matrix.

A number of bioceramics such as sea coral and hydroxyapatite (HA) have been used in comparison to and in combination with DBM in animal models of spine fusion [5, 52, 54]. Ragni and his colleagues evaluated the efficacy of DBM with porous hydroxyapatite (HA) in an anterior lumbar interbody spinal fusion model in rabbits [52, 54]. They reported that HA blocks alone or in combination with DBM had similar radiographic fusion scores to autograft alone or autograft with DBM and BM at 2 months. By 6 months, all groups had stable fusions on dynamic radiographs, with the exception of the group that received no implant. The earliest signs of fusion on dynamic radiographs were achieved in the group implanted with the HA-DBM composite, although, according to the authors, statistical comparisons could not be calculated, because of the insufficient number of observations in the autograft alone group and the group that received no implant [52]. Using a well-characterized and validated rabbit model of posterolateral lumbar spinal fusion, Boden and his co-workers found significantly lower rates of fusion with DBM alone (17%) and biocoral alone (0%) at 5 weeks when compared to autograft alone (62%) [5]. In this study, the addition of bovine-derived bone growth factor extract (bone protein, BP) to DBM, to autograft, and to natural coral resulted in 100% fusions in each of these groups by 5 weeks. Furthermore, the addition of BP to either DBM or biocoral significantly increased the biomechanical strength and stiffness of fusion when compared to BP combined with autograft.

The role of osteoinductive growth factors as an adjunct to enhance spinal fusion is an area of intense experimental investigation. First isolated by Urist from bone in a partially purified form, these growth factors appear to hold the greatest promise for graft alternatives in the challenging environment of the posterolateral spine [69, 71]. A number of investigators have since investigated DBM in conjunction with a variety of osteoinductive growth factors, including bovine-derived osteoinductive protein extract (BP) [4, 5, 6, 65] and recombinant human bone morphogenetic protein 2 (rhBMP-2) [33]. In general, these studies have shown that successful spinal fusion can be achieved using osteoinductive growth factors combined with different carriers, including DBM. Boden et al. demonstrated successful fusion in both the rabbit and primate model of posterolateral spine fusion using BP with a DBM carrier [4, 5, 6]. In the rabbit model, DBM combined with BP demonstrated significantly higher fusion rates as compared to autologous iliac crest graft or to DBM alone. Moreover, the fusion masses in the BP-DBM composite group were significantly stronger and stiffer on biomechanical testing compared to the autograft group with or without the bone protein, perhaps reflecting the impact of the homogeneity of the bone protein-carrier implant on bone remodeling. The more homogeneous fusion mass associated with either DBM or biocoral (i.e., masses consisting of uniform small particles) may be more amenable to bone remodeling and reach biomechanical maturity more quickly than the less homogeneous fusion mass found with autograft (i.e, masses composed of variably sized larger bone pieces) [5]. These authors also noted a dose-dependent response to BP, with 100% fusion at the higher concentration (300 μg BP) and 50% fusion at the lower concentration (100 μg BP), indicating that a threshold must be overcome before bone formation is induced [5]. An eight-fold increase in BP concentration (μg bone protein/g DBM carrier) was required to induce adequate bone formation in the rhesus monkey spine.

In contrast to results indicating improved biomechanical properties when an osteoinductive growth factor is combined with a DBM carrier [4, 5, 6], two studies from different laboratories have reported significantly decreased biomechanical characteristics in the growth factor-DBM carrier groups [33, 65]. Using a unilateral posterior lumbar decompression and contralateral spine fusion model in dogs, Helm and his colleagues [33] compared five groups: autograft alone, autograft with DBM, autograft with Type

I collagen gel, autograft with DBM and collagen gel, and autograft with rhBMP-2. At 3 months, all groups without DBM demonstrated histological and radiographic evidence of fusion, with the rhBMP-2+ autograft group showing the largest fusion mass. Furthermore, all groups with DBM (including the autograft with DBM group) demonstrated markedly lower rates of fusion and decreased biomechanical strength and stiffness compared to groups that did not contain DBM. These disparate findings may be partially explained by differences in the methods used to process the DBM [3]. These authors utilized a demineralization process [13] that differs from the process as originally promulgated by Urist [71] and from the one utilized in the series of studies conducted by Boden and his colleagues [4, 5, 6, 65]. Moreover, the animal model of spinal fusion utilized by these authors (i.e, unilateral decompression and contralateral intralaminar fusion) is relatively unique, making extrapolation of their findings to the more common posterolateral intertransverse process model of spinal arthrodesis difficult.

Silcox et al. found mixed results in a novel experiment designed to evaluate the efficacy of the bovine-derived bone growth factor (BP) in a nicotine rabbit spinal fusion model [65]. This model involves the continuous infusion of nicotine via a subcutaneous implanted miniosmotic nicotine pump, and has been shown to yield a nonunion rate of 100% as compared to the nonunion rate in the nonnicotine model of 35% using autologous iliac crest graft [64]. Silcox et al. reported 100% fusion at 5 and 10 weeks in the BP with autograft group as compared to 64% fusion in the BP with DBM group and 0% fusion with autograft alone. In contrast to previous studies [4, 5, 6], the biomechanical properties of the BP-DBM composite group were significantly lower than the BP-autograft group, with the authors noting a marked degree of graft resorption and an absence of fusion mass formation in 20% (2/10) of the animals in the BP-DBM group.

In summary, a number of well-controlled studies in a validated model of posterolateral spinal fusion have demonstrated that certain formulations of DBM can function as viable bone graft alternatives. The combination of osteoinductive growth factors with suitable osteoinductive and osteoconductive carriers, such as DBM, appears to be an especially potent promoter of spinal fusion in both lower- and higher-order animal models.

Bone morphogenetic proteins

Lovell et al. determined the efficacy of partially purified bovine BMP (bBMP) in a four-level alternating thoracic fusion model (T6–T13) in canines [40]. Four variations were used, including local autograft with bBMP, local autograft with a polylactic acid carrier for bBMP, local autograft alone and decortication alone. Fusions were assessed radiographically and histologically. The bBMP and autograft groups had the highest fusion rate (71%) compared with the other conditions (29%, 14% and 0% respectively). The bBMP/autograft combination produced a larger fusion mass with a more rapid fusion rate than that of autogenous spinous process graft alone.

Through genetically modified cell lines, recombinant bone morphogenetic protein has been produced as singular molecular species in unlimited quantities. Recombinant human BMP (rhBMP) does not cause a host-versus-graft immune response, and is free of infectious agents and contaminants.

Recombinant human osteogenic protein (rhBMP-7, rhOP-1) was evaluated as a bone graft substitute for spinal fusion in a canine posterior lumbar fusion model by Cook et al. [18]. Within 12 weeks, solid fusions were obtained with 2.0 mg of the growth factor, compared with 26 weeks in the autogenous iliac bone graft group. Magin evaluated rhBMP-7 in a sheep lumbar interbody fusion model [44]. An L4-L5 fusion was performed in three groups of ten sheep each. The first group received autograft, the second received deproteinized bovine hydroxylapatite, and the third group received rhBMP-7 on a collagen carrier. Radiographs demonstrated solid fusions in eight of ten sheep in the rhBMP-7 group at 4 months; at 6 months, equal volumes of bone were seen in both the autograft group and the rhBMP-7 group. According to histology and histomorphometry 6 months postoperatively, the rhBMP-7 group showed the highest bone density in the area of the fusion.

Schimandle et al. used rhBMP-2 in a rabbit model of lumbar intertransverse process arthrodesis and compared it with fusions obtained with autogenous bone graft [62]. Different doses and different carriers for rhBMP-2 were used in this study. All rabbits in the experimental group achieved solid spinal fusion as assessed by manual palpation and radiographs, whereas only 42% of the autograft control group achieved fusion. Rabbits implanted with high-dose rhBMP-2 had more mature fusions with greater trabecular bone formation than those rabbits implanted with low-dose rhBMP-2. Sheehan et al. examined the spinal fusion enhancement potential of rhBMP-2 in a unilateral posterolateral canine spine fusion model [63]. Their four experimental groups consisted of the following: autogenous bone graft alone, autogenous bone graft plus collagen, no implant, and autogenous bone, collagen and rhBMP-2. Radiographic assessment, three-dimensional computed tomographic volumetric analysis and biomechanical testing were performed. The average fusion volume and flexion and extension biomechanical properties were significantly greater in the rhBMP-2/autograft/collagen group as compared to the other groups. The results of this study indicated that the most advantageous spinal fusion implant matrix consisted of rhBMP-2, autogenous bone graft and collagen. Sandhu et al. evaluated rhBMP-2 using a canine posterior lumbar intertransverse process fusion model, and found that at 3 months, solid single-level fusion was achieved, with similar volumes of de novo bone across a wide range of doses [59]. Fusion was not achieved in animals with autogenous iliac crest graft alone. The same group then studied whether decortication was essential for successful fusion in the presence of rhBMP-2. Traditionally, achieving successful spinal fusion relies on the exposure of bone marrow through decortication of the posterior elements, hence releasing osteoinductive proteins. The authors hypothesized that the use of an implanted osteoinductive protein (rhBMP-2) would obviate the need for exposure and release of the growth factors. A canine model was utilized with L4-L5 transverse process fusions performed with and without decortication and with varying doses of rhBMP-2. Their results indicated no statistical differences in clinical and radiographic fusion rates between decorticated and undecorticated groups.

Boden et al. examined the efficacy of minimally invasive, video-assisted lateral intertransverse process arthrodeses using rhBMP-2 delivered in a collagen sponge carrier in two different animal models [8]. There were three arms to this study. In the first arm, they used a rabbit model to develop the minimally invasive technique, which then was modified for a primate (rhesus monkey) model. The second arm consisted of three parts:

1. A group of rabbits that underwent standard open-muscle splitting approach using rhBMP-2 and collagen
2. A video-assisted control group that underwent video-assisted lateral intertransverse arthrodesis with collagen implant only, and
3. A video-assisted BMP group that underwent video-assisted lateral intertransverse arthrodesis with rhBMP-2 and collagen as graft material

The third and final arm consisted of rhesus monkeys that underwent video-assisted lateral intertransverse arthrodesis with rhBMP-2 and collagen after laminectomy of L4-L5. All experimental animals implanted with rhBMP-2 went on to solid fusion. The results of this study thus indicated that video-assisted intertransverse process arthrodesis was a feasible and effective method of lumbar spine fusion in the rabbit and rhesus monkey.

Anterior spinal column fusion using rhBMP-2 has also been investigated. Sandhu et al. implanted cylindrical and threaded titanium intervertebral body fusion devices containing rhBMP-2 without autograft in a sheep anterior lumbar interbody fusion model [58]. They demonstrated consistent and rapid interbody intervertebral osseous fusion through the fixation device in 100% (six of six) cases. On the other hand, only 33% (two of six) control animals implanted with the fusion cage containing autograft alone achieved solid fusion. In the same model, Sandhu et al. added rhBMP-2 to porous tantalum cylindrical cages and showed that significantly greater bone ingrowth occurred in the porous macrostructure compared with cages that had not been combined with the rhBMP-2 [60]. Similarly, Cunningham et al. performed three-level anterior thoracic fusions in a sheep model with a threaded cylindrical fusion cage containing either rhBMP-7 or autogenous bone graft derived from the iliac crest [20]. They found fusion rates for the two study groups to be comparable (63%).

Non-human primate models

There is evidence to suggest that the concentration of cells receptive to the growth factors decreases as the evolutionary complexity of the animal increases. Hence, osteoinductive agents may demonstrate desirable effects in a lower species but not in a higher species. As a result, non-human primate models have been investigated in an attempt to mimic the physiologic processes in humans.

Cheung et al. assessed the efficacy of rhBMP-7 used with autologous corticocancellous bone to accelerate intertransverse lumbar fusion in a primate model [16]. Twelve monkeys were divided into two groups; one group receiving autograft soaked in a solution of rhBMP-7 and the second receiving autograft soaked in the carrier solution alone. Fusion was assessed by monthly radiographs and after sacrifice at 5 months, by gross inspection, histological examination and mechanical testing. There was no statistical difference in fusion rate histologically or biomechanically between the two groups (16% in the autograft group vs 66% in the rhBMP-7 group). The authors concluded that the potent osteoinductive characteristics of rhBMP-7 in lower animals did not translate to primates.

Boden et al. examined a purified bovine osteoinductive bone protein extract in the posterior lumbar spines of adult male rhesus monkeys [7]. Animals that were implanted with 3000 µg or more of the growth factor achieved single-level intertransverse process fusion. Spines implanted with lesser doses of the osteoinductive factor did not proceed to fusion. At the same institution, using the same intertransverse process fusion models, Boden et al. found rhBMP-2 to result in a 100% fusion rate with all three different doses tested [11]. The carrier alone and autograft treated control animals did not result in any fusions (0%). At the same institution, Boden et al. also investigated laparoscopic anterior spinal arthrodesis with rhBMP-2 in a primate model [9]. The rhBMP-2 was carried on a collagen sponge in a threaded titanium interbody cage for anterior L7-S1 fusion. Solid fusion was achieved in all five of the animals that had been implanted with the growth factor, as demonstrated histologically. Successful fusion did not occur in either of the two animals that were implanted with the collagen sponge alone. Hecht et al. studied the efficacy of rhBMP-2 in a rhesus macaque monkey anterior interbody fusion model, using cylindrical freeze-dried allograft bone dowels [31]. These dowels were filled with either rhBMP-2-soaked collagen sponges or autogenous bone graft from the iliac crest. Radiographic signs of fusion were demonstrated as early as 8 weeks after implantation, with complete fusion, as evidenced by radiology and histology, by 6 months. There was also evidence by this time of resorption of the allograft and replacement of de novo bone. These changes were not found in the control group, consisting of cortical dowels filled with autogenous bone graft.

Delivery vehicles for BMP

Although the osteoinductive capacity of recombinant BMP has been demonstrated in several models, the optimal method for delivering the protein to inducible cells has not yet been established. BMPs are soluble molecules that, when implanted alone, diffuse too rapidly to allow osteoinduction to occur. In general, a suitable carrier must consist of the following properties: it should provide controlled release of the protein, adequate exposure to inducible cells, be biocompatible with host tissue and have an architecture conducive to the rapid ingrowth of newly formed bone. For posterolateral spine fusions, a load-bearing delivery vehicle is not required, particularly when load bearing spinal fixation devices are also used. The delivery vehicles for this indication are responsible for primarily exposing the osteoinductive protein to induce pluripotent stem cells residing in local mesenchymal tissue and maintaining space for subsequent bone formation of the fusion mass. In contrast, load-bearing carriers are required for certain indications, such as anterior interbody fusion.

Fischgrund et al. evaluated the use of rhBMP-2 with various types of carrier media and the effect of rhBMP-2 with autogenous bone graft in a canine spine fusion model [26]. Bilateral intertransverse spine fusions were performed in six canines at L1-L2, L3-L4 and L5-L6 using autogenous iliac crest bone graft at each level. Hence, the 18 segmental fusion sites were randomly assigned one of six fusion methods:

1. Autogenous bone graft alone
2. Autogenous bone graft+rhBMP-2
3. Autogenous bone graft+collagen "sandwich"+rhBMP-2
4. Autogenous bone graft+collagen morsels+rhBMP-2
5. Autogenous bone graft+polylactic glycolic acid (PLGA) sponge "sandwich"+rhBMP-2, and
6. Autogenous bone graft+open-pore polylactic acid morsels+rhBMP-2

Their results indicated that the addition of rhBMP-2 significantly increased bone graft volume as assessed by computerized tomography (CT), but no significant difference was noted in carrier media for rhBMP-2. However, the use of PLGA as a carrier was associated with a higher rate of fusion mass bone void formation.

Martin et al. compared different combinations of rhBMP-2 dosages and carriers in an adult male primate (rhesus) model [46]. The main findings of this study were that rhBMP-2 could induce bone in the non-human primate and that, when protected from the "squeezing" influence of soft-tissues, collagen carriers allowed more bone induction at lower doses of rhBMP-2. Similarly, Boden et al. used the same model to evaluate various doses of rhBMP-2 in a ceramic (hydroxyapatite-tricalcium phosphate, HA-TCP) carrier as a complete bone graft substitute [11]. The theory behind using a ceramic carrier was that, although resorbable collagen sponges have shown promise in rabbit and canine models of spine fusion, it was too compressible for the paraspinal muscles in rhesus monkeys, as demonstrated by Martin and co-workers (see above). Twenty-one adult rhesus monkeys underwent laminectomies at L4-L5, followed by bilateral intertransverse process arthrodesis via a classic midline incision or minimally invasive video-assisted posterolateral approach. On each side, a 5-cm^3 implant of either autogenous bone graft or 60:40 HA-TCP was placed. The ceramic carrier was loaded with a varying range of doses of rhBMP-2. Fusion was not achieved in the autogenous bone graft alone group, whilst all the experimental animals in the HA:TCP group, irrespective of the dose of rhBMP-2 loaded, achieved solid fusion. These results prove that HA:TCP can be a suitable carrier for rhBMP-2 in a primate posterolateral spine fusion model.

Considerable work in the field of cytokine delivery is still needed. Development and refinement of an appropriate carrier that releases growth factors in a dose-dependent, predictable and continuous fashion is needed. The development of such a carrier may be the most crucial step prior to widespread clinical use.

Gene therapy models and BMP

Recently, there has been interest in exploring the efficacy of regional gene therapy for spine fusions [35]. Preliminary results of this technique in preclinical animal work is exciting; however, there are several issues that remain to be settled before one can advocate the widespread use of gene therapy for spinal fusion. In theory, the effect of transduced cells continuously producing growth factors at the desired site until a solid fusion results is attractive; however, dosage and carrier issues still remain to be settled.

Riew et al. attempted to prolong the bone-inducing effect of bone morphogenetic protein-2 using an adenoviral vector carrying the human BMP-2 gene to transduce marrow-derived mesenchymal stem cells in New Zealand White rabbits [56]. In their model, they isolated and expanded bone marrow mesenchymal cells (MSC) from the resected ribs. Immunocytochemistry was used to show that approximately 80% of MSCs could be genetically modified to over-express BMP-2 protein by treatment with an adenoviral vector encoding human BMP-2 (Adv-BMP-2). A similar efficiency of gene transfer was demonstrated with the control vector encoding a marker gene *E.coli* ß-galactosidase (Adv-ß-gal).

Four weeks after rib harvest, the rabbits underwent spinal fusion at L5-L6. Genetically modified mesenchymal stem cells loaded onto collagen sponges were placed between the transverse processes of L5 and L6, with Adv-BMP-2 transduced MSCs placed on the left side and the Adv-ß-gal on the right.

After the 2nd postoperative week, all rabbits were examined radiographically weekly. Of the five study rabbits, one showed radiographic evidence of new bone formation on the side implanted with Adv-BMP-2, 5 weeks after surgery. No new bone was noted on the control Adv-ß-gal side. No new bone formation was observed on either side in the other four study rabbits. Rabbits were sacrificed 7 weeks after the operation, and histologic examination of the rabbit with new bone revealed mature bone with a trabecular structure. Histology was unremarkable in the control side. The authors thus concluded that it was possible to transduce mesenchymal stem cells with hBMP-2 gene so the transformed cells could produce BMP-2 in vivo that would exert an osteoinductive effect. These initial results, however, warranted further work on the longevity and efficiency of the gene transfer.

In a related study, Alden et al. investigated the effect of percutaneous spinal fusion using BMP-2 with adenovirus-mediated gene transfer techniques in an athymic (immunocompromised) rat model [1]. The 12 rats were divided into three groups of four rats each. All groups underwent paraspinal percutaneous injection with 7.5 µl of virus via a Hamilton microsyringe inserted through a 19-G guide needle placed at the junction of the spinous process and the lamina on each side. The groups were as follows:

1. Adv-BMP-2 bilaterally
2. Adv-BMP-2 on the right, Adv-ß-gal on the left, and
3. Adv-ß-gal bilaterally

CT scans of the lumbosacral junction were obtained at weeks 3, 5, 8, and 12. Twelve weeks following injection, the rats were sacrificed and studied histologically.

Examination of CT scans at each time point revealed new bone formation adjacent to the spinous processes and laminae at each of the Adv-BMP-2 injected sites, but no changes were observed at the Adv-ß-gal control sites. Histology of the Adv-BMP-2 sites 12 weeks following injection revealed extensive endochondral bone formation within the paraspinal musculature, with well-developed vascular channels and areas of cartilage as well as trabecular bone and mature marrow elements. New bone formed was in direct continuity with the adjacent laminae, inferior facets and the spinous process. No new bone formation was detected in the Adv-ß-gal control animals. The authors concluded that in vivo endochondral bone formation was possible using direct adenoviral construct injection into the paraspinal musculature, and suggested that this approach could potentially be used for spine fusion in the future.

Wang et al. transfected marrow cells with an adenoviral vector to produce BMP-2 in a rat intertransverse spinal fusion model [74]. Bone marrow was harvested from syngeneic Lewis rats and expanded in tissue culture. These cells were genetically modified using Adv-BMP-2. The transfected cells were then soaked onto a guanidiun extracted, deactivated demineralized bone matrix carrier and implanted into the rat spine between the transverse processes of L4 and L5. Fifty-six rats were divided into a total of seven groups:

1. Adenovirus-modified BMP-2 producing marrow cells
2. Recombinant BMP-2 protein
3. Demineralized bone matrix alone
4. Cells transfected with a control gene
5. Decortication of the transverse processes alone
6. Autogenous iliac crest bone graft, and
7. Normal (not genetically modified) bone marrow cells with demineralized bone matrix

Outcome assessment to determine fusion was performed by inspection, plain radiographs, manual palpation and histologic evaluation.

At 4 weeks, all rats that had been implanted with adenovirus-modified BMP-2 producing marrow cells demonstrated 100% fusion. All rats (100%) that had been implanted with recombinant BMP-2 alone also had complete arthrodesis by 4 weeks. All other groups did not demonstrate fusion at 8 weeks. The data of this study confirmed that regional gene therapy utilizing BMP-2 producing bone marrow cells produced by adenoviral gene transfer could be successfully used in a rat model of intertransverse spine fusion, opening further avenues for its potential use in humans.

Conclusions and future directions

The studies reviewed above represent a few examples of the exemplary work being conducted in the arena of bone morphogenetic proteins and spinal fusion research. The initial findings of clinical trials using rhBMP-2 have been published, and the spectacular results indicate that the widespread use of BMPs in spine fusion may become a reality fairly soon [12]. However, several questions remain to be answered. The exact dose required for each specific fusion site (posterolateral vs anterior interbody) remains to be comprehensively determined in humans. Furthermore, optimal site-specific carriers are still in the developmental stage. The use of collagen-soaked cortical bone dowels for anterior interbody fusions seem promising in this regard. The overall cost of the device to be implanted will also factor into the use of BMPs for spinal fusion in the future.

One interesting development recently has been the isolation and delivery of an upstream transcription factor that upregulates the expression of multiple BMPs and other factors at the fusion site for sustained protein release [10]. This has been shown to have a powerful recruitment effect on other growth factors and cells to form bone in a rat lumbar spine fusion model. Development of this avenue is underway, and the future controversies on the use of BMPs will include the question of whether it is safer, more cost-effective and more efficacious to use a single large dose at the fusion bed or to use gene therapy mediated techniques for fusion. Relevant factors will include number of levels requiring fusion, metabolic health of the patient, immunological status, osteoporosis and age-mediated decrease in responding pluripotent cells.

Before one can make any definitive arguments, not only is further basic research required to elaborate the biological functioning of each of the BMPs, but further carefully designed, prospective, randomized clinical trials are essential to validate their potential use in the spine.

References

1. Alden TD, Pittman DD, Beres EJ, Hankins GR, Kallmes DF, Wisotsky BM, Kerns KM, Helm GA (1999) Percutaneous spinal fusion using bone morphogenetic protein-2 gene therapy. J Neurosurg [Spine 1] 90:109–114
2. Aldinger G, Herr G, Kusswetter W, Reis HJ, Thielemann FW, Holz U (1991) Bone morphogenetic protein: a review. Int Orthop 15:169–177
3. Block JE, Russell JL (1998) Spine fusion with demineralized bone. J Neurosurg 88:354–356
4. Boden SD, Schimandle JH, Hutton WC (1995) Lumbar intertransverse process spine arthrodesis using a bovine-derived osteoinductive bone protein. J Bone Joint Surg Am 77:1404–1417
5. Boden SD, Schimandle JH, Hutton WC (1995) 1995 Volvo Award in Basic Sciences. The use of an osteoinductive growth factor for lumbar spinal fusion. II. Study of dose, carrier, and species. Spine 20:2633–2644
6. Boden SD, Schimandle JH, Hutton WC (1995) An experimental lumbar intertransverse process spinal fusion model: radiographic, histologic, and biomechanical healing characteristics. Spine 20:412–420
7. Boden SD, Schimandle JH, Hutton WC (1996) Evaluation of a bovine-derived osteoinductive bone protein in a nonhuman primate model of lumbar spinal fusion. Trans Orthop Res Soc 21:118
8. Boden SD, Moskovitz PA, Morone MA, Toribitake Y (1996) Video-assisted lateral intertransverse process arthrodesis – validation of a new minimally invasive lumbar spinal fusion technique in the rabbit and nonhuman primate (rhesus) models. Spine 21: 2689–2697
9. Boden SD, Martin GJ, Horton WC, Truss TL, Sandhu HS (1998) Laparoscopic anterior spinal arthrodesis with rhBMP-2 in a titanium interbody threaded cage. J Spinal Disord 11:95–101
10. Boden SD, Titus L, Hair G, Liu Y, Viggeswarapu M, Nanes MS, Baranowski C (1998) 1998 Volvo Award in Basic Sciences: lumbar spine fusion by local gene therapy with a cDNA encoding a novel osteoinductive protein (LMP-1). Spine 23:2486–2492
11. Boden SD, Martin GJ, Morone MA, Ugbo JL, Moskovitz PA. (1999) Posterolateral lumbar intertransverse process spine arthrodesis with rhBMP-2/hydroxyapatite-tricalcium phosphate (HA-TCP) following laminectomy in the non-human primate. Spine 24: 1179–1185
12. Boden SD, Zdeblick TA, Sandhu HS, Heim SE (2000) The use of rhBMP-2 in interbody fusion cages. Definitive evidence of osteoinduction in humans: a preliminary report. Spine 25:376–381
13. Bolander M E, Balian G (1986) The use of demineralized bone matrix in the repair of segmental defects. Augmentation with extracted matrix proteins and a comparison with autologous grafts. J Bone Joint Surg Am 68: 1264–1274
14. Burwell R.G (1985) The function of bone marrow in the incorporation of a bone graft. Clin Orthop 200:125–141
15. Chalmers J, Gray DH, Rush J (1975) Observations on the induction of bone in soft tissues. J Bone Joint Surg Br 57:36–45
16. Cheung KMC, Leong JCY, Liu SL, et al (1999) Augmentation of intertransverse spinal fusion in primates using OP-1. Presented at the 26th Annual Meeting of the International Society for the Study of the Lumbar Spine, Kona, Hawaii
17. Cook SD, Baffes GC, Wolfe MW, Sampath TK, Rueger DC, Whitecloud TS (1994) The effect of recombinant human osteogenic protein-1 on healing of large segmental bone defects. J Bone Joint Surg Am 76:827–838
18. Cook SD, Dalton JE, Prewett AB, Whitecloud TS (1995) In vivo evaluation of demineralized bone matrix as a bone graft substitute for posterior spinal fusion. Spine 20:877–886
19. Croteau S, Rauch F, Silvestri A, Hamdy RC (1999) Bone morphogenetic proteins in orthopedics: from basic science to clinical practice. Orthopedics 22:686–695
20. Cunningham BW, Kotani Y, McNulty PS, Cappuccino A, Kanayama M, Fedder IL, McAfee PC (1998) Video-assisted thoracoscopic surgery versus open thoracotomy for anterior thoracic spinal fusion. A comparative radiographic, biomechanical, and histologic analysis in a sheep model. Spine 23: 1333–1340
21. Dahners LE, Jacobs RR (1985) Long bone defects treated with demineralized bone. South Med J 78:933–934
22. Damien CJ, Parsons JR (1991) Bone graft and bone graft substitutes: a review of current technology and applications. J Appl Biomater 2:187–208
23. Edwards JT, Diegmann MH, Scarborough NL (1998) Osteoinduction of human demineralized bone: characterization in a rat model. Clin Orthop 357: 219–228
24. Einhorn TA, Lane JM, Burstein AH, Kopman CR, Vigorita VJ (1984) The healing of segmental bone defects induced by demineralized bone matrix: a radiographic and biomechanical study. J Bone Joint Surg Am 66:274–279
25. Ferguson D, Davis WL, Urist MR, Hurt WC, Allen EP (1987) Bovine bone morphogenetic protein (bBmp) fraction-induced repair of craniotomy defects in the rhesus monkey (Macaca speciosa). Clin Orthop 219:251–258
26. Fischgrund JS, James SB, Chabot MC, Hankin R, Herkowitz HN, Wozney JM, Shirkhoda A (1997) Augmentation of autograft using rhBMP-2 and different carrier media in the canine spine fusion model. J Spinal Disord 10:467–472
27. Frenkel SR, Moskovitch R, Spivak J, Zhang ZH, Prewett AB (1993) Demineralized bone matrix. Enhancement of spinal fusion. Spine 18:1634–1639

28. Gepstein R, Weiss RE, Saba K, Hallel T (1987) Bridging large defects in bone by demineralized bone matrix in the form of a powder. J Bone Joint Surg Am 69:984–992
29. Gerhart TN, Kirker-Head CA, Kriz MJ, Holtrop ME, Hennign GE, Hipp J, Schelling SH, Wang E (1993) Healing segmental femoral defects in sheep using recombinant human bone morphogenetic protein. Clin Orthop 293:317–326
30. Guizzardi S, Di Silvestre M, Scandroglio R, Ruggeri A, Savini R (1992) Implants of heterologous demineralized bone matrix for induction of posterior spinal fusion in rats. Spine 17: 701–707
31. Hecht B, Fischgrund J, Herkowitz H, Penman L, Toth J, Shirkhoda A (1999) The use of recombinant human bone morphogenic protein 2 (rhBMP-2) to promote spinal fusion in a nonhuman primate anterior interbody fusion model. Spine 24:629–636
32. Heckman JD, Boyan BD, Aufdemorte TB, Abbott JT (1991) The use of bone morphogenetic protein in the treatment on non-union in a canine model. J Bone Joint Surg 73:750–764
33. Helm GA, Sheehan JM, Sheehan JP, Jane JA, diPierro CG, Simmons NE, Gillies GT, Kallmes DF, Sweeney TM (1997) Utilization of type I collagen gel, demineralized bone matrix, and bone morphogenetic protein-2 to enhance autologous bone lumbar spinal fusion. J Neurosurg 86:93–100
34. Hulth A, Johnell O, Henricson A (1988) The implantation of demineralized fracture matrix yields more new bone formation than does intact matrix. Clin Orthop 234:235–249
35. Khan SN, Hidaka C, Sandhu HS, Girardi FP, Cammisa FP, Diwan AD (2000) Gene therapy for spine fusion. Orthop Clin North Am 31:473–484
36. Lane JM, Cornell CN, Werntz JR, Sandhu HS (1991) Clinical application of biosynthetics. In: Friedlaender GE, Goldberg V (eds) Bone and cartilage allografts. American Academy of Orthopaedic Surgeons, Park Ridge, pp 279–294
37. Lee SC, Shea M, Battle MA (1994) Healing of large segmental defects in rat femurs is enhanced by rhBMP-2 in a PLGA matrix: a torsional and densitometric assessment. Trans Orthop Res Soc 19:206
38. Lindholm TS, Nilsson OS, Lindholm TC (1982) Extraskeletal and intraskeletal new bone formation induced by demineralized bone matrix combined with bone marrow cells. Clin Orthop 171:251–255
39. Lindholm TS, Ragni P, Lindholm TC (1988) Response of bone marrow stroma cells to demineralized cortical bone matrix in experimental spinal fusion in rabbits. Clin Orthop 230:296–302
40. Lovell TP, Dawson EG, Nilsson OS, Urist MR (1989) Augmentation of spinal fusion with bone morphogenetic protein in dogs. Clin Orthop 243:266–274
41. Lowery GL, Maxwell KM, Karasick D, Block JE, Russo R (1995) Comparison of autograft and composite grafts of demineralized bone matrix and autologous bone in posterolateral fusions: an interim report. Innov Tech Biol Med 16:1–8
42. Lucas PA, Syftestad GT, Goldberg VM, Caplan AI (1989) Ectopic induction of cartilage and bone by water-soluble proteins from bovine bone using a collagenous delivery vehicle. J Biomed Mater Res 23 [A1 Suppl]:23–39
43. Luyten FP, Cunningham NS, Vukicevic S, Paralkar V, Ripamonti U, Reddi AH (1992) Advances in osteogenin and related bone morphogenetic proteins in bone induction and repair. Acta Orthop Belg 58 [Suppl 1]:263–267
44. Magin M (1999) BMP-7 (rhOP-1) is able to enhance lumbar vertebral interbody fusion. Results of a sheep trial and clinical impact. Presented at the 26th Annual Meeting of the International Society for the Study of the Lumbar Spine, Kona, Hawaii
45. Martin G, Boden SD, Morone MA, Titus L (1999) New formulations of demineralized bone matrix as a more effective graft alternative in experimental posterolateral lumbar spine arthrodesis. Spine 24:637–645
46. Martin GJ, Boden SD, Morone MA, Moskovitz PA (1999) Posterolateral intertransverse process spinal fusion arthrodesis with rhBMP-2 in a non-human primate. Important lessons learned regarding dose, carrier, and safety. J Spinal Disord 12:179–186
47. Mizutani H, Urist MR (1982) The nature of bone morphogenetic protein (BMP) fractions derived from bovine bone matrix gelatin. Clin Orthop 171: 213–223
48. Morone MA, Boden SD (1998) Experimental posterolateral lumbar spinal fusion with a demineralized bone matrix gel. Spine 23:159–167
49. Nilsson OS, Urist MR, Dawson EG, Schmalzried TP, Finerman GAM (1986) Bone repair induced by bone morphogenetic protein in ulnar defects in dogs. J Bone Joint Surg Br 68:635–642
50. Oikarinen J (1982) Experimental spinal fusion with decalcified bone matrix and deep-frozen allogeneic bone in rabbits. Clin Orthop 162:210–218
51. Ragni PC, Lindholm TS (1989) Bone formation and static changes in the thoracic spine at uni- or bilateral experimental spondylodesis with demineralized bone matrix (DBM). Ital J Orthop Traumatol 15:237–252
52. Ragni P, Lindholm S (1991) Interaction of allogeneic demineralized bone matrix and porous hydroxyapatite bioceramics in lumbar interbody fusion in rabbits. Clin Orthop 272:292–299
53. Ragni PC, Lindholm TS, Lindholm TC (1987) Vertebral fusion dynamics in the thoracic and lumbar spine induced by allogenic demineralized bone matrix combined with autogenous bone marrow. An experimental study in rabbits. Ital J Orthop Traumatol 13:241–251
54. Ragni P, Ala-Mononen P, Lindholm TS (1993) Spinal fusion induced by porous hydroxyapatite blocks (HA). Experimental comparative study with HA, demineralized bone matrix and autogenous bone marrow. Ital J Orthop Traumatol 19:133–144
55. Reddi AH (1995) Bone morphogenetic proteins, bone marrow stromal cells, and mesenchymal stem cells. Maureen Owen revisited. Clin Orthop 313:115–119
56. Riew KD, Wright NM, Cheng S-L, Avioli LV, Lou J (1998) Induction of bone formation using a recombinant adenoviral vector carrying the human BMP-2 gene in a rabbit spinal fusion model. Calcif Tissue Int 63:357–360
57. Sandhu H (2000) Anterior lumbar interbody fusion with osteoinductive growth factors. Clin Orthop 371:56–60
58. Sandhu HS, Kabo JM, Turner AS, Liu D, Kanim LEA, Toth JM (1996) rhBMP-2 augmentation of titanium fusion cages for experimental anterior lumbar fusion. Proceedings of the 11th Annual Meeting of the North American Spine Society, p 47
59. Sandhu HS, Kanim LEA, Kabo JM, Toth JM, Zeegen EN, Liu D, Delamarter RB, Dawson EG (1996) Effective doses of recombinant bone morphogenetic protein-2 in experimental spinal fusion. Spine 21:2115–2122
60. Sandhu HS, Toth JM, Turner AS (1997) Anterior spinal fusions with tantalum "foam" interbody fusion cages. Presented at the 24th Annual Meeting of the International Society for the Study of the Lumbar Spine, Singapore, June 2–6
61. Sassard WR, Eidman DK, Gray PM (1994) Analysis of spine fusion utilizing demineralized bone matrix. Orthop Trans 18:886,887

62. Schimandle JH, Boden SD, Hutton WC (1995) Experimental spinal fusion with recombinant human bone morphogenetic protein-2 (rhBMP-2). Spine 20: 1326–1337
63. Sheehan JP, Kallmes DF, Sheehan JM, Jane JA, Fergus AH, diPierro CG, Simmons NE, Makel DD, Helm GA (1996) Molecular methods of enhancing lumbar spine fusion. Neurosurgery 39:548–554
64. Silcox DH, Daftari T, Boden SD, Schimandle JH, Hutton WC, Whitesides TE (1995) The effect of nicotine on spinal fusion. Spine 20:1549–1553
65. Silcox DH, Boden SD, Schimandle JH, Johnson P, Whitesides TE, Hutton WC (1998) Reversing the inhibitory effect of nicotine on spinal fusion using an osteoinductive protein extract. Spine 23:291–296
66. Simmons DJ, Calhoun JH, Zimmerman B, et al (1994) Effect of recombinant human bone morphogenetic protein 2 (rhBMP-2) on the healing of cortical bone in the rabbit tibia. Proc Orthop Res Soc 40:507
67. Tiedeman JJ, Garvin KL, Kile TA, Connolly JF (1995) The role of a composite demineralized bone matrix and bone marrow in the treatment of osseous defects. Orthopedics 18:1153–1158
68. Tuli SM Singh AD (1978) The osteoinductive property of decalcified bone matrix: an experimental study. J Bone Joint Surg Br 60:116–123
69. Urist MR (1965) Bone: formation by autoinduction. Science 150:893–899
70. Urist MR, Dawson E (1981) Intertransverse process fusion with the aid of chemosterilized autolyzed antigen-extracted allogeneic (AAA) bone. Clin Orthop 154:97–113
71. Urist MR, Silverman BF, Buring K, Dubuc FL, Rosenberg JM. (1967) The bone induction principle. Clin Orthop 53:243–283
72. Urist MR, Mikulski A, Lietze A (1979) Solubilized and insolubilized bone morphogenetic protein. Proc Natl Acad Sci 76:1828–1832
73. Urist MR, DeLange RJ, Finerman GAM (1983) Bone cell differentiation and growth factors. Science 220:680–686
74. Wang JC, Yoo S, Kanim LE, et al (1999) Transformation of marrow cells with an adenoviral vector to produce BMP-2. Presented at the 34th Annual Meeting of the Scoliosis Research Society, San Diego, 20–23 September

Thomas Steffen
Thierry Stoll
Tudor Arvinte
Robert K. Schenk

Porous tricalcium phosphate and transforming growth factor used for anterior spine surgery

Abstract Harvesting autologous bone graft from the iliac crest is associated with considerable secondary morbidity. Bone graft substitutes such as porous ceramics are increasingly used for spinal surgery. This paper presents the results of an animal study in which β-tricalcium phosphate (β-TCP) bone substitutes were used for anterior spinal surgery in sheep and baboons. The presented baboon study also investigated the effect of impregnating the ceramic material with transforming growth factor (TGF). In the first study, using the sheep model, a stand-alone instrumented anterior fusion was performed. The animals were randomized into three treatment groups: autologous bone, β TCP granules, and sham group. The results were analyzed biomechanically and histologically at three survival intervals: 8, 16 and 32 weeks. An additional animal group was added later, with ceramic pre-filled implants. In the second study, a baboon model was used to assess the osteointegration of a 15-mm-diameter porous β-TCP block into the vertebral body. The experiment was partially motivated by a new surgical procedure proposed for local bone graft harvest. Three treatment groups were used: β-TCP plug, β-TCP plug impregnated with TGF-β3, and a sham group with empty defect. The evaluation for all animals included computer tomograms at 3 and 6 months, as well as histology at 6 months. In the sheep model, the mechanical evaluation failed to demonstrate differences between treatment groups. This was because massive anterior bone bridges formed in almost all the animals, masking the effects of individual treatments. Histologically, β-TCP was shown to be a good osteoconductor. While multiple signs of implant micromotion were documented, pre-filling the cages markedly improved the histological fusion outcomes. In the baboon study, the β-TCP plugs were completely osteointegrated at 6 months. For the group that used ceramic plugs impregnated with TGF-β3, no incremental advantage was seen as a result of this particular application. However, TGF-β3 is a potent growth factor at a very low dose. Not only does it speed up the ceramic material resorption, but it is also responsible for massive regional new bone formation. More experiments are required to better understand the biological effects of this growth factor in relation to bone formation, and to be able to take clinical advantage of them.

Keywords Tricalcium phosphate · Bone substitute · Transforming growth factor β · Interbody spinal fusion · Anterior surgery · Sheep · Baboon

T. Steffen (✉)
Orthopaedic Research Laboratory,
Royal Victoria Hospital,
Division of Orthopaedic Surgery,
McGill University,
687 Pine Avenue West, Room L4.69B,
Montreal, QC, Canada H3A 1A1
e-mail: tsteffen@orl.mcgill.ca,
Tel.: +1-514-8421231 ext 5276,
Fax: +1-514-8431699

T. Stoll
Mathys Medical Ltd.,
Bettlach, Switzerland

T. Arvinte
Exploratory Formulation,
Biotechnology Development
and Production, Novartis Pharma AG,
Basle, Switzerland

R.K. Schenk
Department of Oral Surgery,
School of Dental Medicine,
University of Berne, Switzerland

Introduction

Porous synthetic ceramics

Bone transplantation is a frequent procedure in spinal surgery. Autologous bone is most frequently harvested from the iliac crest, but this requires additional surgery to be performed, adds cost, and is associated with an increase in postoperative morbidity [1, 23, 27]. In addition, autologous bone graft is only available in limited quantities. Bone allograft, on the other hand, would be available in larger quantities, but bears the potential risk of infectious disease transmission [15] or immunologic response, with possible graft resorption.

Ceramic graft materials have now become available in a wide variety of chemical compositions [5]. They are attractive, because there is an infinite supply, the sterilization and shelf storage of the materials is easy, and there is no risk of disease transmission or immunogenic response. Today, the most frequently used inorganic ceramic materials in a clinical setting are tricalcium phosphate (TCP) and hydroxyapatite (HA). They have somewhat different ratios of calcium and phosphorus, but in essence they mimic closely the inorganic phase of bone, which makes up 60–70% of mammalian bone material. Both HA and TCP can act as a scaffold for osteogenic cells. It is important that the scaffold material is open porous [25]. The ability of host bone to gradually in-grow into the synthetic graft material depends on this open porosity. The graft resorption depends on its mineral composition. Whereas HA hardly resorbs at all [8, 21], TCP slowly degrades in vivo, and eventually gets completely replaced with remodeled host bone [6, 8].

Transforming growth factors

Transforming growth factor-βs are a family of multifunctional cytokines that modulate various cellular processes [10, 11]. The TGF-β family includes TGF-βs, activin, and bone morphogenetic proteins (BMPs). TGF-βs play a major role in tissue repair, their main function being to control cell proliferation and differentiation [12, 16]. Five isoforms of TGF-β are known, which show a high level of sequence homology and have similar biological activities, but different potencies [7]. The therapeutic potential of the isoforms expressed in mammalians – TGF-β1, TGF-β2, and TGF-β3 – have been investigated for a variety of indications such as wound healing, prevention of oral mucositis, and bone and cartilage repair.

The use of growth hormones from the TGF-β family for the biochemical enhancement of bone healing and bone formation is a field of sustained research. TGF-β1 was shown to induce bone closure of skull defects [3] and to stimulate bone on-growth, and enhances bone healing in tricalcium-phosphate-coated implants [13, 24], accelerating the healing in the vicinity of the implant [14].

One important element in the bone healing, as well as the wound healing effects of TGF, may be the strong angiogenesis-inducing properties of these molecules. At the site of injury, angiogenic factors are immediately released from macrophages and tissue. Endothelial cells stimulated by the angiogenic factors migrate and form new blood vessels at the injured site [19].

Anterior spinal surgery animal studies

In this paper, we present two animal studies that both used porous β-TCP bone graft substitute in an anterior surgical procedure of the lumbar spine. The first one was done using the sheep model for an anterior stand-alone interbody fusion, performed with a titanium implant spacer filled with granular β-TCP material. We later added to the anterior fusion model a ceramic pre-filled titanium cage, in order to improve postoperative filling with graft substitute. The preliminary results of this modified model are also presented in this paper.

The second experiment used the baboon model for a partial vertebral defect model. It was motivated by a formerly proposed and biomechanically validated surgical procedure for regional autologous bone harvest from a vertebral body next to the fusion [20]. The goal was to avoid the usual iliac crest bone harvest, but still be able to use autologous bone graft, the material of first choice for obtaining successful spinal fusion. The proposed procedure uses the small amount of bone that can be obtained from a neighboring vertebral body, to fill the cage with autologous graft. The resulting defect, mechanically more stable than the instrumented disc space, can then easily be plugged with a bone substitute. An appropriately sized porous β-TCP block was used to fill the cylindrical defect. The block's osteointegration was then followed over time. A second treatment group was included in this baboon study, utilizing the same β-TCP scaffold, but impregnated with TGF-β3.

Materials and methods

Instrumented anterior interbody spinal fusion

Fifty-four skeletally mature female Dorset sheep of approximately 45 kg body weight were used for this study. They were divided into three survival groups of equal size, which were sacrificed at 8 weeks, 16 weeks and 32 weeks, respectively. A retroperitoneal approach to the anterior spine was used for exposure of three consecutive disc levels. The step by step surgical technique for retroperitoneal spinal surgery in sheep has been described earlier in great detail [2]. The L2/L3 and L4/L5 disc levels were both prepared for implant insertion by removing the disc material and cartilage from the bony endplates using sharp preparation. The L3/L4 disc remained intact. A custom sized and shaped titanium cage [21] was specifically designed and produced for this study, in ac-

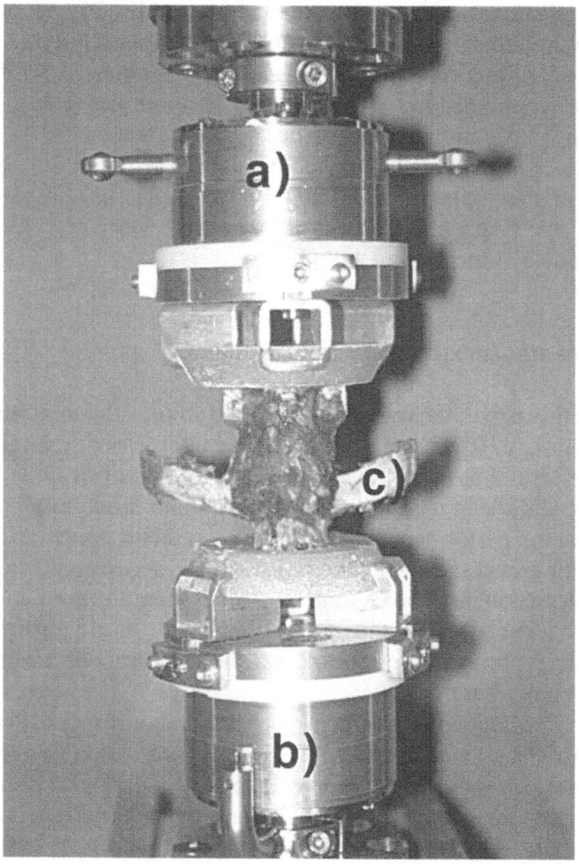

Fig. 1 Mounted sheep specimen to assess the segmental stability in axial rotation, showing the upper (*a*) and lower (*b*) custom-made three-clamp fixation grips, and the specimen with ends embedded in acrylic cement (*c*). The grips can freely angulate in all directions, and can easily be blocked in any starting position

cordance with the distinct sheep anatomy (convex-concave shaped disc space). It had a hollow central part filled with different graft materials, dependent on the particular treatment group. The animals for each of the three survival groups were assigned to the treatment groups in a block randomized fashion. The first treatment group had the cage filled with autologous cortico-cancellous mercerized bone from the sheep's iliac crest (gold standard), the second one used 0.7–1.4-mm-diameter β-TCP porous granules (chronOS, Mathys, Bettlach, Switzerland) to fill the cage, and the third group had an empty cage placed (sham). There were a total of 12 instrumented levels available per survival interval and treatment group for subsequent analysis.

All sheep underwent regular radiographic controls following surgery to search for possible implant migration, failure or bone osteolysis. After sacrifice, the lumbar spine was harvested en bloc and stored at minus 20°C until mechanical testing. To quantify the instrumented levels' bending stiffness in all three cardinal planes, excess soft tissue was removed from the vertebral body ends, and single motion segments were potted in shallow methylmethacrylate fixation blocks (Fig. 1). Once attached to the testing machine (MTS Mini Bionix 856, MTS, Eden Prairie Minn.), three cycles of stepwise loading in 1-Nm steps, from –6 Nm to +6 Nm, were applied to each direction: axial rotation, flexion/extension, and axial bending. The load-displacement curves were plotted for each sample, and the ranges of motion and neutral zones were measured from the third loading cycle. The mechanical testing was followed by microscopic assessment of all instrumented levels using acrylic specimen embedding for non-decalcified bone sections. Cuts in the mid-sagittal direction through the cage were obtained using a diamond saw, grounded, hand polished, and stained with toluidine blue. A qualitative five-step grading system was used for fusion assessment of each level.

As part of a later experiment, six additional sheep were operated on using an identical surgical protocol. The cage filling technique for the ceramic bone substitute, however, was modified. Based on the experience we had with granular β-TCP material, a pre-filled cage was used instead. The thermal treatment used to fabricate the porous TCP ceramics was applied with the titanium implant embedded in the solution. This technique produced a "ready-to-use" titanium implant, completely filled with a molded TCP insert. A ceramic pre-filled cage was placed in each animal, along with an autologous control, with the segmental levels block randomized to either treatment method. The survival period for this particular experiment was set at 20 weeks. No biomechanical evaluation was performed, only a histological work-up.

Vertebral body block filling

Nine male baboons (Papio anubis) of approximately 25 kg body weight were operated using a retroperitoneal surgical approach. The animals were randomized into three treatment groups of equal size. The anterior aspects of the L2 and L4 vertebrae were exposed. A manual core drilling tool, guided over a centrally placed K-wire, was used to remove a bone cylinder of 15 mm diameter and approximately 15 mm in length from the L2 and L4 vertebrae. The posterior vertebral body wall always remained intact. A total of 18 bone plugs were removed. For each animal, both levels underwent identical treatment. Based on the treatment group chosen, the defect was either left unplugged (sham group) or plugged with either a 15-mm-diameter cylindrical porous β-TCP implant or a β-TCP implant loaded with TGF-β3. In the present study, the TCP blocks were impregnated with a TGF-β3 solution and then dried under vacuum. The loading was performed under aseptic conditions. The final concentration of TGF-β3 adsorbed onto the dry TCP block was 50 µg/ml.

On the anesthetized animal, computed tomographic (CT) scans were obtained at 3 months postoperatively. In addition, bi-planar plain radiographs were obtained at 6 weeks, and 3 and 6 months postoperatively. The baboons were sacrificed at 6 months, and the CT examination was repeated post mortem. The L2 and L4 vertebral bodies were then processed for non-decalcified bone histology. Several frontal cuts through the defect were obtained for each vertebra, grounded and stained with toluidine blue.

Results

Instrumented anterior interbody spinal fusion

The radiographic follow-ups on the sheep rarely showed signs of anterior implant migration. No mechanical implant failure or significant occurrence of bone osteolysis was found. A prominent finding was large anterior bone bridges that characteristically formed at the instrumented levels, especially in the 16-week, and even more notably in the 32-week, survival groups.

For the mechanical testing, the trends found for the ranges of motion (ROM) and the neutral zones (NZ) were very similar, and therefore only the results for ROM are presented (Fig. 2). In all three motion directions tested,

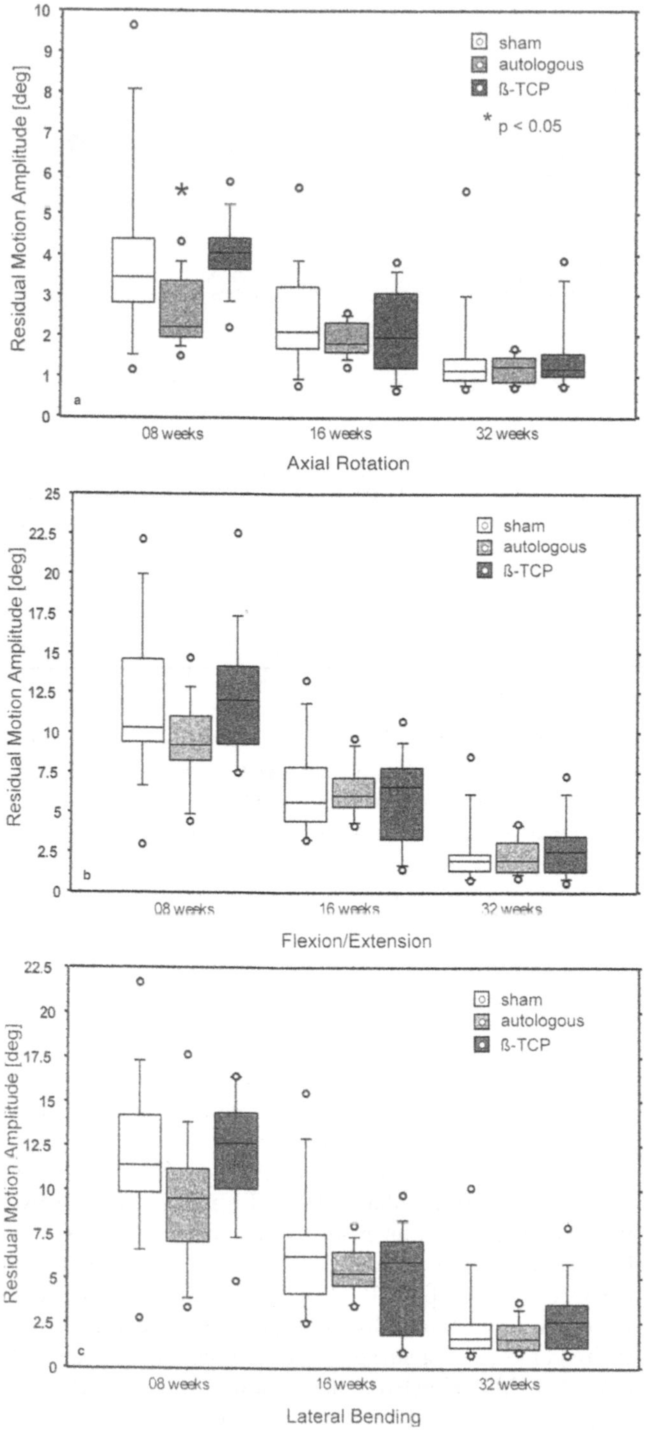

Fig. 2 Segmental ranges of motion (ROM) measured for each survival group in **A** axial rotation, **B** flexion/extension, and **C** lateral bending. Significant differences ($P<0.05$) found between treatment groups are marked with an *asterisk*

the average ROM significantly decreased (ANOVA, $P<0.0001$) for each consecutive survival interval. However, except for the 8-week results in axial rotation, no significant differences (ANOVA, $P>0.05$) were found between treatment groups. In axial rotation, the 8-week group with autologous bone had a significantly smaller ROM compared to both the sham and the β-TCP groups (post-hoc tests, Bonferoni corrected, $P<0.05$).

Table 1 Histological grades assessed for the three survival groups. The number of observations is listed for each treatment group, and the mean grade is calculated (*grading*: I fibrous tissue, II fibro-cartilage, III uncalcified bone matrix, IV woven or parallel-fibered bone, V remodeled cancellous bone)

Group/grade	Sham	Autologous	β-TCP
8 weeks			
I	6	3	3
II	1	2	4
III	3	3	2
IV	2	1	3
V	–	3	–
mean	2.1	2.9	2.4
16 weeks			
I	2	–	2
II	3	1	1
III	7	5	3
IV	1	5	5
V	–	1	2
mean	2.5	3.5	3.3
32 weeks			
I	–	–	–
II	1	–	1
III	4	–	4
IV	4	4	4
V	4	9	4
mean	3.8	4.7	3.8

The histology grading results are summarized in Table 1. A higher grade indicates a better fusion result. At 8 weeks, the grades for the autologous bone group were somewhat better compared to sham and β-TCP groups. At 16 weeks, however, the results of the β-TCP groups were almost as good as the autologous bone group, and better than the sham group. Between 16 and 32 weeks, both the autologous bone and the sham groups showed a remarkable improvement, but the β-TCP group remained almost unchanged. At 32 weeks, the autologous bone clearly demonstrated the best results.

Two additional observations were of interest. Firstly, the cages filled with β-TCP granules often had significant filling defects. But wherever granules were remaining, bone in-growth into the porous ceramic material was regularly seen, starting at 8 weeks following surgery (Fig. 3A). Secondly, more than half the specimens had a fibro-cartilagenous layer running horizontally through a large portion of the cage's inner portion, often spanning the entire cage cross-section. The struts of the cage were often not in direct contact with bone, but separated from bone by a fibrous membrane encapsulating the implant. This finding

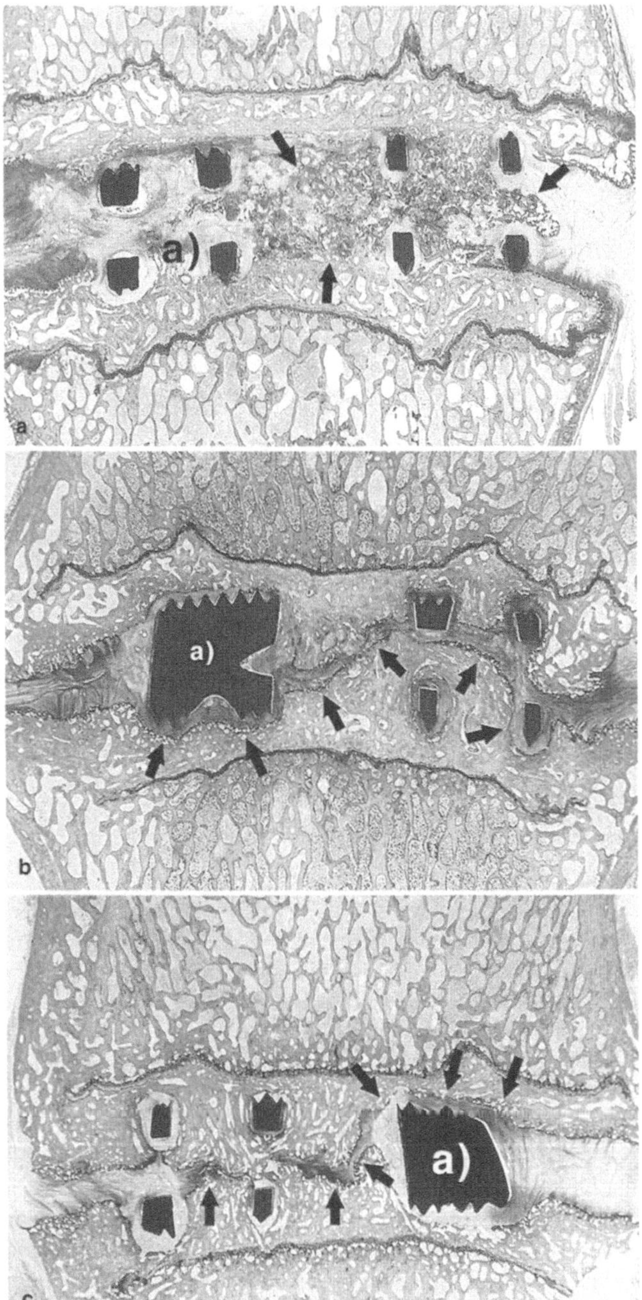

Fig. 3A–C Non-decalcified sagittal cut through the cage middle portion, polished to 70 μm, stained with toluidine blue and visualized at very low power magnification. **A** Cage filled with β-TCP granules at 8 weeks, with posterior filling defects (*a*) and woven and parallel fibered bone invading the porous ceramic granules (*arrows*). **B** β-TCP granules at 32 weeks: the implant strut is encapsulated in fibrous tissue (*a*), and a continuous fibro-cartilagenous tissue layer runs across the cage (*arrows*). **C** Autologous bone at 32 weeks, showing the implant (*a*), and the fibro-cartilagenous tissue layer (*arrows*)

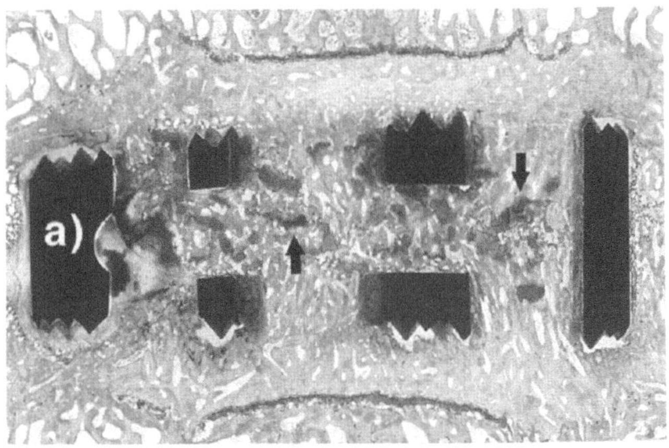

Fig. 4 TCP pre-filled cage at 20 weeks, showing the implant (*a*) and unresorbed porous TCP, completely osteointegrated (*arrows*). New bone is evident, mostly in direct contact with the implant surface (non-decalcified ground section, stained with toluidine blue, low power magnification)

was seen to some extent in all three treatment groups, but mostly in the 16- and 32-week survival groups, and mostly for β-TCP and autologous bone (Fig. 3B,C).

The ceramic pre-filled cages showed a marked improvement in histological fusion outcome compared to the ones filled with granular material (Fig. 4). The fibro-cartilagenous tissue layer running across the cage inside, the fibrous membranes encapsulating the implant, as well as the substantial filling defects observed for granular β-TCP, all were no longer a prevalent finding.

Vertebral body block filling

As confirmed on plain radiographs, none of the vertebral bodies showed a fracture or had a radiologically documented height loss. The CT data recorded at 3 and 6 months were reconstructed for coronal and sagittal projections. The sham group regularly showed minimal bone growth into the defect starting from its posterior wall. Nevertheless, most of the vertebral defect was still filled with soft tissue only. The β-TCP plugs appeared well osteointegrated at 3 and 6 months, with direct bone contact to the entire ceramic plug surface, and its boundaries starting to blur (Fig. 5A). However, the ceramic plug material was clearly visible on CT throughout the 6-months period.

At 3 months, the CT scans of the ceramic plugs impregnated with TGF-β3 suggested a prominent peripheral resorption within the original graft boundaries (Fig. 5B). At 6 months, this resorption zone was filled with dense bone, and the original graft material appeared largely resorbed (Fig. 5B). The baboons that received TGF-β3 impregnated plugs showed massive subperiosteal new bone formation along the entire anterior aspect of the vertebral body, but no new bone formation occurred in the spinal canal or the neuroforaminal regions.

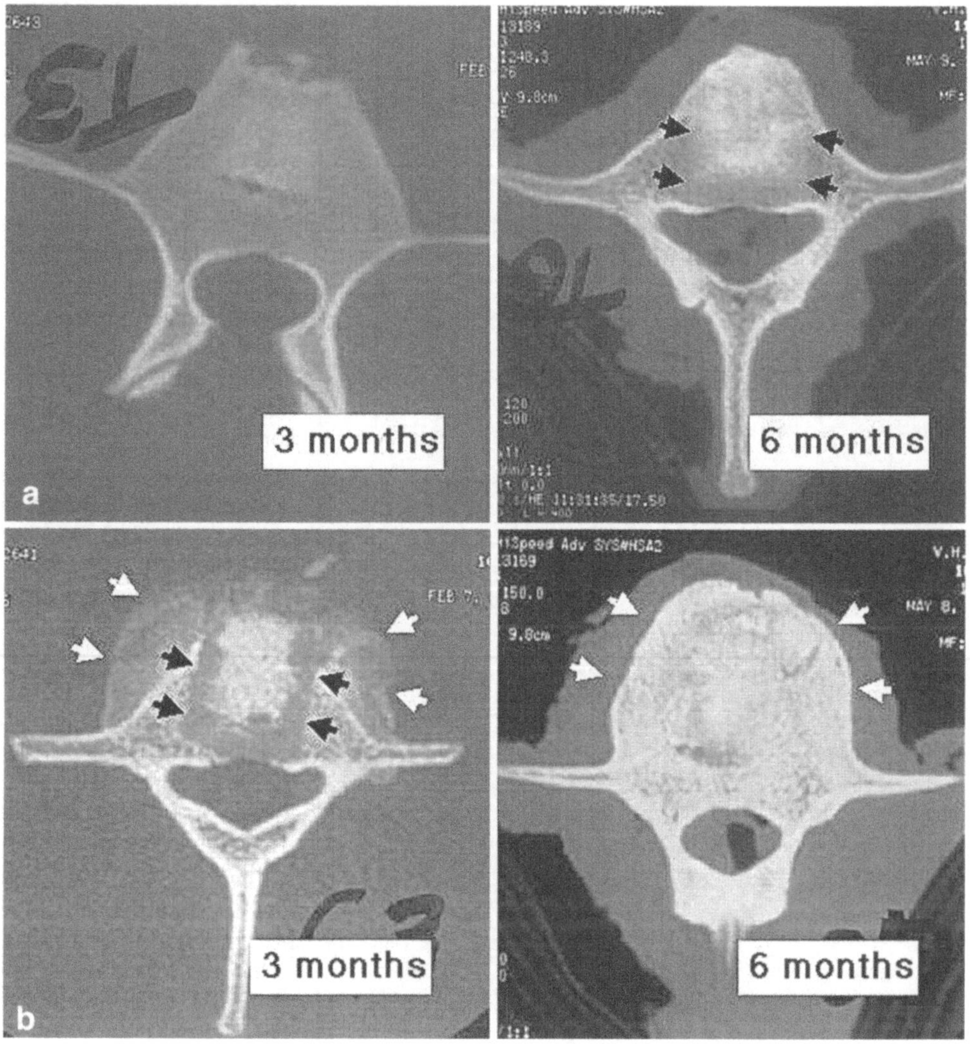

Fig. 5A,B Computed tomographic scan of baboon lumbar spine with a 15-mm-diameter cylindrical defect, plugged with porous ceramic implant at 3 and 6 months following surgery. **A** β-TCP plug with no growth factor. At 6 months the plug was osteointegrated and there was no bone lysis (*black arrows*). **B** β-TCP plug loaded with TGF-β3. At 3 months, large "lytic zones" are evident in the ceramic implant periphery (*black arrows*), which are completely filled with dense bone at 6 months. Massive subperiostal new bone formation had started at 3 months; by 6 months, dense bone with neo-cortex has formed (*white arrows*)

Light microscopy (Fig. 6 A) demonstrated that all β-TCP plugs were osteointegrated, with plenty of direct bone apposition found on the porous mineral surface right to the center of the plugs. However, abundant ceramic material was still left in place. The ceramic plugs loaded with TGF-β3 (Fig. 6B), on the other hand, showed in the peripheral areas of the plug a complete resorption of the ceramic material, replaced with remodeled cancellous bone. Surprisingly, in the central area there was often poorly osteointegrated ceramic material left that showed no signs of resorption.

Discussion

Instrumented anterior interbody spinal fusions have been performed previously in sheep [18]. However, to our knowledge, we are the first to present a sheep model for an anterior spinal fusion instrumented with a non-threaded cage design, in essence preserving the vertebral endplates. A cage design customized to the sheep anatomy was a clear necessity. The sheep model, nevertheless, is not ideal for studying anterior interbody spinal fusion, since surgically altered motion segments habitually respond with massive anterior bone bridges being formed as early as 2 months following surgery. Mechanical testing, consequently, failed to determine effects of different graft material placed inside the cage. The tests rather measured the mechanical effect of those progressively forming anterior bone bridges, regardless of the graft material placed inside the cage.

Histological examination provided greater insight into treatment-related effects. The small β-TCP granules often did not fill the cage well, and may have fallen out of the cage during surgical insertion or soon after. β-TCP was found to be a very osteoconductive material, with bone apposition on the ceramic surface found regularly at 8 weeks. Due to the filling defects, though, the fusion mass forming inside the cage was incomplete.

It also became evident that the instrumented anterior spinal fusion studied in the sheep model was not a mechanically stable construct. Frequent absence of direct

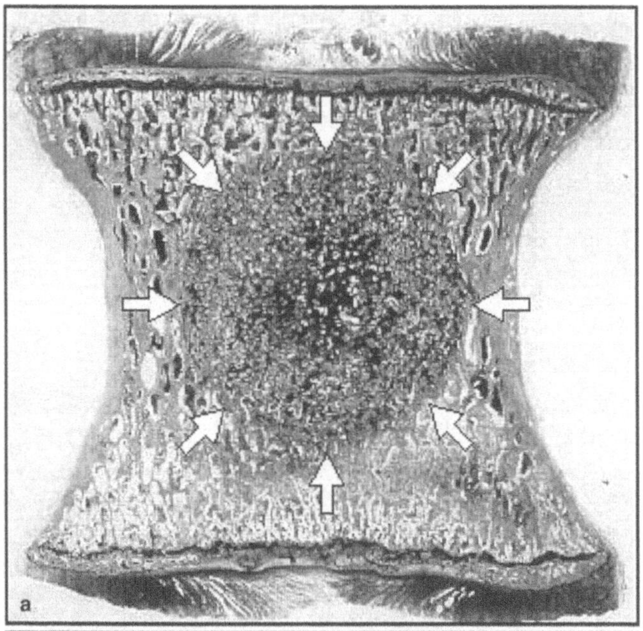

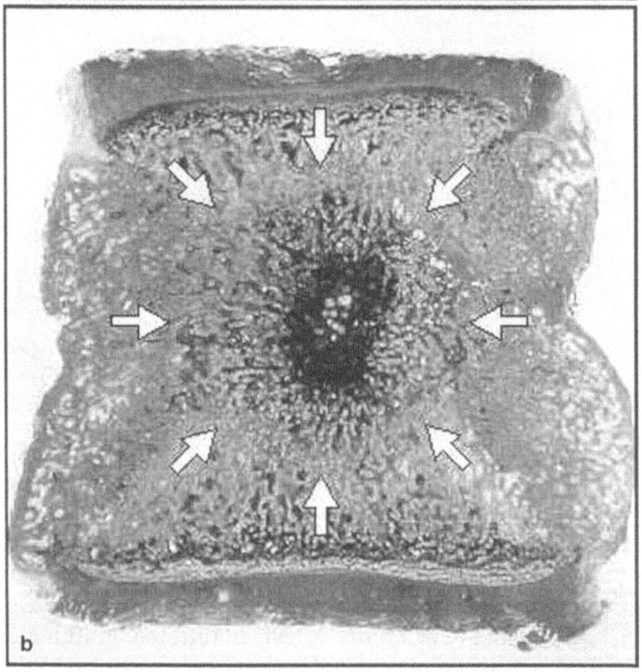

Fig. 6A,B Frontal non-decalcified grounded histological sections through ceramic graft beds 6 months following implantation, stained with toluidine blue, at very low power magnification. **A** β-TCP plug with no growth factor. Original plug boundaries (*white arrows*) are still clearly visible, the β-TCP block is partially resorbed. **B** β-TCP plug loaded with TGF-β3. Original plug boundaries (*white arrows*) have blurred out, the β-TCP block is peripherally resorbed, but a large unresorbed and poorly osteointegrated central portion is left

bone apposition on the titanium implant surface, as well as a frequently observed fibrous tissue layer encapsulating the implant, were indicators of implant micromotion. The fibro-cartilagenous tissue layers seen in all treatment groups were also interpreted as a sign of segmental instability. Alternative interpretations of this phenomenon are a nutritional limitation becoming pertinent in the cage's central area, or the interposition of soft tissue between bone in-growing from either side of the cage. The alternative interpretations were considered less likely, but could not be excluded.

The lack of initial segmental stability of stand-alone anterior lumbar interbody fusion, compared to posterior fusion or circumferential fusion, can clearly be reproduced in human cadaveric studies [22, 26], and is increasingly supported by clinical outcomes, which are unfavorable for stand-alone anterior interbody fusion [9, 17]. Our histological findings in the sheep model corroborate this conclusion.

Using a ceramic pre-filled cage is an interesting option. It appears from our animal study that pre-filling the cage with porous TCP can improve the fusion outcome. Bone substitute filling defects as well as the fibro-cartilagenous tissue layers running through the cage could be avoided. In addition, pre-filled cages can easily be shelved at room temperature and potentially can shorten the surgery time. Whether pre-filled cages will show handling benefits and improve fusion outcome in practice, will have to be to established in clinical studies.

The baboon study was primarily designed to validate the proposed local bone graft harvesting procedure, following anatomical and biomechanical studies in a biological experiment. However, it also constitutes the first biological experiment in a non-human primate combining β-TCP as a carrier with TGF-β3 in a spinal application. The β-TCP plug used without growth factor has already produced very encouraging results. The vertebra's mechanical integrity, disturbed by the iatrogenic bone defect created by locally harvested bone, was considered after 6 months to be functionally completely restored. The plugs were all fully osteointegrated, and the β-TCP block was gradually resorbed. This experiment demonstrates the capacity for porous β-TCP also to serve as an adequate osteoconductor for sizable bone substitute blocks. In this case, up to 7.5 mm successful bone in-growth into a monolithic block (radially toward the center) was confirmed.

For our specific surgical model, the marginal benefits of loading the ceramic plug with a growth factor were not clearly evident. Addition of TGF-β3 certainly affected the ceramic block resorption over time, and also resulted within 3 months in substantial regional new bone formation in the prevertebral space. This new bone, as confirmed histologically at 6 months, was well remodeled and mechanically competent. However, the ceramic plug with no growth factor addition was considered adequate for the purpose of restoring the vertebral body's integrity. In fact, the surgical procedure for harvesting a local bone plug for the adjacent vertebral body, and plugging this defect with a porous ceramic spacer, has now been used clinically, with satisfactory results.

The application of TGF-β3 for bone substitution, nevertheless, appears to be a promising direction to be further investigated. The regional new bone formation in the prevertebral space clearly is to be attributed to TGF-β3, even though the dose used in this study was relatively low. Animal studies showed that in many cases TGF-β induces bone healing at much lower concentrations than other growth hormones tested, including BMPs [13]. In recent human studies showing that recombinant BMP-2 applied in a collagen sponge induced bone formation inside interbody fusion cages, the local concentration of BMP-2 used was 1.5 mg/ml [4].

Impregnating the porous ceramic blocks with TGF-β3 also affected the ceramic material's resorption pattern. Whereas in the plug periphery the resorption was much faster, it was slower in the central areas when compared to the non-impregnated blocks. The large peripheral resorption zone already evident on the 3-month CT scans had, at 6 months, been replaced with dense bone. We interpreted this observation as an effect of the early and massive angiogenesis mediated by TGF-β3, which may have permitted the faster resorption in the plug's periphery, to the extent that it "sealed off" the center of the plug from a timely bone in-growth.

More studies will be required to define the optimal spatial and temporal release characteristics of TGF-β3. This growth factor hormone has proven to be biologically highly potent in the non-human primate, but other surgical applications need to be further explored.

Acknowledgements We are grateful to Dr. M. Bohner, Robert Mathys Foundation, Bettlach, Switzerland, for the development and preparation of the ceramic biomaterials. Prof. A. Olah, Institute for Anatomy, University of Berne, Switzerland, did a wonderful histology on the baboons. The authors also thank the entire team of the Orthopaedic Research Laboratory, McGill University, Montreal, but especially Dr. P. Papin and Dr. R. Reindle for performing the many sheep and baboon surgeries, and Ms. F. Marchesi for essential technical assistance. We also thank Ms. B. Hoffmann from the School of Dental Medicine, University of Berne, for technical assistance in preparing the sheep histology. We are indebted to the animal care teams at the Lady Davis Research Institute, McGill University in Montreal, as well as to the Southwest Foundation for Biomedical Research in San Antonio, Texas. The studies were supported by several grants from the Robert Mathys Foundation, Bettlach, Switzerland.

References

1. Banwart JC, Asher MA, Hassanein RS (1995) Iliac crest bone graft harvest donor site morbidity. A statistical evaluation. Spine 20:1055–1060
2. Baramki HG, Papin P, Steffen T (2000) A surgical approach to the ventral aspect of the lumbar vertebrae in the sheep model. Surg Radiol Anat 22: 25–27
3. Beck LS, Amento EP, Xu Y, et al (1993) TGF-beta 1 induces bone closure of skull defects: temporal dynamics of bone formation in defects exposed to rhTGF-beta 1. J Bone Miner Res 8:753–761
4. Boden SD, Zdeblick TA, Sandhu HS, Heim SE (2000) The use of rhBMP-2 in interbody fusion cages. Definitive evidence of osteoinduction in humans: a preliminary report. Spine 25:376–381
5. Bohner M (2000) Calcium orthophosphates in medicine: from ceramics to calcium phosphate cements. Injury 31: 37–47
6. Buser D, Hoffmann B, Bernard JP, Lussi A, Mettler D, Schenk RK (1998) Evaluation of filling materials in membrane-protected bone defects. A comparative histomorphometric study in the mandible of miniature pigs. Clin Oral Implants Res 9:137–150
7. Cox DA (1995) Transforming growth factor-beta 3. Cell Biol Int 19:357–371
8. Eggli PS, Muller W, Schenk RK (1988) Porous hydroxyapatite and tricalcium phosphate cylinders with two different pore size ranges implanted in the cancellous bone of rabbits. Clin Orthop 232:127–138
9. Gillet P (2000) The value and limits of intervertebral cages in lumbar arthrodesis (in French). Rev Med Liege 55:839–846
10. Hu PP, Datto MB, Wang XF (1998) Molecular mechanisms of transforming growth factor-beta signaling. Endocr Rev 19:349–363
11. Itoh S, Itoh F, Goumans MJ, Ten Dijke P (2000) Signaling of transforming growth factor-beta family members through Smad proteins. Eur J Biochem 267:6954–6967
12. Kingsley DM (1994) The TGF-beta superfamily: new members, new receptors, and new genetic tests of function in different organisms. Genes Dev 8: 133–146
13. Lind M, Overgaard S, Nguyen T, Ongpipattanakul B, Bunger C, Soballe K (1996) Transforming growth factor-beta stimulates bone ongrowth. Hydroxyapatite-coated implants studied in dogs. Acta Orthop Scand 67:611–616
14. Lind M, Overgaard S, Jensen TB, et al (2001) Effect of osteogenic protein 1/collagen composite combined with impacted allograft around hydroxyapatite-coated titanium alloy implants is moderate. J Biomed Mater Res 55:89–95
15. Lord CF, Gebhardt MC, Tomford WW, Mankin HJ (1988) Infection in bone allografts. Incidence, nature, and treatment. J Bone Joint Surg Am 70: 369–376
16. Moses HL, Yang EY, Pietenpol JA (1990) TGF-beta stimulation and inhibition of cell proliferation: new mechanistic insights. Cell 63:245–247
17. Pavlov PW, Spruit M, Havinga M, Anderson PG, van Limbeek J, Jacobs WC (2000) Anterior lumbar interbody fusion with threaded fusion cages and autologous bone grafts. Eur Spine J 9: 224–229
18. Sandhu HS, Turner S, Kabo JM, et al (1996) Distractive properties of a threaded interbody fusion device. An in vivo model. Spine 21:1201–1210
19. Singer AJ, Clark RA (1999) Cutaneous wound healing. N Engl J Med 341:738–746
20. Steffen T, Downer P, Steiner B, Hehli M, Aebi M (2000) Minimally invasive bone harvesting tools. Eur Spine J 9: S114-S118
21. Steffen T, Marchesi D, Aebi M (2000) Posterolateral and anterior interbody spinal fusion models in the sheep. Clin Orthop 371:28–37
22. Steffen T, Tsantrizos A, Fruth I, Aebi M (2000) Cages: designs and concepts. Eur Spine J 9:S89-S94

23. Summers BN, Eisenstein SM (1989) Donor site pain from the ilium. A complication of lumbar spine fusion. J Bone Joint Surg Br 71:677–680
24. Sumner DR, Turner TM, Purchio AF, Gombotz WR, Urban RM, Galante JO (1995) Enhancement of bone ingrowth by transforming growth factor-beta. J Bone Joint Surg Am 77:1135–1147
25. Toth JM, An HS, Lim TH, et al (1995) Evaluation of porous biphasic calcium phosphate ceramics for anterior cervical interbody fusion in a caprine model. Spine 20:2203–2210
26. Tsantrizos A, Baramki HG, Zeidman S, Steffen T (2000) Segmental stability and compressive strength of posterior lumbar interbody fusion implants. Spine 25:1899–1907
27. Younger EM, Chapman MW (1989) Morbidity at bone graft donor sites. J Orthop Trauma 3:192–195

E. M. Erbe
J. G. Marx
T. D. Clineff
L. D. Bellincampi

Potential of an ultraporous β-tricalcium phosphate synthetic cancellous bone void filler and bone marrow aspirate composite graft

E.M. Erbe (✉) · J.G. Marx · T.D. Clineff
L.D. Bellincampi
45 Great Valley Parkway,
Malvern, PA 19355, USA
e-mail: emerbe@aol.com,
Tel.: +1-610-251-0971

Abstract Autogenous cancellous bone is considered to be the best bone grafting material. Autogenous bone grafts provide scaffolding for osteoconduction, growth factors for osteoinduction, and progenitor stem cells for osteogenesis. However, the procurement morbidity, limited availability, and expense associated with the use of autogenous bone grafts are significant disadvantages. Allografts and xenografts lack the osteoinduction and osteogenesis properties of autogenous bone, and they introduce the potential for both transferring disease and triggering a host immune response. Synthetic bone grafts [hydroxyapatite or tricalcium phosphate(TCP)], while good platforms for osteoconduction, lack any intrinsic properties of osteoinduction and osteogenesis. A composite graft that combines synthetic scaffold with autogenous osteoprogenitor cells from bone marrow aspirate (BMA), a low-morbidity procedure, could potentially deliver the advantages of autogenous bone grafts without the disadvantages. A new ultraporous β-TCP construct, engineered using solution-derived nano-particle technology, may prove to be an ideal carrier for BMA in such a composite. The unique, interconnected macroporosity, mesoporosity, and microporosity of this synthetic cancellous bone void filler allows it to wick in cells and nutrients via enhanced capillarity. Preliminary canine data support this expectation, demonstrating bone formation that suggests good penetration of cells and nutrients. These results suggest that BMA cells, absorbed into such a scaffold, may remain viable, thereby potentially making such a composite a true synthetic replacement for autogenous cancellous bone.

Keywords Bone remodeling · Bone biology · Bone marrow aspirate · Cancellous bone · β-TCP

Introduction

Role of cancellous bone

Eighty percent of bone is comprised of dense cortical bone, within which is found the highly porous and vascular cancellous bone (20%). However, the cancellous bone is responsible for 88% of the amount of the normal bone turnover. Cancellous bone has minimal weight-bearing function and is predominantly susceptible to compressive forces; it is a load distributor rather than a weight bearer. It can be considered a scaffold within which pluripotent progenitor stem cells fuel hematopoesis, myelogenesis, and platelet formation.

Bone graft overview

When trauma, infection, congenital malformation, tumor growth, or degenerative diseases threaten bone integrity, bone grafting may be used to encourage the affected bone

Table 1 Advantages and disadvantages of bone grafting materials

Graft material	Description	Properties	Advantages	Disadvantages
Autograft osteoconductive scaffold plus marrow	Bone donor and recipient are one and the same; bone mineral scaffold plus viable cells and cytokines	Osteoconductive (trabecular), osteoinductive, and osteogenic	No host rejection; no disease transmission; retains viable osteoblasts	Significant morbidity and limited quantities of bone associated with harvest (especially if graft is from iliac crest); high cost
Allograft (requires removal of proteins and fat)	Bone donor and recipient are different individuals of same species	Osteoconductive and weakly osteoinductive	Tissue bone banks are generally available; patient needs only one surgical procedure	Potential to produce host immune response and transfer disease; processing removes osteogenic cells
Xenograft (requires removal of proteins and fat)	Bone donor and recipient are of different species	Osteoconductive	Patient needs only one surgical procedure	Potential to produce host immune response and transfer disease; processing removes osteoinductive potential
Synthetics	Hydroxyapatite or tricalcium phosphate, or combinations thereof	Osteoconductive	No patient donation; patient needs only one surgical procedure; no disease transmission	Need to augment with osteogenic cells and osteoinductive materials
β-TCP plus BMA	β-TCP scaffold plus viable cells and cytokines	Osteoconductive, osteoinductive, and osteogenic	Same as for autograft; minimization of donor-site morbidity	Not yet a gold standard

β-TCP, β-tricalcium phosphate; BMA, bone marrow aspirate.

to regenerate and heal. For a bone graft to be successful, three processes that mimic natural events in cancellous bone must take place [2]:

1. Osteoconduction: the apposition of growing bone to the three-dimensional surface of a suitable scaffold provided by the graft
2. Osteoinduction: the biologically mediated recruitment and differentiation of cell types essential to bone formation
3. Osteogenesis: the process of bone formation through cellular activity, which, in turn, is dependent upon the presence of osteoprogenitor stem cells

Orthopedists currently use a variety of materials that enhance these three processes to different degrees (Table 1). [1, 2].

Autograft

Autogenous bone is generally considered the gold-standard graft material [18]. The unique advantage of the autograft is that it contains viable osteoblasts and osteogenic precursor cells that can contribute to the formation of new bone [1]. Unfortunately, this advantage is not fully realized in practice because graft processing results in the death of most of the cellular elements [17]. Those cells that survive must initially receive their oxygen via diffusion; thus considerable anoxic cell death probably occurs before sufficient vascularization has permeated the graft. Revascularization into the internal regions of the autograft is slow and incomplete; the process can be inhibited by

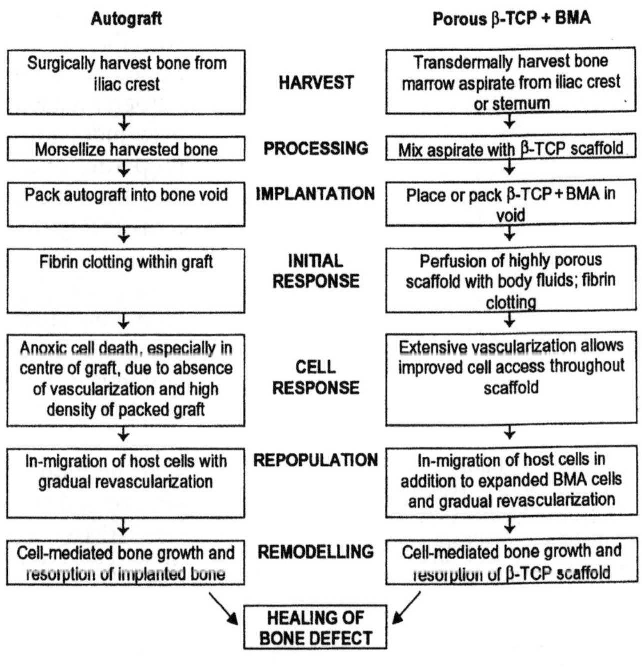

Fig. 1 Processes involved in filling bone voids with either autograft or porous β-tricalcium phosphate (*TCP*) seeded with bone marrow aspirate (*BMA*). Both are expected to support the osteogenesis, osteoconduction, and osteoinduction needed for healing

fibrin clotting in the autograft and by the packing procedure used to place the graft into the surgical site.

Most of the osteogenic cells that repopulate the graft are thought to be extrinsic cells that migrate, along with osteoinductive growth factors, into the graft from the surrounding bone defect site. The repopulation of the bone mineral structure by extrinsic cells drives the healing process, as the trabecular structure of natural cancellous bone serves as the scaffold for cell-mediated resorption and concurrent rebuilding of new bone (Fig. 1).

Complications of iliac crest autograft procurement

Autograft procurement is associated with significant morbidity [17]. An early retrospective study of donor-site morbidity reviewed 243 bone grafts, 90% of which were from the iliac crest [21]. Complications were found to occur at an overall rate of 29.2%. Later studies have reported donor-site complication rates ranging from 4% to 49% [7]. Major complications, which have been reported at rates from 0.7% to 25% [17], include infection, prolonged wound drainage, large hematomas, reoperation, complete pelvic ring failure, enterocutaneous fistula, pain lasting longer than 6 months, sensory loss, subluxation, gait disturbances, sacroiliac joint destabilization, herniation of muscle and abdominal contents, pelvic or iliac fracture, and heterotopic bone formation [4, 7, 8]

Even in the absence of "avoidable" complications, unavoidable problems are associated with autograft procurement. These include limited availability, high cost, temporary disruption of donor-site bone structure, increased operative time, and significantly increased operative blood loss [1, 17, 19].

Autograft alternatives

Allografts

Allografts are bone grafts harvested from another member of the same species. They are processed to remove cells and debris in order to minimize their infectious and immunogenic potential. As a result of this processing, allografts do not contain living cells and are not osteogenic [17]. However, they generally have excellent osteoconductive properties and can exert a somewhat osteoinductive effect on cell in-migration and differentiation.

Xenografts

Because of their immunogenicity, xenograft preparations harvested from another species have generally been impractical for clinical use. To guarantee viral inactivation, not only cells but all proteins must be removed, thus eliminating both osteogenic and osteoinductive potential.

Synthetic bone grafts

By sidestepping both the avoidable and unavoidable problems of autograft use, synthetic bone graft materials

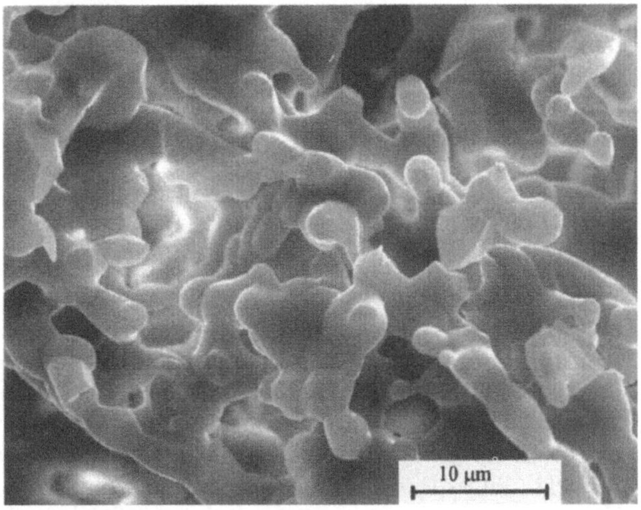

Fig. 2 Micron-sized particles of Vitoss as visualized by scanning electron microscopy. The particles are 1–2 μm. These polycrystalline particles are comprised of crystallites that range from 70 to 100 nm in diameter by X-ray diffraction (XRD) methods

have the potential to greatly expand orthopedic options. Historically, the materials used have been ceramics of hydroxyapatite ($Ca_{10}(PO_4)_6(OH)_2$), tricalcium phosphate ($Ca_3(PO_4)_2$), or combinations of the two. When used alone for grafting, synthetic grafting materials function solely as osteoconductive scaffolding for new bone growth and as bridges to the host bone. The scaffold is then removed by a combination of dissolution and phagocytosis (cell-mediated resorption). Since 1982, β-TCP constructs have been used as synthetic bone void fillers in dentistry and orthopedics without adverse events [6, 13]. Porous β-TCP synthetic cancellous bone void fillers should resemble human cancellous bone in structure and composition. Generally, β-TCPs contain approximately 39% calcium and 20% phosphorus by weight, similar to natural mineral content in bone [12].

Vitoss synthetic cancellous bone void filler differs from previously used β-TCP constructs in that it is characterized by nano-sized particles and an extensive pore size distribution (Fig. 2). Vitoss™ is a porous, low-density construct prepared by lightly fusing particles of β-TCP that average approximately 1–2 μm in diameter. The use of nano-sized β-TCP primary particles increases the microporosity of the structure, resulting in a scaffold of approximately 90% interconnected void space, with pores ranging in size from less than 1 μm to 1000 μm. This large increase in interconnected porosity, relative to other β-TCP constructs, potentially permits a more continuous supply of nutrients, more extensive cellular and tissue ingrowth into the scaffold, and enhanced revascularization, allowing bone repair to take place faster and more completely. In vivo studies have shown that progressively smaller particles improve osteoconductive performance [11]. Since more of its surface area is exposed to the biologic milieu, the scaffold may be resorbed at a higher rate than are denser forms of β-TCP. In fact, nanometer-sized crystallites are small enough for the body to digest with normal cellular activity; this is crucial for resorption during bone remodeling.

Animal Study

A canine study was undertaken to assess the efficacy of Vitoss synthetic cancellous bone void filler. Blocks of Vitoss were used in the repair of cylindrical metaphyseal defects measuring 10 mm×25 mm in canine humeri. Bone ingrowth and scaffold resorption were quantified using standard histomorphometric techniques for specimens examined up to 1 year postimplantation. As early as 3 weeks, Vitoss showed resorption throughout the defect site and some immature bone formation evenly throughout as well (Fig. 3). Remodeling was essentially complete in 6–12 weeks, with bone density in the normal range and with the scaffold almost completely resorbed by the end of that period (Fig. 4). By 24 weeks, the implant trabecular orientation approximated the normal stress patterns of adjacent bone. Histologically and radiographically, the bone within the defects was virtually indistinguishable from the surrounding bone at the 12-, 24-, and 52-week follow-ups. The stress–strain curve of Vitoss is nearly identical to bone at 24 weeks and at 52 weeks (Fig. 5), and X-ray diffraction (XRD) data confirms a 95% match to normal bone at 1 year.

These results indicated that Vitoss might perform better in a number of ways than previously studied ceramics. First, using traditional synthetics, bone formation and osteoconduction took longer and was most prevalent at the periphery of the defect [3, 11]. The only new bone that formed as a result of the osteoconductivity of the porous ceramic was an extension of the outgrowth from the cut ends of the host bone [3]. In contrast, one of the striking things about Vitoss is the pattern of resorption and osteogenesis throughout the implant site. Second, whereas Vitoss was almost completely resorbed in 12 weeks, a ceramic composed of hydroxyapatite and traditional β-TCP showed essentially no resorption over the first 16 weeks after implantation [3]. Third, despite very high porosity, Vitoss synthetic cancellous bone void filler is easily manipulated at surgery, either sculpted as blocks or poured as morsels. In contrast, hydroxyapatite bone substitute was not ideal for the treatment of segmental defects because of its incompressible nature and lack of completely interconnected pores [3].

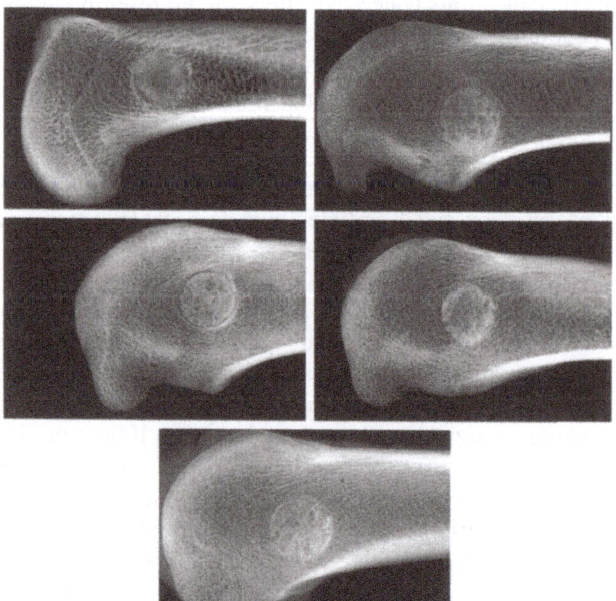

Fig. 3 Radiographs of Vitoss implant from 3 to 52 weeks

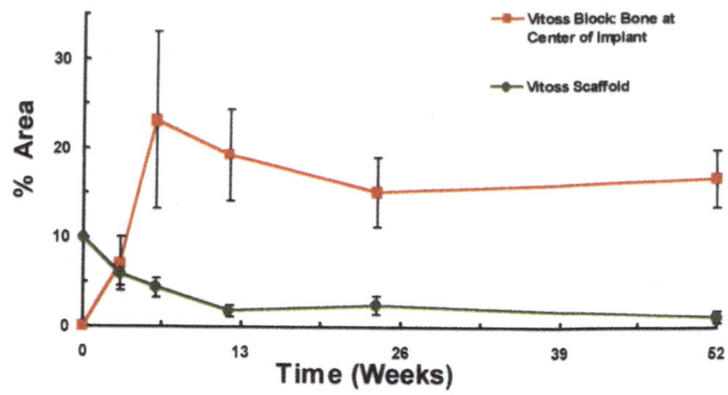

Fig. 4 Results of quantitative histomorphometry

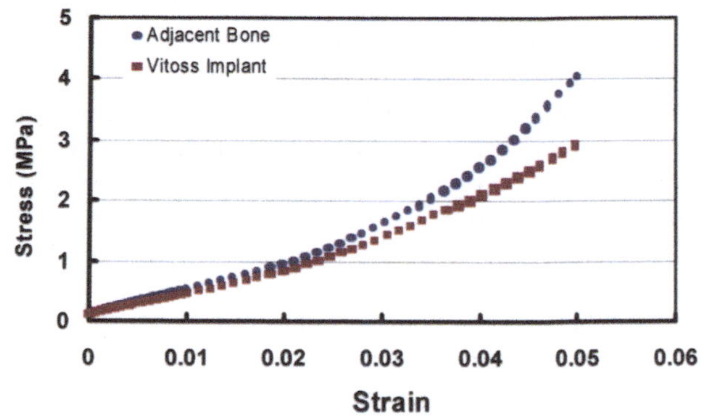

Fig. 5 Results of compression testing of the Vitoss implant compared with adjacent bone at 52 weeks

Composite grafts

A composite graft can be defined as any combination of materials that includes an osteoconductive matrix, an osteogenic material, and an osteoinductive material, thus fulfilling the three requirements for a successful bone graft.

Osteogenic and osteoinductive bone marrow aspirate

Background

If the osteoconductive ceramic scaffold is seeded with bone progenitor cells, the composite graft should become osteogenic and osteoinductive as well, in effect providing a competitive alternative to autografts. The hypothesis is that such a strategy accelerates healing by minimizing the immediate need for chemotaxis and massive proliferation of osteoblast progenitor cells into the defect. With years of experience and wide clinical use, bone marrow aspirate (BMA) is the most practical source of bone progenitor cells [14]. Aspiration of bone marrow cells is a relatively benign procedure, and a number of previous studies demonstrate the positive effect of BMA on bone formation both in vitro and in vivo [5]. Osteoprogenitor stem cells are prevalent in BMA and are able to differentiate into five other cell types (osteoblasts, osteoclasts, adipose cells, chondroblasts, and fibroblasts) and modify their morphologic/functional attributes as needed [15]. This osteogenic potential was maintained as the cells were expanded in culture and enriched for grafting [9].

Bone marrow aspirate and bone composites

Autologous bone marrow aspirated from the iliac crest had a beneficial effect upon osteogenesis when implanted with xenograft bone graft material (Kiel bone) [16], and the addition of BMA to autograft iliac crest bone graft facilitated greater bone formation and successful fusion in a rabbit posterolateral spine fusion model [5]. Furthermore, it was found that xenograft bone and other bone substitutes could be rendered osteogenic by combining them with fresh BMA [20].

Bone marrow aspirate and synthetic composites

A number of studies have used composites of bone marrow and synthetics for bone grafting [3, 10, 11]. Studies on the healing of canine femoral defects with implanted calcium phosphate cylinders loaded with cultured autologous mesenchymal stem cells showed that the addition of such cells augmented the development of new periosteal bone around the implants [3].

Similarly, hydroxyapatite ceramic (HAC) combined with bone marrow stromal cell populations resulted in far more extensive bone defect repair over a 2-month period [11]. However, in both of these studies, even in the cell-loaded scaffold, a higher concentration of new bone began in the periphery. The authors speculate that this is due to better survival of loaded cells within the outermost portions of the HAC cylinder, the area expected to be vascularized faster and more efficiently than more internal regions. They note that this may be related to the design and structure of the implant device. The animal study with Vitoss, which showed bone formation throughout with an ultraporous β-TCP scaffold, would support this hypothesis.

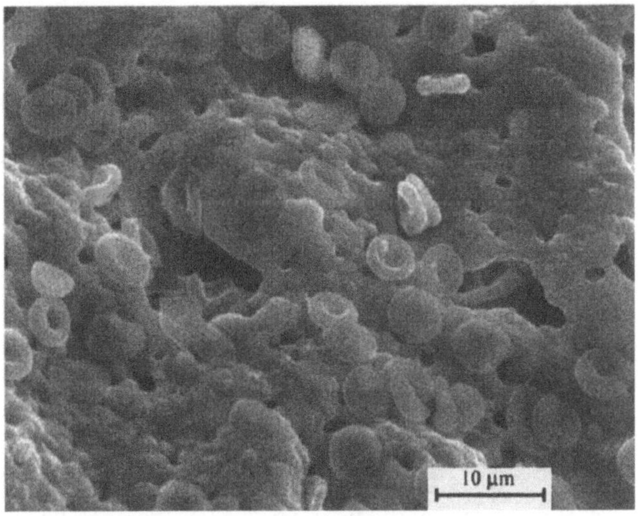

Fig. 6 Scanning electron image showing a large number of canine erythrocytes (approximately 4–5 μm diameter) in the center of the β-tricalcium phosphate scaffold. ×2000

Bone marrow aspirate and ultraporous β-tricalcium phosphate synthetic cancellous bone void filler composite

The newest generation of ultraporous β-TCP constructs have unique biomechanical properties that may make them particularly well suited for use with BMA in a composite graft. The extremely broad range of pore sizes (<1 μm to 1000 μm) and the sponge-like interconnected microporosity endow the scaffold with excellent wicking and hydrophilic properties. These attributes allow the migration of bone-forming cells, phagocytic cells, growth factors, and nutrients into the scaffold, enhancing the processes of new bone development and scaffold resorption. The unique structure of β-TCP would, therefore, be conducive to rapid vascularization and nourishment of the seeded bone marrow, including bone-forming cells. In this respect, a β-TCP/BMA composite may even be superior to the autograft, in which most cellular elements suffer from anoxic cell death due to delayed revascularization (Fig. 1). One of the striking features of grafting with ultraporous β-TCP, compared with using other synthetic constructs, is the formation of bone that occurs throughout the implant, suggesting good penetration of cells and nutrients (Fig. 6).

Conclusion

Synthetic bone substitutes have the potential to increase graft availability, to eliminate autograft procurement morbidity, and to avoid the risk of disease transmission associated with allografts and xenografts. Vitoss synthetic cancellous bone void filler, an ultraporous construct (90% interconnecting, multidirectional pores) of pure β-TCP, is a new bone graft synthetic based on proprietary solution-derived nanoparticle construction. Interconnected microporosity may accelerate remodeling by facilitating in-migration and retention of osteogenic cells and nutrients via enhanced capillarity. Preliminary canine data demonstrate significant bone formation and resorption, supporting this hypothesis. Thus Vitoss would seem a logical delivery vehicle for BMA-derived osteoinductive growth factors and osteogenic bone precursor cells. Studies evaluating an ultraporous β-TCP/BMA composite as a true autogenous bone graft substitute are under way.

References

1. Arrington ED, Smith WJ, Chambers HG, Bucknell AL, Davino NA (1996) Complications of iliac crest bone graft harvesting. Clin Orthop Related Res 329:300
2. Bauer TW, Muschler GF (2000) Bone graft materials: an overview of the basic science. Clin Orthop 371:10
3. Bruder SP, Kraus KH, Goldberg VM, Kadiyala S (1998) The effect of implants loaded with autologous mesenchymal stem cells on the healing of canine segmental bone defects. J Bone Joint Surg [Am] 80:985
4. Connolly JF, Guse R, Tiedeman J, Dehne R (1991) Autologous marrow injection as a substitute for operative grafting of tibial nonunions. Clin Orthop 266:259
5. Curylo LJ, Johnstone B, Petersilge CA, Janicki JA, Yoo JU (1999) Augmentation of spinal arthrodesis with autologous bone marrow in a rabbit posterolateral spine fusion model. Spine 24: 434
6. Doursounian L, Cazeau C, Touzard R-C (1999) Use of tricalcium phosphate ceramics in tibial plateau fracture repair: results of 15 cases reviewed at 38 months (available at: http://bhd.online.fr/framesus.htm)
7. Dösoglu M, Orakdögen M, Tevrüz M, Gögüsgeren MA, Mutlu F (1998) Enterocutaneous fistula: a complication of posterior iliac bone graft harvesting not previously described. Acta Neurochir (Wien) 140:1089
8. Fernando TL, Kim SS, Mohler DG (1999) Complete pelvic ring failure after posterior iliac bone graft harvesting. Spine 24:2101
9. Haynesworth SE, Goshima J, Goldberg VM, Caplan AI (1992) Characterization of cells with osteogenic potential from human marrow. Bone 13:81
10. Johnson KD, Frierson KE, Keller TS, Cook C, Scheinberg R, Zerwekh J, Meyers L, Sciadini MF (1996) Porous ceramics as bone graft substitutes in long bone defects: a biomechanical, histological, and radiographic analysis. J Orthop Res 14:351
11. Kon E, Muraglia A, Corsi A, Bianco P, Marcacci M, Martin I et al (1999) Autologous bone marrow stromal cells loaded onto porous hydroxyapatite ceramic accerlerate bone repair in critical-size defects of sheep long bones. J Biomed Mater Res 49:328
12. LeGeros RZ (1991) Calcium phosphates in oral biology and medicine. Basel, p 110
13. McAndrew MP, Gorman PW, Lange TA (1989) Tricalcium phosphate as a bone graft substitute in trauma: preliminary report. J Orthop Trauma 2:333
14. Muschler GF, Boehm C, Easley K (1997) Aspiration to obtain osteoblast progenitor cells from human bone marrow: the influence of aspiration volume. J Bone Joint Surg Am 79:1699
15. Ross MH, Romrell LJ, Kaye GI (1995) Histology: a text and atlas. Williams and Wilkins, Baltimore, p 150
16. Salama R, Weissman SL (1978) The clinical use of combined xenografts of bone and autologous red marrow: a preliminary report. J Bone Joint Surg [Am] 60:111
17. Sandhu HS, Grewal HS, Parvataneni H (1999) Bone grafting for spinal fusion. Orthop Clin North Am 30:685
18. Schulhofer SD, Oloff LM (1997) Iliac crest donor site morbidity in foot and ankle surgery. J Foot Ankle Surg 36: 155
19. Summers BN, Eisenstein SM (1989) Donor site pain from the ilium. J Bone Joint Surg [Br] 71:677
20. Wientroub S, Goodwin D, Khermosh O, Salama R (1989) The clinical use of autologous marrow to improve osteogenic potential of bone grafts in pediatric orthopedics. J Pediatr Orthop 9: 186
21. Younger EM, Chapman MW (2000) Morbidity at bone graft donor sites. J Orthop Trauma 3:192

Erik M. Erbe
Ted D. Clineff
Gina Gualtieri

Comparison of a new bisphenol-a-glycidyl dimethacrylate-based cortical bone void filler with polymethyl methacrylate

Abstract A newly formulated and reinforced bisphenol-a-glycidyl dimethacrylate (bis-GMA) resin (Cortoss/Orthovita, Malvern, Pa.) was compared with Simplex P polymethyl methacrylate (Stryker Howmedica Osteonics, East Rutherford, N.J.) in rabbits for up to 52 weeks and in sheep for up to 78 weeks. As seen in scanning electron microscopy and histology examinations, both implant materials were surrounded by bone at late time periods, with fibrous layers of connective tissue seen in half the Simplex P specimens. No clinically significant safety differences between implant materials were apparent. Interfacial bond strengths between the implant and bone generally increased with time, but were 4.5-fold greater with Cortoss than Simplex P at 24 weeks, and 100-fold greater at 52 weeks. Forces required to displace 316SS rods held in place with Cortoss were consistently greater than forces to displace rods held in place with Simplex P. No statistically significant differences in displacement forces were found between rods held in place with Cortoss polymerized in situ and rods held with prepolymerized Cortoss. Interfacial bond strengths were greater for Simplex P that was polymerized in situ than for prepolymerized polymethyl methacrylate specimens. Cortoss synthetic cortical bone void filler is a good candidate material to fix implants in bone. It has characteristics consistent with long-term safety and has a better ability to bond to bone than Simplex P.

Keywords Bone cement · Bone substitute · Bone regeneration · Polymethyl methacrylate · Bisphenol-a-glycidyl dimethacrylate

E.M. Erbe (✉) · T.D. Clineff · G. Gualtieri
1247 Berwyn-Paoli RD, Berwyn,
PA 19312, USA
e-mail: emerbe@aol.com,
Tel.: +1-610-2510971

Introduction

Bisphenol-a-glycidyl dimethacrylate (bis-GMA) resins have been studied in orthopedic applications since the late 1970s [21]. Various formulations were developed in efforts to reduce the amount of leachable unreacted monomer, to avoid high local temperatures during polymerization, to improve mechanical properties, and to enhance direct bone contact [4, 19]. Current formulations of bis-GMA resins have achieved these goals of improved mechanical, chemical, and biologic properties [14, 18]. One such formulation is Cortoss synthetic cortical bone void filler, a biocompatible, bone-bonding, terpolymer cortical bone substitute containing bisphenol-a-glycidyl dimethacrylate (bis-GMA), bisphenol-a-ethoxy dimethacrylate (bis-EMA), and triethylene glycol dimethacrylate (TEGDMA) resins reinforced with synthetic combeite glass-ceramic particles to stimulate bone apposition at the interface, barium boroaluminosilicate glass for radiopacity and strength, and silica for improved viscosity.

For more than 20 years, polymethyl methacrylate (PMMA) bone cement has been used to reconstruct vertebral bodies that have collapsed as a result of trauma or tumor invasion [8, 9, 12]. Long-term studies report that these treatments are highly durable and that significant failures or secondary fractures related to cement are rare [1, 3, 6, 11, 13, 16, 17]. For at least the last 10 years, PMMA has been placed into vertebral bodies percutaneously using X-ray guidance to treat pain related to osteoporotic compression fractures or tumor invasion [5]. In a series of PVP surgeries extending to more than 300 patients, radiculopathies were found in only 1% of patients with fractures caused by osteoporosis [2]. Low complication rates, including infection, and high success rates for pain relief justify the use of conservative surgical approaches in the treatment of severely painful osteoporotic compression fractures.

Disadvantages of using PMMA cement in spinal procedures include the minimal working time and the radiolucency of the cement. Additional monomer is often added to the cement mixture to extend the working time. To improve radiopacity and visual control, additional contrast materials are blended into the mixture. Such changes in formulation reduce the mechanical properties of the cement [7, 10]. Cortoss synthetic cortical bone void filler has been developed in response to these deficiencies. It has been shown to be an optimal material with which to fix implants in bone, both with respect to its safety profile and to its greater ability to bond to bone in comparison with PMMA.

Cortoss is currently being evaluated clinically as a device to augment stripped-out bone screws. In addition, a multicenter study with more than 200 patients is planned to evaluate Cortoss as a bone void filler for percutaneous vertebral augmentation. The present study compares the biocompatibility and interfacial bond strengths of Cortoss synthetic cortical bone void filler with a commercially available PMMA bone filler implanted into rabbit femurs for up to 52 weeks and in sheep long bones for up to 78 weeks.

Materials and methods

Implant materials

Cortoss (Orthovita, Malvern, Pa.), which is formulated as a two-paste thermoset resin, was mixed in a static mix-tip upon simultaneous expulsion from a dual-chamber cartridge. Once expelled and mixed, the material hardens in approximately 5 min into an off-white composite with sufficient integrity to bear the load of body weight.

Simplex P (Stryker Howmedica Osteonics, East Rutherford, N.J.) is a commercial PMMA bone cement composed mainly of methyl methacrylate and methyl methacrylate-styrene (MMA-styrene). It is formulated with 10% barium sulfate for radiopacity. The manufacturer recommends that it be mixed under a vacuum and centrifuged to remove trapped air bubbles, and these recommendations were followed [20].

Surgery

Experiments with rabbits were performed in the animal facilities of Toxikon Corporation (Bedford, Mass.). Femoral defects (3 mm) were created bilaterally in the lateral cortex of the proximal condyles, the diaphyses, and the distal condyles of 25 New Zealand White rabbits. Implant materials were injected into the defect sites using a 1-cc syringe. On the left side, the two proximal defects were filled with Cortoss and the distal defect was filled with Simplex P. On the right side, the proximal defect was filled with Simplex P and the two distal defects were filled with Cortoss. At 4, 8, 12, and 24 weeks, five animals were euthanized with injectable barbiturate.

Experiments with sheep were performed at the University of Pennsylvania Veterinary School of Medicine (New Bolten, Pa.). Four defects (4.8 mm in diameter×10 mm in depth) were created bilaterally in 22 sheep (1.5–2 years old). Defects in the distal radii were filled with either Cortoss or Simplex P. Defects in the greater tubercle of the proximal humeri were filled with 4.5×10-mm rods of Cortoss or Simplex P polymerized prior to surgery. Defects in the medial ulnae were fitted with 1×12-mm 316SS rods held in place with either Cortoss or Simplex P. Defects in the lateral calcanei were fitted with 316SS rods embedded in prepolymerized 4.5×11-mm dowels of Cortoss or Simplex P. Cortoss and Simplex P were randomized to the right or left side in each animal. Radiographs were taken at the midpoint of the study period and after euthanasia. After recovery from surgery, the sheep were allowed to graze. The sheep were killed at 6, 12, and 24 weeks (six sheep per time period), followed by two at 52 weeks, and two at 78 weeks [15].

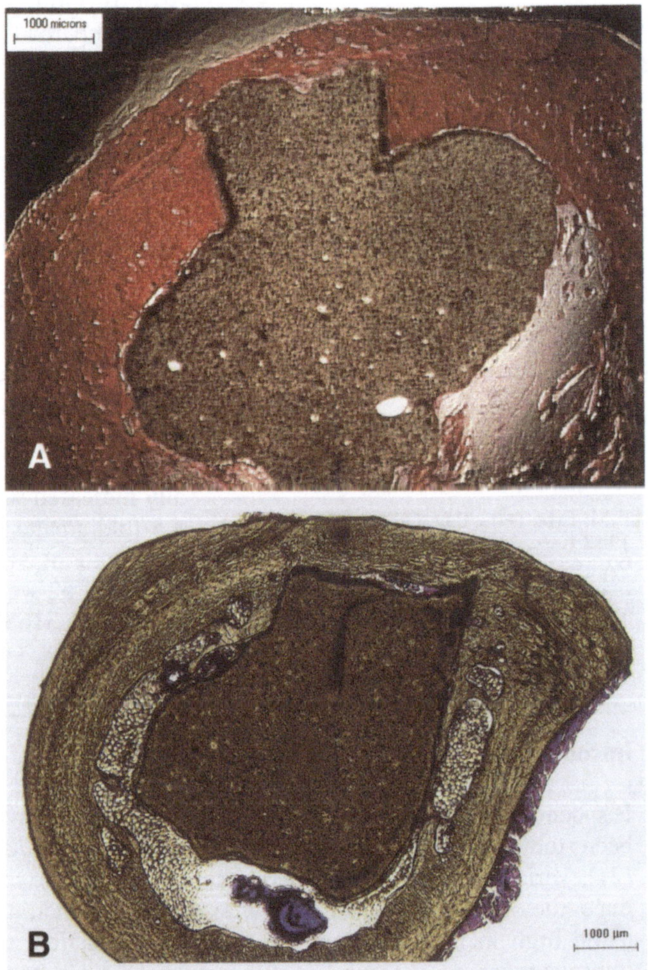

Fig. 1A,B Histological images of rabbit specimens. **A** Cortoss implant with new bone in direct contact at 4 weeks. **B** Cortoss implant surrounded by bone at 24 weeks

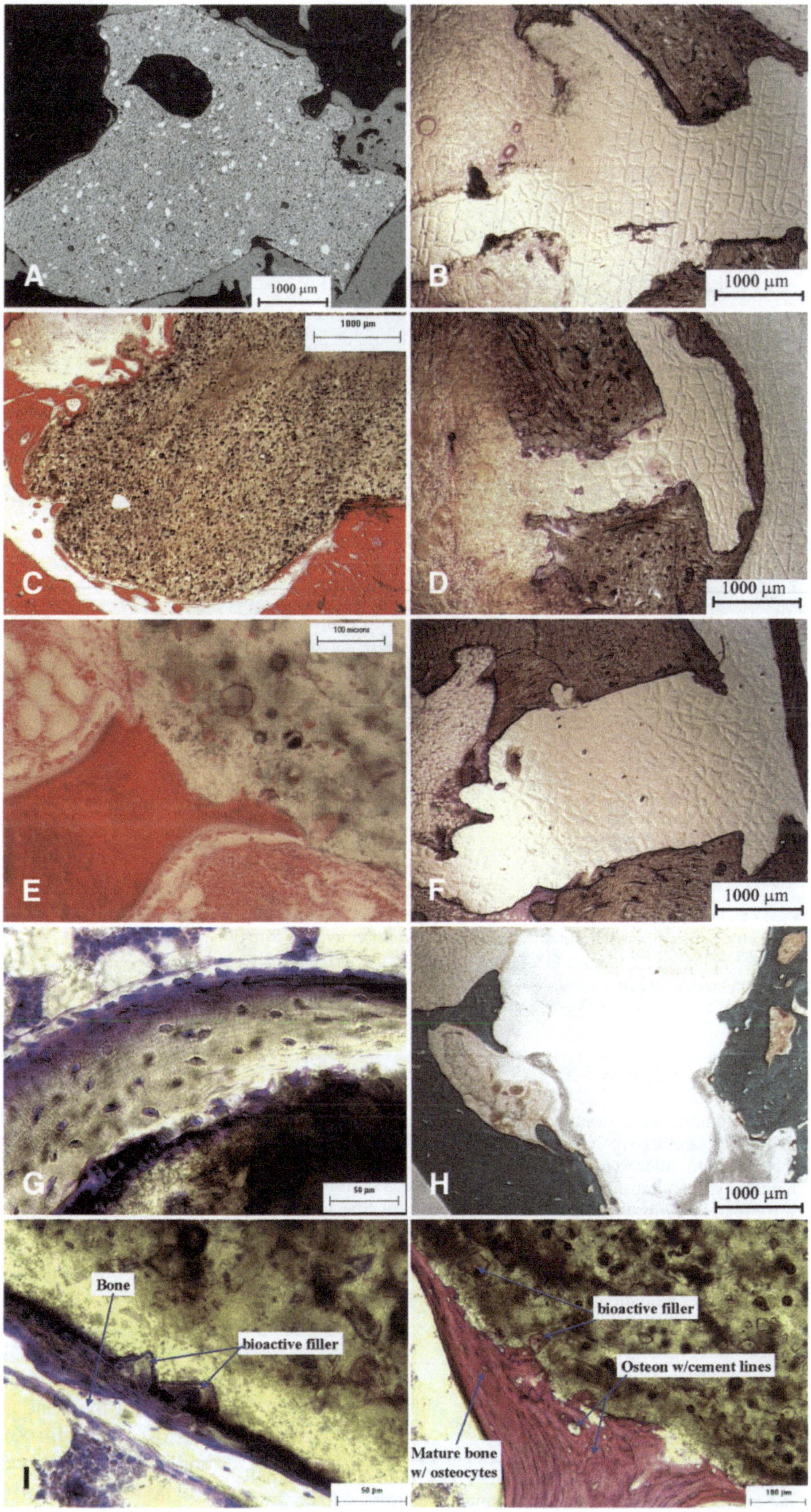

Fig. 2A–I Rabbit histology. **A** Cortoss implant at 4 weeks, **B** polymethyl methacrylate (PMMA) implant at 4 weeks, **C** Cortoss implant at 8 weeks, **D** PMAA implant showing foci of necrosis at 8 weeks, **E** Cortoss implant with new bone formation at 12 weeks, **F** PMMA implant showing some bone formation at 12 weeks, **G** Cortoss implant showing complete apposition of bone at 24 weeks, **H** PMMA implant at 24 weeks, **I** Cortoss implant with apposition of bone at 52 weeks

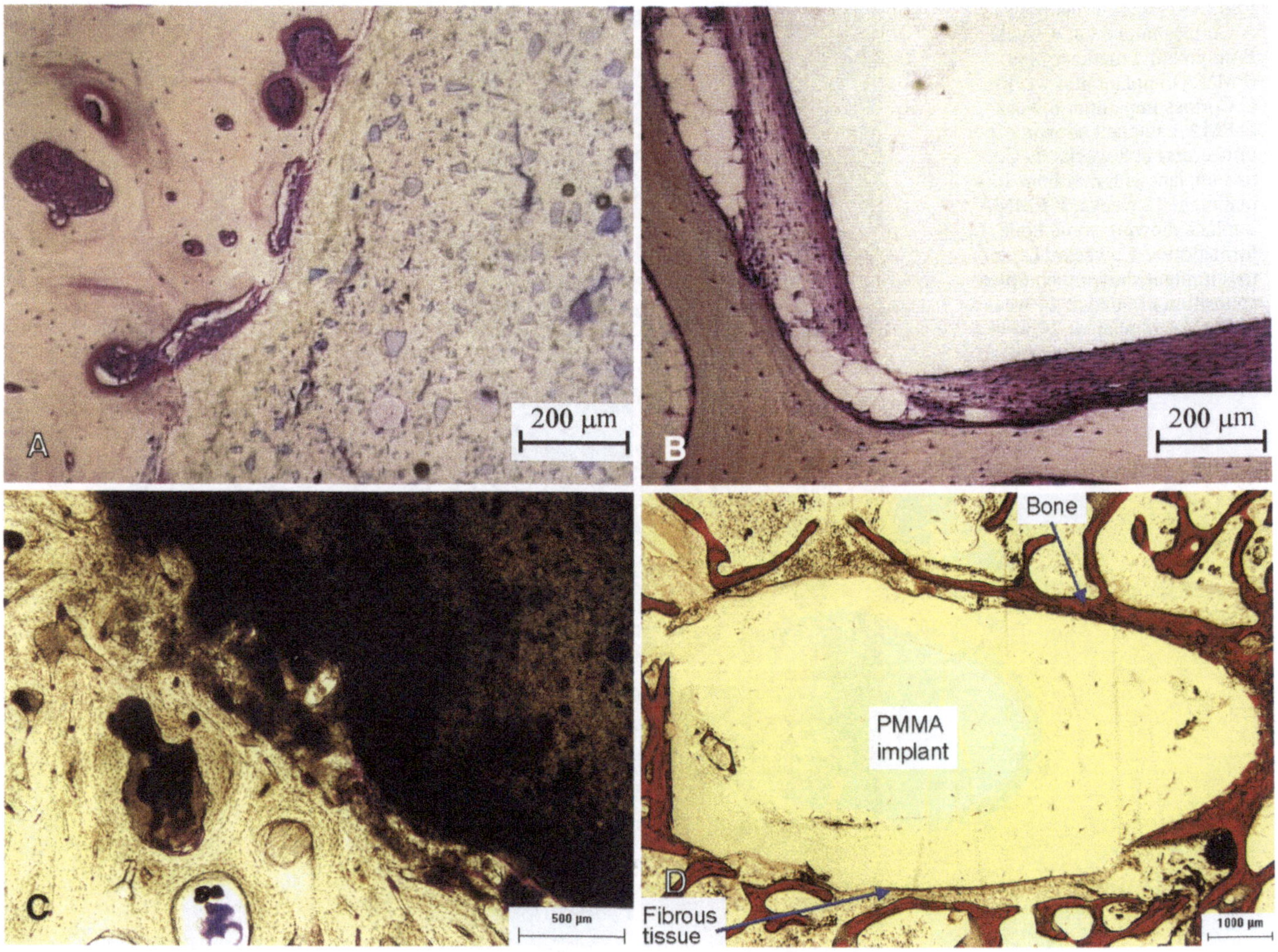

Fig. 3A–D Sheep histology. **A** Cortoss implant polymerized in situ with apposition of bone at 52 weeks, **B** prepolymerized Simplex P implant at 52 weeks, **C** Cortoss implant polymerized in situ in direct contact with bone at 78 weeks, **D** prepolymerized Simplex P implant surrounded by bone and connective tissue at 78 weeks

Microscopic evaluation

Rabbit femora were examined by scanning electron microscopy and energy dispersive X-ray analyses, and, after further processing, by light microscopy. Histology sections were stained with hematoxylin and eosin (H&E) or Paragon. Selected rabbit sections were read in a blinded manner at the Hospital for Special Surgery (New York, NY), the NH Veterinary Diagnostic Lab (Durham, N.H.), and Pathology Associates International (Frederick, Md.).

Sheep sections were stained with either Paragon or H&E prior to histologic evaluation and digital image analysis. Selected sheep sections from the radii and humeri were read in a blinded manner at the NH Veterinary Diagnostic Lab.

Mechanical testing

Specimens from the ulnae and calcanei of the sheep were wrapped in saline-soaked towels and stored at –200°C until the time of pull-out testing [15]. Rods that were manually determined to be firmly in place were pulled from the defect sites at 1 mm/s for 2 mm (Instron model number 8500, Canton, Mass.). Loads were measured using a 5-kN load cell.

Results

Scanning electron microscopy

In histologic images, Cortoss appeared to be in direct contact with new bone at 4 weeks in the rabbit, and was entirely surrounded at 24 weeks (Fig. 1).

Histology

Rabbit

At 4 weeks, periosteal and endosteal bone were seen at both Cortoss- and Simplex P-repaired sites, but a greater proportion of the bone margin appeared to be in contact with Cortoss than with Simplex P. Signs of mild inflammation and multinucleated cells were present to comparable extents for both types of implant at all time points (Fig. 2A,B) [15]. This is not uncommon.

At 8 weeks, peripheral resorption and vascularization were seen with progressing periosteal and endosteal bone formation within sites filled with either implant material. Foreign-body multinucleated giant cells, mild to moderate fibrosis, multinucleated giant cells, lymphocytes, and plasma cells remained to a similar extent in defects filled with either Cortoss or Simplex P (Fig. 2C,D).

New periosteal and endosteal bone was seen around both implant materials at 12 weeks. New bone was seen in areas where blood vessels had grown directly adjacent to Cortoss. Further vascular invasion of Simplex P was generally not seen (Fig. 2E,F).

The amount of bone was greater around Cortoss at 24 weeks than at 12 weeks. Some specimens of Simplex P were observed to lie adjacent to a layer of fibrous connective tissue; approximately half the specimens of Simplex P were adjacent to new bone (Fig. 2G,H). Cortoss appeared to have significant bone apposition by 52 weeks (Fig. 2I).

Sheep

Some endosteal bone formation and slight foreign-body reactions (fibrosis and macrophages) were seen in response to both implant materials at 6, 12, and 24 weeks, with no qualitative differences at early timepoints. At 52 weeks, both Cortoss and Simplex P were surrounded by endosteal bone and inflammatory cell infiltrates. Foreign-body multinucleated giant cells were seen around Cortoss, but were rarely seen around Simplex P at 52 weeks (Fig. 3A,B).

Microradiographic evaluation of sheep specimens

The extent of radiopacity around the perimeter of implants was significantly greater for Cortoss bone void filler polymerized in situ than for Simplex P implants polymerized in situ.

Displacement forces

Displacement forces generally increased with time (Fig. 4). Rods were more firmly held in place with Cortoss than with Simplex P at all time periods ($P \leq 0.01$). At 24 weeks, the force required to displace rods in prepolymerized Cortoss was 4.5 times as high as the force needed to displace rods in Simplex P ($P \leq 0.01$). Failure occurred at the bone/resin interface.

For rods fixed with bone void fillers that polymerized in situ, displacement forces for Cortoss generally exceeded those of Simplex P. However, the difficulty in normalizing the interfacial area due to varying interdigitation of Cortoss and PMMA made exact comparisons difficult.

For rods fixed with bone void fillers that were prepolymerized, displacement forces for Cortoss exceeded those of Simplex P at 52 and 78 weeks (Fig. 4).

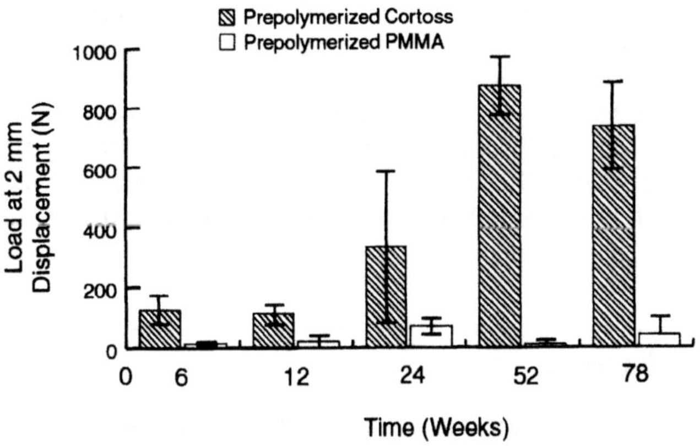

Fig. 4 Displacement forces versus time. Rods were fixed in place in situ with either Cortoss or PMMA

For 316SS rods held in place with Cortoss, displacement forces did not depend upon whether the Cortoss was allowed to polymerize in situ or before surgery. There were no statistically significant differences between displacement forces of 316SS rods held in place with Cortoss that was polymerized in situ and those held in place by prepolymerized Cortoss.

Discussion

New periosteal and endosteal bone was formed within defect sites filled with either Cortoss or Simplex P, but the initial response was greater with Cortoss than with Simplex P. Subsequently, the periphery of Cortoss implants was invaded by new blood vessels that supported reparative osteogenesis; Simplex P was generally unreactive in terms of bone formation. Although both Cortoss and Simplex P were seen to be surrounded by bone in the long term (52 weeks in sheep, 24 weeks in rabbits), half the Simplex P specimens were separated from bone by a layer of fibrous connective tissue at 24 weeks.

Cortoss and Simplex P were different, however, in their abilities to bond to bone. Whereas the forces required to displace 316SS rods generally increased with time for both materials, displacement forces were greater for rods held in place with Cortoss than with Simplex P at every time point examined throughout this study, up to 78 weeks. At 24 weeks, the force required to break the bond between bone and Cortoss was 330 N versus 70 N for Simplex P, a relative strength difference of 4.5. The greater stability of the bone/Cortoss interface is attributed to a faster initial bone response and a greater degree of mineralization around Cortoss, as evidenced by digital analyses of radiographs.

Conclusions

Cortoss bone void filler has been shown to engender a biocompatible tissue response, resulting in significant apposition of new bone around the filler at 24 weeks in rabbits and at 52 weeks in sheep. Further, Cortoss increased the interfacial bone strengths between implants and bone by a factor of 4.5 after 24 weeks. Thus, it is concluded that this study presents supportive data concerning the safety and efficacy of Cortoss bone void filler, and that Cortoss is a promising candidate for clinical testing in applications requiring improved mechanical bone bonding between implants and host bone.

Acknowledgements The authors gratefully acknowledge Barb Dallap and Dean Richardson for their technical support of the sheep study.

References

1. Bini SA, Gill K, Johnston JO (1995) Giant cell tumor of bone. Curettage and cement reconstruction. Clin Orthop 245
2. Chiras J, Depriester C, Weill A, Sola-Martinez MT, Deramond H (1997) [Percutaneous vertebral surgery. Techniques and indications]. J Neuroradiol 24:45
3. Dreinhöfer KE, Rydholm A, Bauer HC, Kreicbergs A (1995) Giant-cell tumours with fracture at diagnosis. Curettage and acrylic cementing in ten cases. J Bone Joint Surg Br 77:189
4. Freeman MAR, Bradley GW, Revell PA (1982) Observations upon the interface between bone and polymethylmethacrylate cement. J Bone Joint Surg Br 64:489
5. Galibert P, Deramond H, Rosat P, Le Gars D (1987) [Preliminary note on the treatment of vertebral angioma by percutaneous acrylic vertebroplasty]. Neurochirurgie 33:166
6. Gitelis S, Mallin BA, Piasecki P, Turner F (1993) Intralesional excision compared with en bloc resection for giant-cell tumors of bone. J Bone Joint Surg Am 75:1648
7. Harper EJ (1998) Bioactive bone cements. Proc Inst Mech Eng [H] 212:113
8. Harrington KD (1981) The use of methylmethacrylate for vertebral-body replacement and anterior stabilization of pathological fracture-dislocations of the spine due to metastatic malignant disease. J Bone Joint Surg Am 63:36
9. Harrington KD (1986) Metastatic disease of the spine. J Bone Joint Surg Am 68:1110
10. Jasper LE, Deramond H, Mathis JM, Belkoff SM (1999) The effect of monomer-to-powder ratio on the material properties of cranioplastic. Bone 25:27S
11. Komiya S, Inoue A (1993) Cementation in the treatment of giant cell tumor of bone. Arch Orthop Trauma Surg 112:51
12. McAfee PC, Bohlman HH, Ducker T, Eismont FJ (1986) Failure of stabilization of the spine with methylmethacrylate: a retrospective analysis of twenty-four cases. J Bone Joint Surg Am 68:1145
13. O'Donnell RJ, Springfield DS, Motwani HK, Ready JE, Gebhardt MC, Mankin HJ (1994) Recurrence of giant-cell tumors of the long bones after curettage and packing with cement. J Bone Joint Surg Am 76:1827
14. Okada Y, Kawanabe K, Fujita H, Nishio K, Nakamura T (1999) Repair of segmental bone defects using bioactive bone cement: comparison with PMMA bone cement. J Biomed Mater Res 47:353
15. OrthoVita. Data on file. 1999.
16. Pals SD, Wilkins RM (1992) Giant cell tumor of bone treated by curettage, cementation, and bone grafting. Orthopedics 15:703
17. Persson BM, Ekelund L, Lovdahl R, Gunterberg B (1984) Favourable results of acrylic cementation for giant cell tumors. Acta Orthop Scand 55:209
18. Raveh J, Stich H, Schawalder P, Ruchti C, Cottier H (1982) Biocement – a new material. Results of its experimental use for osseous repair of skull cap defects with lesions of the dura mater and liquorrhea, reconstruction of the anterior wall of the frontal sinuses and fixation of alloimplants. Acta Otolaryngol (Stockh) 94:371
19. Saha S, Pal S (1984) Mechanical properties of bone cement: a review. J Biomed Mater Res 18:435
20. Stryker Howmedica. The formula for success. Stryker® Howmedica website. http://www.howmedica.com/simplex/pages/intro.html (accessed August 24, 2000)
21. Vainio J (1978) Non-metallic fixatives in orthopedic surgery: some aspects of their present and future properties. Arch Orthop Trauma Surg 92:169

E. Munting
A. Faundez
E. Manche

Vertebral reconstruction with cortical allograft: long-term evaluation

E. Munting (✉) · A. Faundez · E. Manche
Department of Orthopaedics,
Saint Luc University Hospital,
Avenue Hippocrate 10,
1200 Brussels, Belgium
e-mail: munting@orto.ucl.ac.be,
Tel.: +32-2-7642979,
Fax: +32-2-7648904

Abstract Reconstruction of large anterior vertebral column defects is indicated in a number of pathological conditions including tumor, infection, trauma and post-traumatic deformity. Several substitutes and techniques are available for the functional restoration of the vertebral column. Vascularized bone transfers, autografts, allografts or xenografts have been used, as well as metal or ceramic implants. All of these bear potential advantages and drawbacks in terms of associated morbidity of graft harvesting, disease transmission, mechanical failure, implant incorporation and overall long-term clinical outcome. In the present paper we report our experience with the use of freeze-dried, gamma-irradiated, cortical allograft for the reconstruction of large, anterior segmental defects of the spine, involving at least one vertebral body with its two adjacent discs. Cortical allografts were used in 67 cases operated for a variety of conditions. No case of disease transmission, infection or long-term mechanical graft failure occurred in our entire series, with a mean follow-up of 31 months. Fusion and mechanical stability was reliably obtained. Specific advantages include the absence of donor site morbidity, the possibilities for exact trimming to the size of the defect, superior mechanical strength as compared to available autograft, and reliable fusion with the host bone with partial bone remodeling, preventing fatigue failure. We conclude that freeze-dried, irradiated cortical allografts are safe and effective for anterior reconstruction of the spine.

Keywords Spine · Cortical · Allograft · Anterior · Fusion

Introduction

Spinal reconstruction following trauma, tumor, infection, congenital abnormalities, degenerative diseases or dysplastic diseases of bone is possible with several types of materials: autograft, allograft or artificial implants. Each type of implant has its theoretical advantages and drawbacks in terms of effectiveness and ease of use.

The goals of surgical management of vertebral destruction remain the same whatever the technical means used for reconstruction. They include restoration of the normal morphology of the spine with adequate mechanical resistance and appropriate space for the neural structures. Normal spinal function should be obtained after surgery and maintained in the long term. Short-term results are mostly dependent on technical factors: decompression if needed, adequate spinal morphology, and solid osteosynthesis. The long-term maintenance of a good immediate postoperative result is dependent on a solid and lasting mechanical continuity between the host bone and the reconstructed area. Solid bony fusion appears to be the most reliable means to achieve this goal, but fibrous union may also provide a long-term favorable clinical outcome [6]. Durable fixation by a mechanical interlock between the host bone and an artificial implant is an alternative solution that has demonstrated its efficacy in other applications like joint reconstruction.

Autograft yields very high rates of fusion, as long as mechanical stability is provided along with appropriate preparation of the adjacent end plates. However, in anterior vertebral reconstruction involving at least one vertebral body and its adjacent discs in the thoracic or lumbar spine, the size of the defect to be filled necessitates the harvesting of a large amount of autograft, often associated with a significant morbidity at the graft harvesting site(s) [3]. Furthermore, the mechanical resistance of such a large reconstruction with autograft is usually not sufficient to allow full weight bearing without a corset until several months after surgery, and is associated with a risk of graft fracture.

The safety and effectiveness of allografts, regarding disease transmission, mechanical resistance, and fusion, has often been questioned [4, 12]. Several authors have reported good long-term results with the use of cortical ring allografts for anterior interbody fusion [5, 9, 10, 11], but reports about the long-term results of reconstruction with cortical allograft of large, structural defects involving at least one vertebral body with its adjacent discs are limited [8, 11].

In the present paper we report our experience with freeze-dried, irradiated, cortical allografts used for the reconstruction of large anterior segmental defects of the spine in various conditions.

Materials and methods

Patient description

From April 1989 to December 1999, vertebral resection including at least one vertebral body with the two adjacent discs was carried out 67 times in 64 patients, followed by reconstruction with cortical allograft.

Indication for corpectomy (n=57) or vertebrectomy (n=10) included a variety of conditions (Table 1). Trauma or post-traumatic kyphosis, primary tumor and metastatic disease were the most frequent indications.

The location was in the cervical spine in 12 cases, in the thoracic spine in 19 cases, at the thoraco-lumbar junction in 21 cases and in the lumbar spine in 14 cases. In one case, a total sacrectomy was carried out. Age at surgery ranged from 3 to 74 years (mean: 45, median: 47).

Table 1 Indications for vertebral reconstruction

Trauma: burst fracture	13
Post-traumatic kyphosis	14
Metastatic disease	16
Primary tumor	10
Degenerative disease	4
Congenital deformity	5
Pott's disease	2
Radionecrosis	2
Ankylosing spondylitis	1

Cortical allograft

Segmental cortical allografts are obtained from the UCL St-Luc Academic Hospital Bone Bank. The bones are procured during multiorgan harvesting according to the most recent standards of the American Association of Tissues Banks [1].

Long bones are cut and freed of all soft tissues. Further physical and chemical treatment includes washing, lipid extraction in chloroform and methanol, prion inactivation, freeze drying, packaging and sterilization by 2.5-Gy gamma irradiation.

For reconstruction in the thoracic and lumbar spine, grafts obtained from the femoral shaft were mostly used, whereas for the cervical spine, segments of the radius, ulna or fibula are used. During surgery, after careful preparation of the end plates above and below the defect, the gap is precisely measured with a paper template. A segment of diaphysis is exactly cut according to the template.

Filling of the medullary cavity of the allograft: use of autograft

In 41 cases, the medullary cavity of the cortical allograft was filled with autologous bone, locally available. Either rib fragments or, in traumatic or degenerative cases, cancellous bone from the vertebral body that had to be resected was used. Cancellous allograft can be used instead. In five cases of metastatic disease, acrylic cement was injected into the medullary cavity of the allograft.

Osteosynthesis

Anterior plating was used in cervical reconstruction. In the thoracic spine, either no osteosynthesis or anterior plating or posterior fixation was used. In the thoraco-lumbar and lumbar spine, posterior osteosynthesis was carried out and associated with anterior plating in 15 cases. In one pediatric case, only anterior plating was used after L3 vertebrectomy. In most cases, arthrodesis and instrumentation was limited to the level above and below. Only in some cases of total vertebrectomy or extended associated pathology was the fusion extended more than one level above and below the resection.

Extent of reconstruction

One-level resection with adjacent discs was carried out in 59 cases. Reconstruction on two or more levels was performed nine times in the thoracic or lumbar spine.

Radiological assessment

Solid and rigid mechanical continuity between the host site and the reconstruction implant appears to be the paramount factor for long-term success. When using bone grafts, this is synonymous with bony fusion. However, the radiological aspect does not always allow solid fusion to be confirmed or negated. Therefore, we must also consider a number of indirect criteria suggesting strong and stable incorporation of the graft.

Radiological aspects strongly suggesting solid fusion include:

- Graft remodeling
- Graft density modifications
- Apparent bony continuity in all radiological incidences

Indirect criteria for solid and stable reconstruction include:

- Absence of loss of correction or progressive deformity
- Absence of radiolucency around osteosynthesis screws
- No hardware breakage

Favorable clinical outcome associated with the previous arguments is a supplementary positive element.

Negative arguments include:

- Lasting local pain
- Graft resorption
- Progressive deformity

Modifications in the adjacent vertebrae must be evaluated, like bone density modifications, resorption, and compression fractures. The radiographic documents were evaluated by two independent observers (E.Ma. and A.F.).

Results

No infection was encountered in this series of vertebral reconstructions.

Seven patients died within 6 months after surgery from systemic disease; four of these had regained good function. Six patients were lost to follow-up after less than 4 months and could not be evaluated regarding fusion or outcome. Therefore, 54 cases were evaluated, with a mean radiological follow-up of 31.1 months (range 4–120 months, median 24 months). The radiological follow-up in this series is reported in Table 2.

Fusion was rated as certain in 33 cases (Fig. 1), and as most likely in 10 cases. Of the 11 remaining cases, 1 patient had a true pseudarthrosis with loss of correction and 5 had a fibrous union without loss of correction or graft displacement. Radiographic follow-up was less then 9 months in 3 of these. Five grafts with cement could not be well evaluated regarding fusion. None had a loss of correction. Significant graft resorption occurred in one case without clinical consequence.

In six cases, an early loss of correction was observed because of insufficient fixation. This led, in five cases, to addition or extension of posterior instrumentation in order to restore stability. Of note is the fact that the initial displacement of the graft did not preclude fusion in any case (Fig. 2).

One patient with a chordoma of the second lumbar vertebra had to be re-operated for recurrent disease, 19 months after the index surgery. Secondary posterior fixation had to be carried out 2 weeks after the index surgery because of a fracture of the vertebral body below. This had resulted in some graft displacement. Despite this and the fact that the patient underwent high-dose radiotherapy on the surgical site, the allograft appeared perfectly incorporated and strongly united to the adjacent vertebral bodies. En bloc resection involving the graft/host junctions was carried out, allowing microscopic analysis of the material. Extensive incorporation was documented with bone remodeling involving the periphery of the allograft (Fig. 3).

After several months of normal function, progressive sinking into the vertebra below occurred in two patients who had received high-dose radiotherapy postoperatively. This led to repeat surgery in one case.

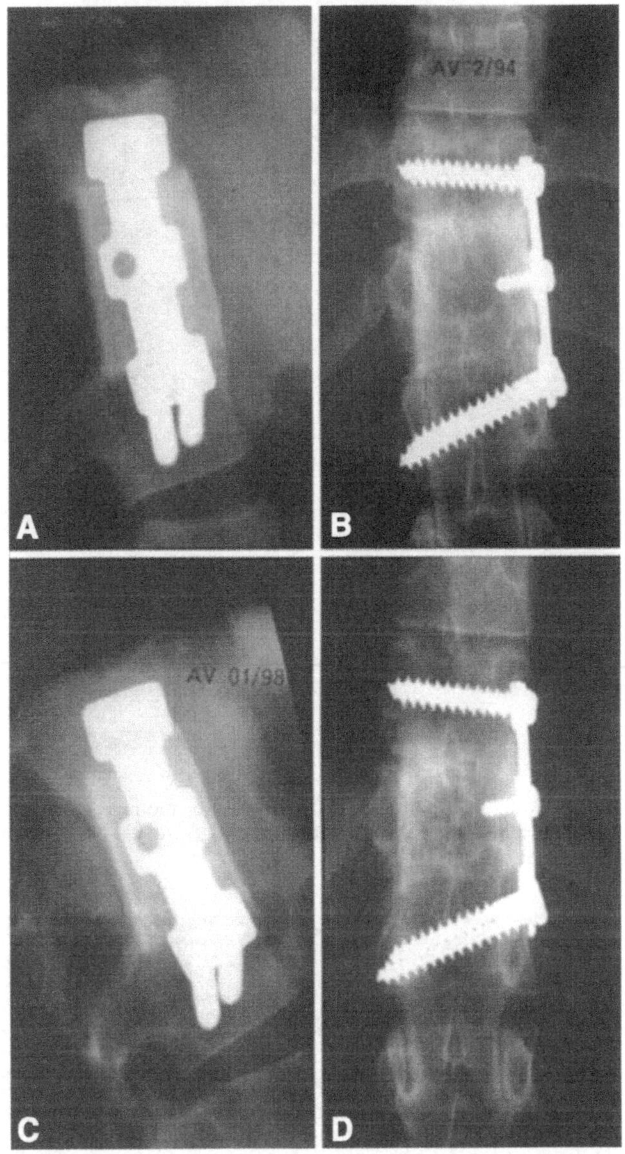

Fig. 1A–D Four-year evolution of a cortical allograft inserted for a post-traumatic kyphosis after a neglected T12 burst fracture. **A,B** Eight months after surgery, **C,D** 55 months after surgery. Note the graft remodelling on both lateral (**A,C**) and anteroposterior (**B,D**) views

Table 2 Length of radiological follow-up

Months	No. of patients
0–6	6
7–12	8
13–24	17
25–36	8
37–48	4
48–60	4
>60	7

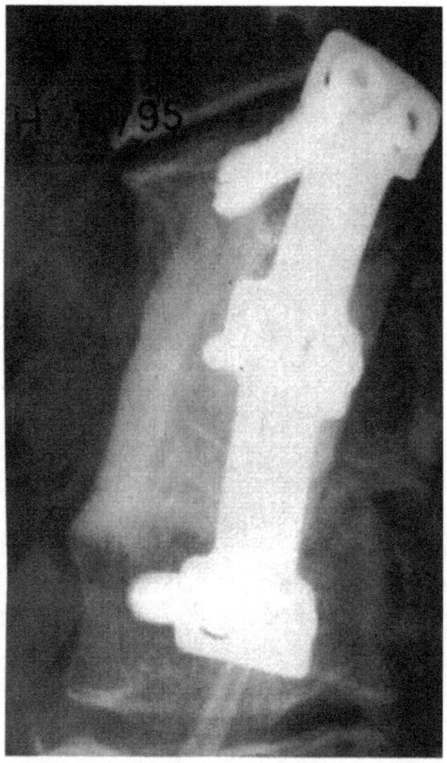

Fig. 2 Graft incorporation documented 16 months postoperatively, despite early displacement of the graft treated by posterior instrumentation

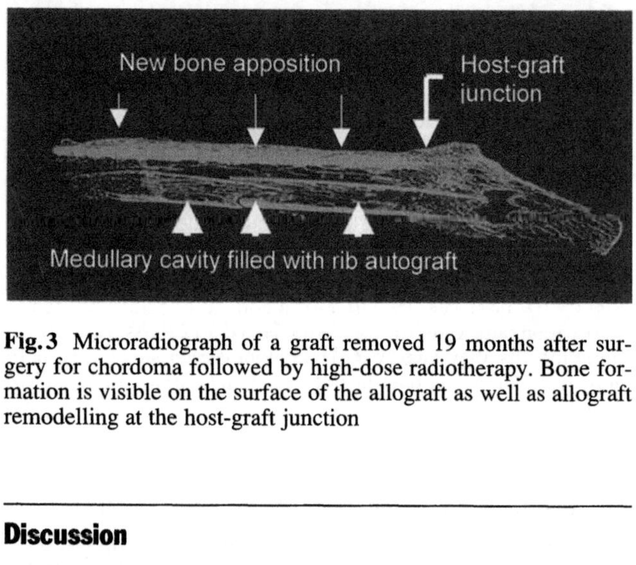

Fig. 3 Microradiograph of a graft removed 19 months after surgery for chordoma followed by high-dose radiotherapy. Bone formation is visible on the surface of the allograft as well as allograft remodelling at the host-graft junction

Discussion

According to the results of this study, washed, lipid-extracted, freeze-dried, gamma-irradiated cortical allografts appears to be an effective material for reconstruction of large anterior vertebral defects related to a variety of pathological conditions.

So long as it is obtained from a bone bank implementing all the recommendations of the European Association of Musculo-skeletal Tissue Banks or equivalent bodies in other parts of the world, this material appears perfectly safe in terms of disease transmission. In our whole series of patients where anterior cortical allograft was used for either vertebral reconstruction or interbody fusion, which represents a further 80 cases, we had no single case of documented or suspected infection or transmission of disease.

The biology of bony incorporation of the allograft may be affected by the different physical and chemical procedures the material is submitted to, including washing, lipid extraction, conservation means and, in particular, sterilization. This may explain some less favorable results that have been reported with some types of allograft [2, 4]. The anterior location, associated with a weight-bearing situation, appears as a favorable factor regarding the incorporation of a cortical allograft [7]. While resorption of cancellous allograft has been reported with a rather high frequency, this observation is seldom reported with cortical allografts [2]. Of course the surgical technique is an important variable, which is often difficult to evaluate and may significantly affect the results. Careful preparation of the end plates until the appearance of dense, bleeding subchondral bone and appropriate osteosynthesis is mandatory.

The large surface area of the cylindrical cortical allograft in contact with the host bone is another favorable feature regarding fusion. The addition of locally available autograft in the medullary cavity and around the graft is obviously contributive to fusion promotion. Fusion is, however, reliably obtained without the addition of autograft, but the medullary cavity should be filled with cancellous allograft, or cement, in patients with a short life expectancy, in order to provide a large surface area for load transmission at the graft-to-host interface.

Secondary displacement or loss of correction, which occurred in some cases, was the consequence of technical errors such as insufficient osteosynthesis or graft misplacement. According to our experience, one level above and one level below transpedicular fixation is sufficient in the lumbar spine if the posterior elements are preserved along with the anterior longitudinal ligament. In cases of total vertebrectomy or disruption of the anterior and posterior elements, instrumentation should be front and back, or if only posterior, it should be extended two levels above and below the resection.

The morphological analysis of a graft harvested 19 months after an implantation that was followed by high-dose radiotherapy indicates that the allograft becomes fully incorporated and undergoes a slow and partial remodeling process by creeping substitution (Fig. 3). This is further suggested by the repeated radiographic appearance of graft remodeling in the present series, which is also reported by other authors [8, 11] (Fig. 1, Fig. 2). The partial revascularization and bone remodeling of the graft contributes to prevention of fatigue fracture of the reconstructed area.

Conclusions

We conclude from our experience over more than 10 years of using freeze-dried, gamma-irradiated cortical allografts, that these implants do fulfil the specification chart for functional restoration of the vertebral column after large anterior resection of a vertebral segment, in terms of implant safety, effective vertebral column reconstruction and long-term outcome. Fusion is reliably obtained, but the surgical technique must be very rigorous for the preparation of the host bone bed as well as for the graft sizing and the osteosynthesis.

References

1. American Association of Tissues Banks (1999) Standards for musculo skeletal tissue banking. American Association of Tissues Banks, Arlington
2. An HS, Lynch K, Toth J (1995) Prospective comparison of autograft vs allograft for adult posterolateral lumbar spine fusion: differences among freeze-dried, frozen, and mixed grafts. J Spinal Disord 8:131–135
3. Banwart JC, Asher M, Hassanein S (1995) Iliac crest bone graft harvest donor site morbidity. Spine 20:1055–1060
4. Buttermann GR, Glazer PA, Bradford DS (1996) The use of bone allograft in the spine. Clin Orthop 324:75–85
5. Coric D, Branch CL, Jenkins JD (1997) Revision of anterior cervical pseudarthrosis with anterior allograft fusion and plating. J Neurosurg 86: 969–974
6. Finkelstein JA, Chapman JR, Mirza S (1999) Anterior cortical allograft in thoracolumbar fractures. J Spinal Disord 12:424–429
7. Gill K, O'Brien JP (1993) Observation of resorption of the posterior lateral bone graft in combined anterior and posterior lumbar fusion. Spine 18: 1885–1889
8. Govender S, Parbhoo AH (1999) Support of the anterior column with allografts in tuberculosis of the spine. J Bone Joint Surg Br 81:106–109
9. Liljenqvist U, O'Brien JP, Renton P (1998) Simultaneous combined anterior and posterior lumbar fusion with femoral cortical allograft. Eur Spine J 7:125–131
10. Martin GJ, Haid RW, MacMillan M, Rodts GE, Berkman R (1999) Anterior cervical discectomy with freeze-dried fibula allograft. Overview of 317 cases and literature review. Spine 24:852–858
11. Molinari RW, Bridwell KH, Klepps SJ, Baldus C (1999) Minimum 5 year follow-up of anterior column structural allografts in the thoracic and lumbar spine. Spine 24:967–972
12. Swank ML, Lowery GL, Bhat AL, McDonough RF (1997) Anterior cervical allograft arthrodesis and instrumentation: multilevel interbody grafting or strut graft reconstruction. Eur Spine J 6:138–143

M. E. Janssen
C. Lam
R. Beckham

Outcomes of allogenic cages in anterior and posterior lumbar interbody fusion

Abstract Interbody lumbar fusions provide a proven logical solution to diseases of the intervertebral discs by eliminating motion of the segment. Historically, there are many techniques to achieve spinal fusion in the lumbar spine. These include anterior, posterior, and foramenal approaches, often in combination with various internal fixation devices. The surgeon's choice of the approach and mechanical or biological implant is dependent on the patient's specific pathology and anatomy, in addition to the experience and training of the surgeon in similar conditions. In the past decade, new mechanical spine implants/spacers have been designed to provide restoration of disc height and improve stabilization of the spine. The ability to radiographically assess the "biology" of bone incorporation in these mechanical (metal) spacers has become a significant limitation.

The femoral ring allograft (FRA) and the posterior lumbar interbody fusion (PLIF) spacers have been developed as "biological cages" that permit restoration of the anterior column with machined allograft bone biological cages. Test results demonstrate that the FRA and PLIF spacers have a compressive strength of over 25,000 N. The pyramid-shaped teeth on the surfaces and the geometry of the implant increase the resistance to expulsion at clinically relevant loads (1053 and 1236 N). The technique of anterior column reconstruction with both the FRA and the PLIF biological cages have been previously reported.

Clinical outcomes and experience with the FRA spacer (137 patients) and the PLIF spacer (13 patients) were reported on and did not reveal any evidence of bone cage resorption or infectious inflammatory process. There was clinical migration with one PLIF spacer, which was later revised with an anterior approach and a FRA spacer. The radiographic outcomes demonstrated that 94% arthrodesis was achieved with the biological spacer and additional posterior instrumentation. The clinical success of every spine fusion procedure is dependent on many factors such as the extent of the instability, the pathology, type of graft used, the patient's pathology/anatomy and lifestyle.

Keywords Biological cages · Femoral ring allograft spacer · Posterior lumbar interbody fusion spacer · Interbody lumbar fusion · Arthrodesis

M.E. Janssen · C. Lam (✉) · R. Beckham
Center for Spinal Disorders, P.C.,
8515 Pearl Street, Suite 350,
Denver, Colorado 80229, USA
e-mail: spinecntr@aol.com,
Tel.: +1-303-287-2800,
Fax: +1-303-287-7357

Introduction

Spinal arthrodesis is a generally accepted procedure for the management of patients with a variety of spinal disorders. The primary goal for spinal fusion is to eliminate the instability of the spine, often caused by trauma, deformity, tumor, inflammation or infection, and common degenerative deterioration of the motion segments. In many clinical situations, the optimal solution in restoring the spine's integrity is through surgical intervention. There are many techniques of spinal fusion applicable to the lumbar spine. Posterior (PLIF) and anterior lumbar interbody fusion (ALIF) have been developed and employed to address these concerns alone or in combination with various internal fixation devices. The anterior column is often reconstructed with metallic intervertebral cages or biological implants (allograft or autograft bone) [16, 31].

The success of every spine fusion procedure depends on the phenomenon of bone healing. Whether the healing process occurs depends on many factors, including the type of biological graft, host factors, technique, and the rigidity of the particular surgical construct. Bone grafts serve two main functions: they provide for the synthesis of new bone originating from the host cells (osteogenesis), and they can serve as mechanical/structural support [31]. Graft bone cells have been shown to survive initial transplantation if properly handled to synthesize new bone.

Many studies have compared allografts with autografts in spinal arthrodesis for a variety of pathologic conditions. In adults, autografts are generally superior to allografts for achieving bone fusion. However, under certain circumstances, it may be advantageous to use an allograft. The usage of a structural allograft precludes the need for harvesting a graft from the patient and eliminates the morbidity associated with donor site complications [31]. These complications may include infection, pain, blood loss, secondary fracture, instability at the donor site, and possible neural damage. A recent retrospective study involving the Smith-Robinson technique compared the results of fibular allograft interbody fusions in 23 patients with tricortical iliac autograft fusions in 25 patients [5, 17]. The results indicate that there was no significant difference in the fusion rates in autogenic bone grafting compared with allogenic bone grafting.

Preservation techniques can maintain the graft's mechanical properties and its ability to stimulate osteogenesis while eliminating its antigenicity [14]. Frozen allografts are still somewhat immunogenic. Revascularization and remodeling are delayed compared with fresh autografts, but resorption and osteoconduction occur more rapidly and completely in these grafts. Freeze-drying reduces the immunogenicity of allografts even more, but alters their mechanical properties, resulting in a weaker structure. Although the initial inflammatory stage is diminished after transplantation of frozen or freeze-dried allografts, resorption and ultimately new bone formation will occur slowly.

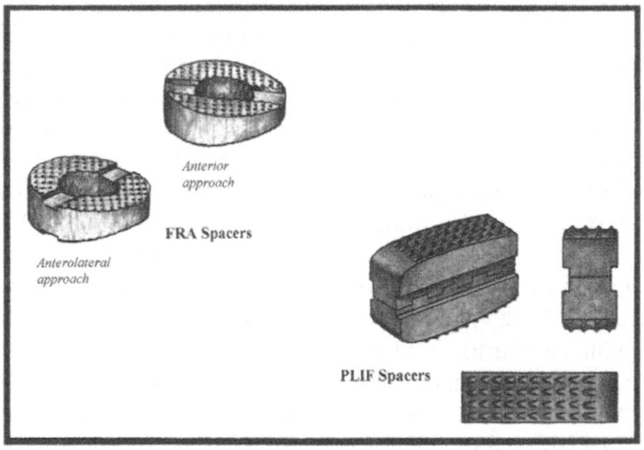

Fig. 1 Femoral ring allograft (*FRA*) and posterior lumbar interbody fusion (*PLIF*) spacers

This paper aims to provide a review of the two newly developed biological cages, the femoral ring allograft (FRA) spacer and the posterior lumbar interbody fusion (PLIF) spacer (Fig. 1). To aid in the understanding of the clinical outcome of these devices, this paper will review the biomechanics, development, and the screening process of these unique "biological cages."

History

As we reflect on past centuries and where science has led us in the study of the spine, we can begin to envision what is in store for the next century. Take, for example, Mercer, who in 1936 stated, "The ideal operation for fusing the spine would be an interbody fusion, but the surgical difficulties encountered in performing such a feat would make the operation technically impossible" [24]. Even among supporters of interbody fusion, enthusiasm for the technique remained sedate until the 1940s. Over the years, many variations of PLIF have been invented to facilitate the fusion process while maintaining stability of the spine. Capener first described ALIF for spondylolisthesis in 1932 [6]. Today, spinal fusion can be accomplished by various techniques such as posterior procedures with and without internal fixation, anterior procedures with and without internal fixation, and combined anterior and posterior column procedures, which may include PLIF or ALIF for anterior column support [31].

During the last decade, an increasing number of studies have looked at the morphology, physiology, biomechanics, and immunology of the various components of the spine [26]. Today, there are several options available to spine surgeons for correcting spinal instabilities and achieving physiological anterior column support, including autograft, allograft, synthetics, and metallic fusion cages. Fresh autologous cancellous bone is considered the best choice for osseous reconstruction because of its optimal biological behavior and histocompatibility [12]. However, autologous bone has inadequate initial mechanical strength for interbody loading and may collapse and/or extrude [10, 13, 18]. Significant morbidity is also associated with anterior structural graft harvesting of the ilium and may result in infection, chronic pain, incisional hernias, vascular injuries, and iliac wing fractures [30]. The use of allograft is a safe, simple, and inexpensive method of harvesting bone. Through continued clinical research, devices are being manufactured from cortical bone similar to metal fusion cages, providing built-in lordosis and endplate gripping "teeth" for additional stability. Two of these biological devices are the PLIF spacer for PLIF and the FRA spacer for ALIF.

Various aspects of intervertebral disc disease have been proposed as definitive indications for PLIF. Collis' indications are lumbar pain with or without sciatica, a degenerative disc with or without a protrusion, a midline disc protrusion, post-lumbar laminectomy/disectomy syndrome, a recurrent soft tissue protrusion, spondylolisthesis (grade I or II), a reverse spondylolisthesis, or any combination of the preceding seven conditions [8]. The advantages of PLIF are (a) the large surface area for fusions provided by the vertebral bodies, (b) the fusion is in compression across the vertebral bodies, and (c) the potential for partial restoration of disc space height. In addition, because the patient is already exposed for decompression, it eliminates the need for another incision [1]. The disadvantages of PLIF include the high degree of technical demands and the possibility of extrusion of the graft. However, using internal fixation devices probably can decrease this risk. Dural tears are more likely when this extensive exposure is undertaken, and scarring of the anterior portion of the dural sac is more common.

Historically, the indications for and role of anterior spinal surgery of the lumbar spine have been controversial. At present, the specific indications for ALIF include symptomatic post-traumatic kyphosis with or without neurologic sequelae, iatrogenic lumbar kyphosis (flatback syndrome), and painful lumbar degenerative scoliosis with disc disease. In addition, relative indications for anterior internal fixation and fusion include repair of failed posterior fusion, instability secondary to wide laminectomy and posterior decompression, high-grade spondylolisthesis or spondyloptosis, and spinal osteotomy [27].

ALIF has the same potential benefits as PLIF. First, the graft will be in compression, and there is a large area for fusion. In addition, more bone can be placed between the vertebral bodies in ALIF than in PLIF, and the disc height appears to be only temporarily increased. Other advantages include a reduced operative time and blood loss, non-interference with the potentially painful posterior elements of the lumbar spine, and avoidance of scarring within the spinal canal [1]. However, ALIF does have several drawbacks. First, it requires a separate incision. With a transperitoneal approach, there is risk of abdominal adhesions and incisional hernias. Damage to the major vessels is a rare complication. In males, ALIF also carries the risk of impotence or retrograde ejaculation. Isolated ALIF has also been associated with a high pseudoarthrosis rate. For this reason, we routinely combine anterior fusion with posterior intertransverse fusion, often under the same anesthesia, and with internal fixation. This combination achieves the maximum biomechanical stability, neural element decompression, and recruitment of motion segment bone-grafting surface area.

Anatomy and biomechanics of interbody fusion

Interbody fusions provide a logical solution to diseases of the intervertebral disc. The definition of "success" in spine care is controversial and can vary from the perspectives of the patient, family, employer, insurance company, attorney, primary care physician, and the treating surgeon. A fusion is often considered "clinically" successful if (a) there is increased or maintained bone density within the cage implant due to the presence of mature bony trabeculae bridging the interbody space, (b) there is an absence of a "halo" around the implant (resorption), (c) there is a sclerotic line between the cage and vertebral endplate, due to bone remodeling and new bone formation, (d) resorption of anterior vertebral traction spurs or anterior progression of the graft within the disc space occurs, and (e) there is a lack of movement on flexion/extension views [16]. Pseudoarthrosis, or failure of fusion, is suggested by persistent pain, progression of deformity, loss of disc height, vertebral displacement, hardware failure, haloing,

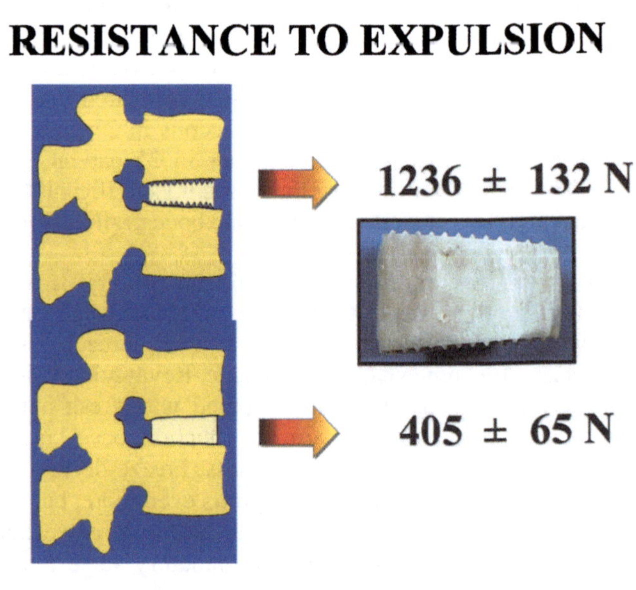

Fig. 2 The "teeth" on the femoral ring allograft (FRA) increase the resistance to implant pullout

migrations, or resorption of the bone graft with movement on flexion/extension views.

The FRA/PLIF biological cages are innovative lumbar interbody allografts, manufactured by the Musculoskeletal Transplant Foundation in conjunction with SYNTHES Spine. They come in a variety of sizes to precisely fit the disc space of each individual patient. Each FRA/PLIF spacer is machined from allograft into a wedge-shaped ring with "teeth." The teeth grip the adjacent vertebrae, thereby increasing the stability of the spacer (Fig. 2). The FRA spacer also has a hollow center that can be filled with autograft, allograft bone filler, a synthetic bone substitute, or bone morphogenic protein (BMP). This "bone void filler" may enhance or accelerate the biological fusion process of the spacer. An ideal implant must be capable of withstanding the axial compressive forces of the body. In addition, it must be able to displace the compressive force without inducing a great deal of motion in the adjacent segment while also promoting arthrodesis [20].

The anterior column of the spine absorbs 80% of axial compressive force, while the posterior structures absorb the remaining 20%. A study by Brown and colleagues [3] of motion segments of the lumbar region with static compressive loads indicated that the first component to fail was the vertebral body. This occurred as a result of the fractured endplates. These findings suggest that the vertebral body's strength is dependent on intact endplates.

Tests were conducted on the PLIF and FRA spacers to ensure that they could withstand the loads on the lumbar spine. The ultimate compressive strength of a vertebral body is 8000 N [25]. Test results show that the PLIF and FRA spacers have a compressive strength of over 25,000 N. A successful interbody fusion will restore every mechanical function of the functional spinal unit except motion. The bone graft must bear substantially all of the body's weight above the fusion level(s) while it is being incorporated [4]. The goal of any spinal fusion procedure is to maintain the correction, avoid hardware or graft failure, and obtain a solid fusion.

In addition to compressive strength, resistance to implant expulsion is a major factor in the design of intervertebral spacers. The PLIF spacer is designed with "saw teeth" to increase resistance to pullout. Pullout testing was conducted to ensure that the spacer was able to resist expulsion. The maximum shear force that a human disc can withstand is about 150 N [29]. An axial preload (450 N) [29] and a shear load were applied to the implant to determine the pullout strength. The results show that the PLIF spacer has a pullout strength of (1053±80 N), more than three times the pullout strength of a comparable design without teeth (234±38 N). Testing was conducted on the FRA spacer to ensure that it was capable of resisting expulsion at clinically relevant loads. The resistance of the implant being expelled from the disc space was determined by pushout testing. A clinically relevant load (450 N) [29] and side load was applied to the implant to increase resistance to pushout. Test results show that the FRA spacer has a pushout strength (1236±132 N) three times that of a comparable femoral wedge (405±65 N).

Biological fusion cages

Over the years, many variations of fusion cages have been invented to facilitate the fusion process while maintaining stability of the spine. Metal cages are widely utilized for anterior column reconstruction, with the goal of achieving spinal arthrodesis. The disadvantages of these metallic cages include subsidence and the inability to assess the "biology" of the intervertebral segment. Other potential problems include sizing of the implant, loosening, migrations, and theoretical metallic ion absorption [23]. In the last few years, several interbody cages of different designs have been developed for use through an anterior and posterior approach. The aim was to provide mechanical support to the segment being fused with biocompatible implant material and to allow the use of autogenous bone to promote fusion. Theoretically, these new biological implants give more lasting restoration of disc height and better stabilization to the spine.

There are five processes involved in the incorporation of the graft. The first stage of the graft is the inflammatory process, which occurs within hours after implantation. Inflammation is followed by revascularization, osteogenesis, remodeling, and finally mechanical stability [14]. During the inflammatory stage, the body's defenses elicit an immune response, causing inflammatory cells such as neutrophils and fibroblasts to invade the graft [14]. Rejection of the graft often occurs during revascularization where the host is highly sensitive to the graft's antigen [14]. During revascularization, possible complications may occur, including graft necrosis and occlusion of the host vessels. Osteogenesis, the synthesis of new bone by the host, begins shortly after the immediate postoperative period. This process involves the mesenchymal cells proliferating and eventually differentiating into chondrocytes and later into osteoblasts. "Osteoconduction" refers to the graft's ability to induce osteogenesis, which can persist for several months following surgery. Remodeling and mechanical stability follow, producing a functional and efficient graft [12]. Because allografts are capable of eliciting a more aggressive immune response, freeze-drying, cryopreservation, and other preservation techniques are used to delay the inflammatory and revascularization process.

Surgical technique and clinical outcomes

Femoral ring allograft spacer

The FRA spacer instruments are designed for use with this "biological cage" for a straight anterior or anterolat-

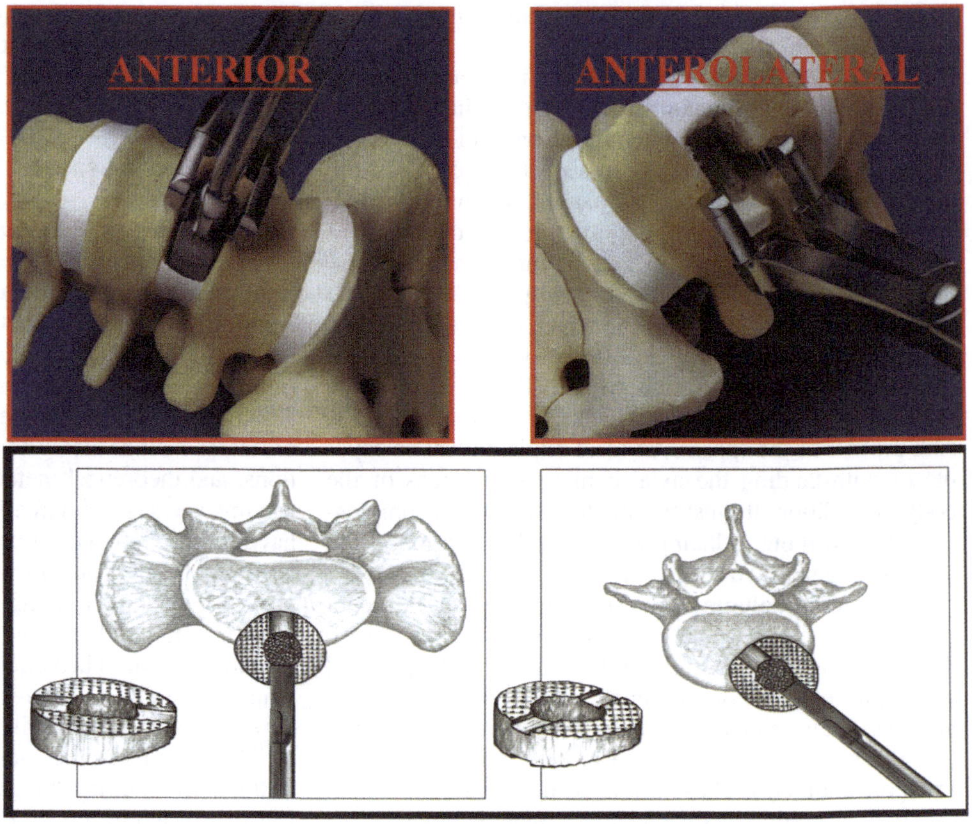

Fig. 3 Anterior and anterolateral approach using a femoral ring allograft (FRA) spacer

eral approach (Fig. 3). A preoperative planner can aid in determining the size of the adjacent intervertebral discs and allow the implant to be firmly seated with a secure fit between the endplates.

For a direct anterior insertion/approach, the midline of the intervertebral disc is exposed and evacuated with removal of the superficial layers of the cartilaginous endplates to expose the bleeding bone (Fig. 4a,b). Adequate preparation is essential to facilitate the vascular supply to the biological cage. Distractor blades are inserted into the disc space to restore the disc height, open the neural foramen, and stabilize the biological cage (Fig. 4a,b). The implant size is determined using the trial spacers. The implant corresponding to the correct trial spacer (Fig. 4c) is prepared, and bone graft material (either autograft, demineralized bone matrix, bone morphogenic protein, or allograft) can be inserted into and around the biological implant and in contact with the endplates (Fig. 4d) [19].

For an anterolateral insertion/approach, the center of the implant and the distractor sit 30° offset from the anterior vertebral midline. This approach is commonly used at the L2–L5 vertebral segments and requires less soft tissue dissection and mobilization of vascular midline structures. The anterior longitudinal ligament need not be sacrificed in this approach. The trial size and biological cage are inserted at a 30° offset from the midline (Fig. 3).

A total of 179 FRA cages were utilized for anterior column reconstruction in 137 patients from March 1998 to July 2000. There were 89 men and 48 women. The age range of the patients was from 19 to 73 years, with the average age being 45 years. Sixty-five patients from this group also exhibited co-morbidities including smoking (n=46), obesity (defined as >20% of the ideal body weight, n=12), and diabetes (n=7) (Table 1).

The most common preoperative diagnoses were internal disc disruption with disc resorptive syndrome, instability/spondylolisthesis, recurrent disc herniation with instability, degenerative scoliosis, vertebral osteomyelitis, and previous posterolateral arthrodesis that required additional anterior column support. Anterior "stand-alone" devices were used in about 25% (33/137) of the patients, while the majority of the patients (104/137) had additional posterior instrumentation. Additional posterior pedicle screw fixation was utilized in 49 patients, and translaminar screws (n=55) were more frequently used (Table 2). The additional posterior instrumentation in general is widely accepted by orthopedic surgeons to provide rigidity, improve fusion rates, reduce postoperative morbidity, and correct deformity [27]. Pedicle screws were used in patients who had spondylolisthesis, instability, or previous wide decompressive procedures. Patients with pedicle screws more often reported increased myofascial pain most likely secondary to greater soft tissue dissection and surgical exposure. Translaminar screws can be inserted with less dissection and tend to result in less postoperative morbidity. However, there was no difference in the fusion

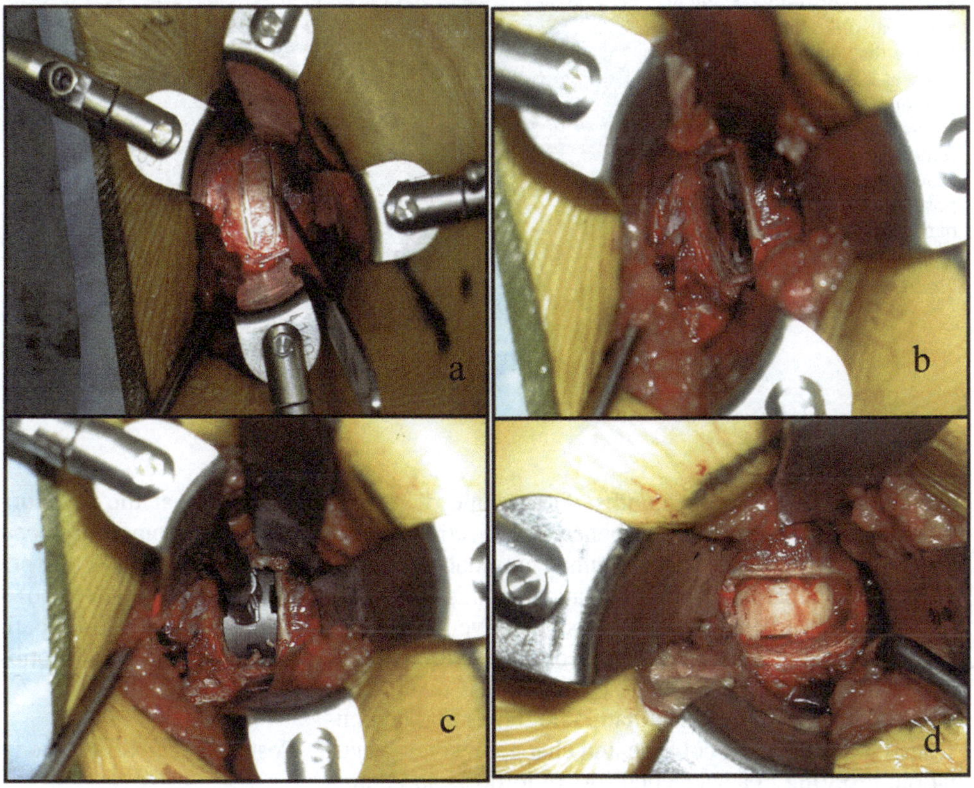

Fig. 4a–d Surgical technique using a femoral ring allograft (FRA) spacer

Table 1 Patient characteristics

	FRA spacer (n=137)	PLIF spacer (n=13)
Mean age (years)	45	54
Females (n)	48	8
Males (n)	89	5
Smokers (n)	46	4
Obese patients (n)	12	0
Diabetic patients (n)	7	0

FRA, femoral ring allograft; PLIF, posterior lumbar interbody fusion.

rate whether pedicle screws or translaminar screws were used in this series.

The majority of the patients (n=98) received one biological FRA spacer, while 39 required two-level biological cages, and only one patient received three-level implants (Table 2). The most common motion segment fused was L5–S1. Patients had either autograft (n=117) taken from the patient's iliac crest, demineralized bone matrix (n=13), or some other graft material (n=2) packed into and around the FRA spacer to promote a biological environment for arthrodesis. No differences in fusion rates were observed in patients that received autogenous bone versus patients with demineralized bone matrix. Additional postoperative orthosis was not indicated in any of the anterior column support patients. The radiographic outcomes were favorable for the majority (94%) of the patients and therefore demonstrate that arthrodesis was achieved with the biological bone spacer (Fig. 5a–c). These results support the theory that additional posterior column fixation predictably achieves a greater incidence of successful anterior interbody fusion. The longest follow-up in this series of patients was 36 months, with an

Table 2 Method of arthrodesis

	ALIF alone (n=33)	ALIF with posterior fusion (n=104)	PLIF with posterior fusion (n=13)
FRA spacers (n)	35	144	–
PLIF spacers (n)	–	–	30
Pedicle screw fixation (n)	0	49	12
Translaminar screw fixation (n)	0	55	1
One-level fusion (n)	27	71	11
Two-level fusion (n)	4	35	2
Three-level fusion (n)	0	1	0

ALIF, anterior lumbar interbody fusion; PLIF, posterior lumbar interbody fusion.

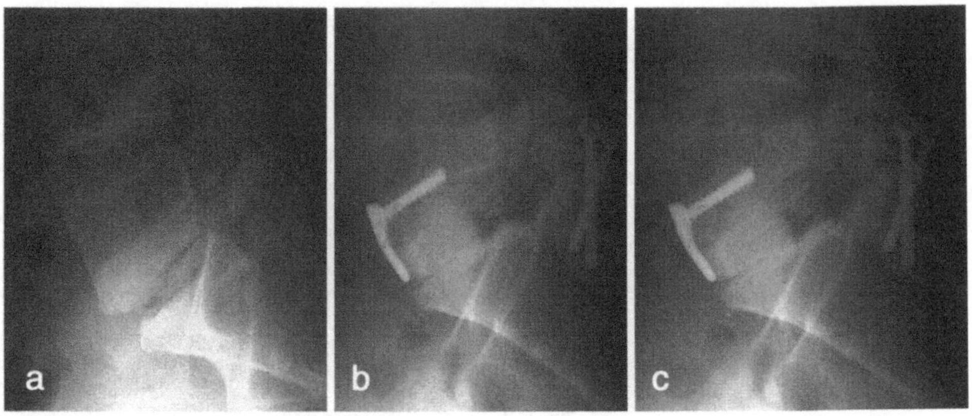

Fig. 5 **a** Preoperative X-ray of a 40-year-old man with degenerative disc disease and instability at L5–S1. **b** X-ray (1 month after surgery) of an anterior interbody fusion with femoral ring allograft (FRA) spacer insertion in addition to posterior fusion with translaminar screw fixation. **c** X-ray 6 months after surgery showing successful fusion with the FRA spacer in L5–S1

average follow-up of 18 months. At the time of review, there had been no evidence of bone graft rejection/resorption, migration, or infection (human immunodeficiency virus, HIV; hepatitis). Only one patient in this series had to be revised early, because of a postoperative radiculopathy that was felt to be secondary to over-distention resulting in neuropraxia to the right S1 nerve that resolved in about 6 months. One patient had radiographs that demonstrated a L4–L5 graft collapse and change in screw angulation, resulting in a segmental loss of lordosis and deformity.

Three patients requiring an anterior interbody fusion had clinical failure of the intradiscal electrothermal therapy (IDET) procedure, and in one patient pseudoarthrosis was suspected (on plain radiographs) but solid arthrodesis was confirmed on additional imaging techniques (CT scan) (Fig. 6). Five patients treated solely with the anterior approach required additional posterior fusions with instrumentation (5/33), secondary to either persistent pain, lucency of the implant, or motion with dynamic X-rays. Intra-operative fracture of the implant (the smallest size) occurred early in the series in five patients. These patients required removal of the fractured biological spacer and replacement at the time of the initial surgical procedure. This most commonly occurred when the trial spacer was not inserted completely prior to the implant or there was a geometrical mismatch of the endplates to the biological cage. No remaining patients demonstrated any radiographic evidence of motion or failure of consolidations.

Posterior lumbar interbody fusion spacer

The PLIF spacer is a contoured, wedge-shaped cortical allograft that comes in five anterior heights: 9–17 mm, in 2-mm increments. The surface of the spacer contains a saw-tooth pattern on the superior and inferior surfaces to minimize migration (Fig. 1). Two implants are inserted into the same disc height to ensure maximum stabilization.

There are two major techniques that may be used to distract, size, and insert the implants: distraction with the PLIF distractor or distraction with the PLIF trial spacer. The surgical technique used depends on the patient's local anatomy, the pathology, and the surgeon's preference [19]. The majority of the posterior elements, including the

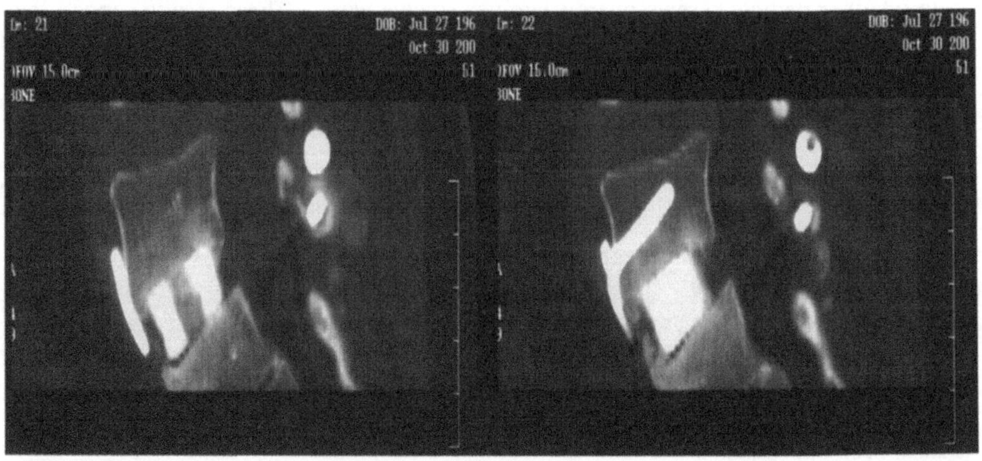

Fig. 6 A 35-year-old woman had a femoral ring allograft (FRA) spacer in which pseudoarthrosis was suspected on plain films. However, this computed tomography (CT) scan showed that the patient had a solid fusion at the level of surgery

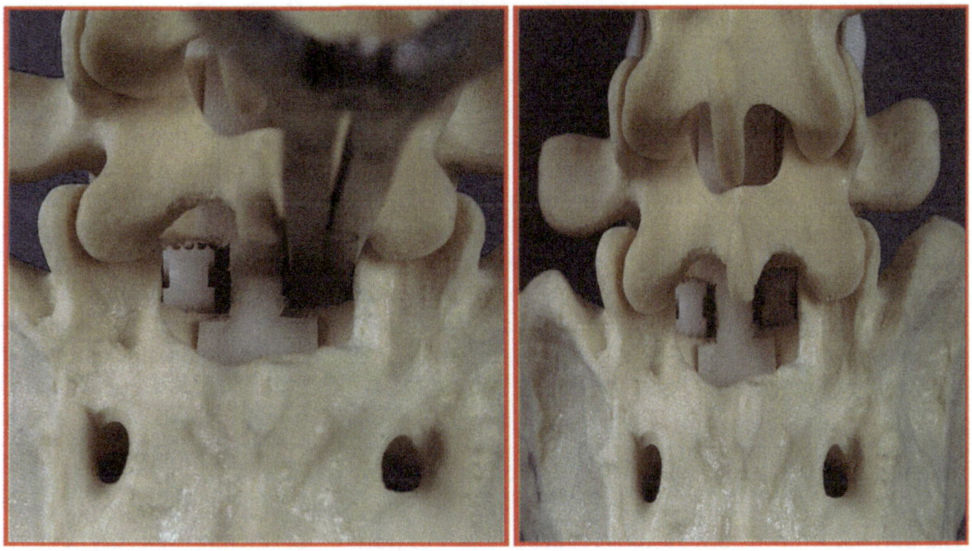

Fig. 7 Surgical technique using a posterior lumbar interbody fusion (PLIF) spacer

facets, do not have to be sacrificed for delivery of this geometry of biological implants (Fig. 7). The PLIF trial spacer ensures accurate sizing of the PLIF spacer. Once the site has been prepared for device insertion, the PLIF distractor blades are inserted completely into the disc space so that the ridges at the end of the blade rest on the vertebral body and are lateral to the dura. The PLIF distractor distracts the vertebrae to obtain maximum implant height, while the PLIF trial spacer is inserted into the contralateral disc space to ensure the accurate sizing of the PLIF spacer. Fluoroscopy and tactile judgment can assist in confirming the fit and placement of the trail spacer. If the trial spacer is either too loose or too tight, the next size is used to achieve the desired secure fit. Once the correct sizing is obtained, the trial spacer can be removed and the biological implant is introduced (using the implant holder) in the correct orientation into the contralateral disc space (Fig. 7). Autogenous cancellous bone or bone substitute (demineralized bone matrix, BMP, or allograft) is also placed in the anterior and medial aspect of the vertebral disc space *prior* to placement of the second implant.

For the surgical technique utilizing the PLIF trial spacer, it is necessary to begin with the trial spacer determined during preoperative planning. It is first inserted horizontally and then rotated vertically to size and distract the disc space. The implant corresponding to the correct trial spacer is chosen and introduced in the correct orientation into the contralateral disc space. The trial spacer is removed and the second implant is inserted. It is advisable to recess the implant 2–4 mm beyond the posterior rim of the vertebral body [19]. Additional posterior instrumentation may also be used to enhance the fusion rate and decrease the risk of anterior column allograft migration.

Thirty implants were inserted into 13 patients between January 1999 and July 2000. Five were men and eight were women, ranging in age from 32 to 70 years (average age, 54 years) (Table 1). The follow-up on these preliminary patients averaged 18 months (range, 6–24 months). The indications for surgical implantation included recurrent disc herniation, spondylolisthesis with foraminal stenosis, and instability. The most common levels fused were L4–L5 and L5–S1. All of the patients were treated

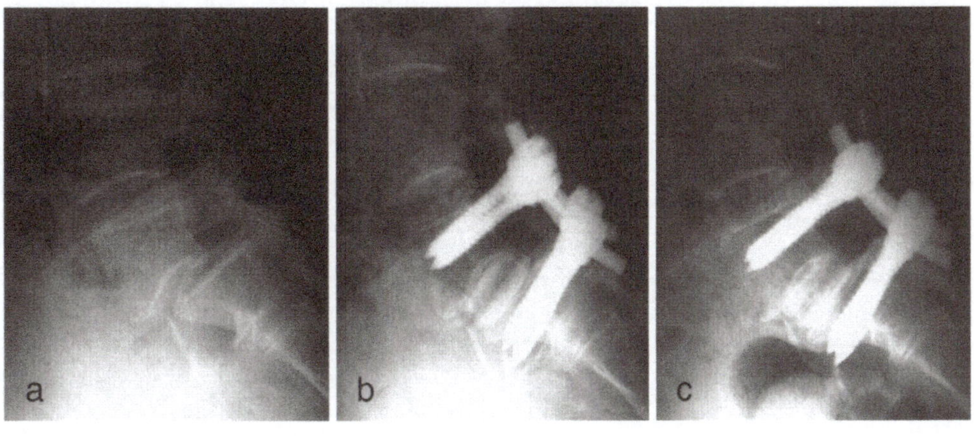

Fig. 8 **a** Preoperative X-ray of a 69-year-old woman with spondylolisthesis, instability, and bilateral pars fracture. **b** X-ray (1 month after surgery) of a posterior interbody fusion with posterior lumbar interbody fusion (PLIF) spacer insertion and pedicle screw fixation. **c** X-ray 6 months after surgery showing a successful fusion with the PLIF spacer in L5–S1

with additional posterior segmental instrumentation including pedicle screw fixation (n=12) or translaminar screw fixation (n=1) (Table 2). In this series of patients, there were four (33%) smokers, but results did not show any differences in the fusion rates of smokers versus nonsmokers. There were no additional co-morbidities observed in this selected patient population (Table 1). One patient developed anterior migration of a single PLIF spacer that required revision and an anterior approach and reconstruction, with a good clinical outcome. The clinical outcome of this posterior device is promising, with minimal incidence of migration, dislodgment, infection, pseudoarthrosis, or iatrogenic instability (Fig. 8a–c).

Discussion

The purpose of interbody fusions (either anterior or posterior) are to decrease motion and increase function in relation to the existing pathology. Unfortunately, these are difficult parameters to measure objectively because people have different ways of evaluating pain and their perceptions of realistic goals from a spine surgical procedure. The criteria we used to evaluate our results were therefore based on radiographic fusions because they offered the most objective evaluation. Mature fusion appears on X-rays films at a postoperative interval of 6–9 months (Fig. 9a–c).

The combined anterior and posterior column reconstruction used in this study seemed to produce better success rates than those obtained by "stand-alone" anterior interbody arthrodesis. Previous studies have shown that, in general, the technical success rate (indicated by obtaining fusion) is greater than the clinical success rate (indicated by decrease in pain) [7, 11, 28]. Although the radiographic fusion rates in the current study were higher than 90%, the clinical results were variable and often influenced by such factors as litigation, co-morbidities, disability, and secondary gain issues.

Our results were consistent with Brodke et al. [2] and Enker and Steffee [9] that concurrent use of instrumentation increases interbody fusion success by increasing rigidity at the fusion site. Pedicle screw fixation restores segmental stability and minimizes graft retropulsion. Lorenz and coworkers [22] reported 100% fusion for posterolateral fusion with segmental pedicle screw fixation, compared with 58.6% without instrumentation. Laminar-based systems have also been employed to enhance fusion rates. In comparing laminar- and pedicle-based instrumentation systems, Gurr et al. [15] demonstrated superior axial, torsional, and flexural rigidity with pedicle-based segmental instrumentation systems. Although pedicle

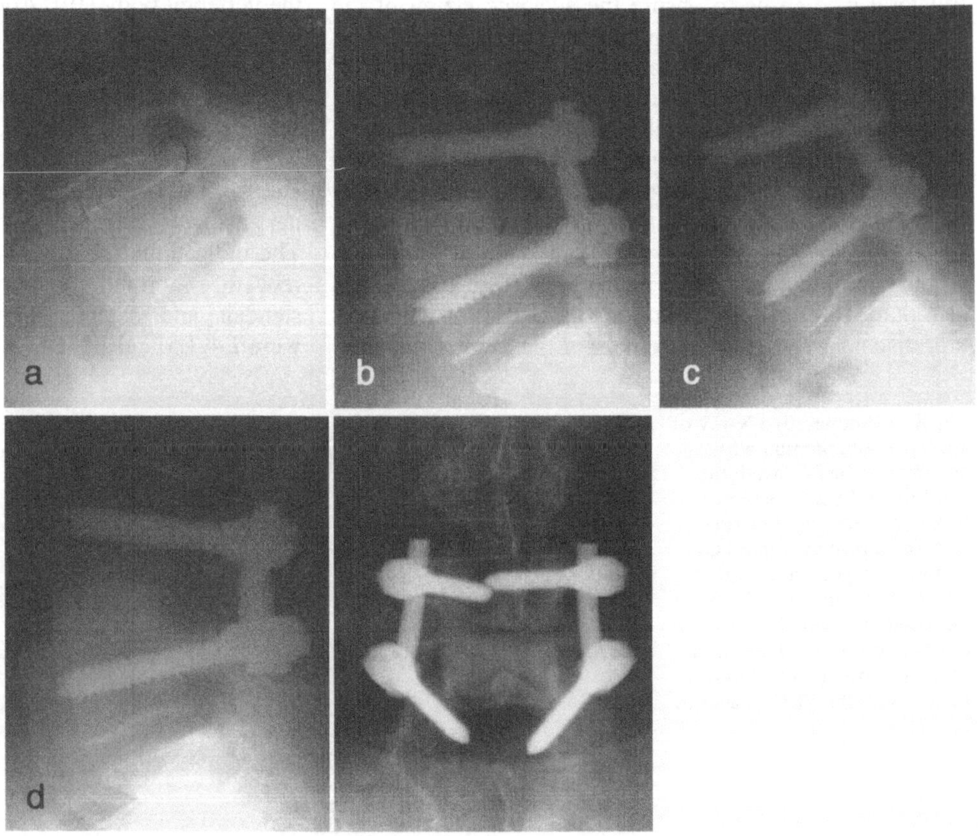

Fig. 9 **a** Preoperative X-ray of a 59-year-old woman with degenerative disk disease, L4–L5 facet arthropathy, and spondylolisthesis. **b** 24-month lateral view X-ray of a femoral ring allograft (FRA) spacer in L4–L5 with pedicle screw fixation. **c** 24-month flexion view. **d** 36-month extension and anteroposterior views

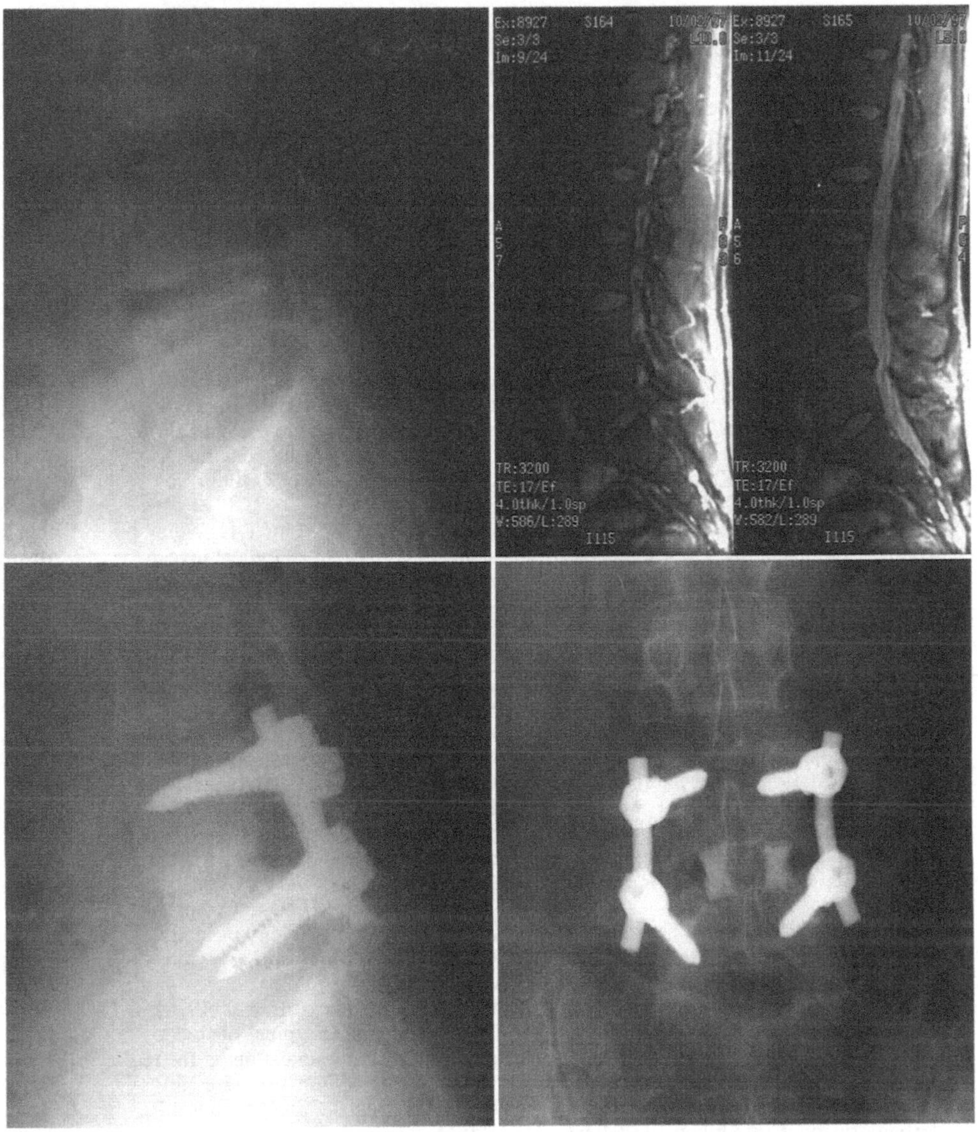

Fig. 10 Both of these implants facilitate preservation of the endplates and anatomic restoration of the sagittal alignment to provide the optimal "biological" environment to obtain arthrodesis

screws are proven to be more effective for stabilization in patients with degenerative disc disease or instability, our results do not show any differences in fusion rates between the pedicle and translaminar screws. However, for the treatment of spondylolisthesis or Par's defect, the pedicle screws were equally successful when used with FRA spacers or PLIF spacers (Fig. 10).

In a study carried out by Loguidice and colleagues [21], nonsmokers had a 14% incidence of pseudoarthrosis. Those smoking up to one pack per day had a 17% incidence of pseudoarthrosis, while those smoking more than one pack per day had a 36% incidence of pseudoarthrosis. However, the 50 smokers in our study who had either anterior or posterior interbody arthrodesis did not exhibit a greater incidence of pseudoarthrosis than the nonsmokers.

The success of every spine fusion procedure hinges on the biological phenomenon of bone healing. Whether this biological process occurs, however, is dependent on many factors. The extent of the instability problem being addressed, type of bone graft chosen, type of surgical construct created, and even the patient's own anatomy and lifestyle can affect the success of a fusion procedure. Although a number of studies have examined the outcome of interbody fusions, the results of many studies have been contradictory. It needs to be realized that there are many varieties of surgical techniques and healing processes, and expected outcomes may vary considerably regardless of recent research.

Conclusion

Bone has been used in a variety of shapes and configurations for interbody reconstruction for decades. More recently, the preparation and machining of allograft bone allows it to be used and to function similarly to other metal mechanical spacers. FRA and PLIF biological cages are designed along with a set of instruments that allow the surgeon to perform these procedures using a minimally invasive approach. Both of these implants facilitate preservation of the endplates and anatomic restoration of the sagittal alignment to provide the optimal "biological" environment in order to obtain arthrodesis (Figs. 9a-c, 10).

This biological process of fusion can be monitored with conventional techniques, unlike common metallic anterior column implants. Our clinical experience in these 150 patients is encouraging. Future development of additional BMP may increase the arthrodesis rate, reduce the time to consolidation, and alter the need for rigid posterior instrumentation.

References

1. Bridwell KH, Dewald RL et al (eds) (1991) Degenerative conditions. The textbook of spinal surgery. Lippincott, Philadelphia
2. Brodke DS, Dick JC, Kunz DN, McCabe R, Zdeblick TA (1997) Posterior lumbar interbody fusion: a biomechanical comparison, including a new threaded titanium cage. Spine 22: 26–31
3. Brown T, Hanson R, Yorra A (1957) Some mechanical tests on the lumbosacral spine with particular reference to the Intervertebral discs. J Bone Joint Surg [Am] 39:1135
4. Brantigan JW, Cunnigham BW et al (1993) Compression strength of donor bone for posterior lumbar interbody fusion. Spine 18:1213–1221
5. Buttermann GR, Glazer PA, Bradford DS (1996) The use of bone allografts in the spine. Clin Orthop Rel Res 324: 75–85
6. Capner N (1932) Spondylolisthesis. Br J Surg 19:374–386
7. Carpenter CT, Dietz JW, Leung KYK et al (1996) Repair of pseudoarthrosis of the lumbar spine. J Bone Joint Surg [Am] 78:712–720
8. Collis JS (1995) Total disc replacement: a modified posterior lumbar interbody fusion. Clin Orthop 193:64–67
9. Enker P, Steffee AD (1994) Interbody fusion and instrumentation. Clin Orthop Rel Res 300:90–101
10. Evans JH (1985) Biomechanics of lumbar fusion. Clin Orthop 193:38–46
11. Franklin GM, Haug J, Heyer NJ et al (1994) Outcome of lumbar fusion in Washington State workers' compensation. Spine 19:1897–1904
12. Glowacki J (1991) Cellular responses to bone-derived materials. Bone and cartilage allografts: biology and clinical applications. Presented at the American Academy of Orthopedic Surgeons
13. Goel VK, Kim YE, Lim T-H, Weinstein JN (1989) An analytical investigation of the mechanics of spinal instrumentation. Spine 14:1003–1011
14. Goldberg VM, Stevenson S, Shaffer JW (1991) Biology of autografts and allografts. Bone and cartilage allografts: biology and clinical applications. Presented at the American Academy of Orthopedic Surgeons, pp 3–12
15. Gurr KR, McAfee PC, Shih C (1988) Biomechanical analysis of anterior and posterior instrumentation systems after corpectomy. J Bone Joint Surg 70 [Am]:1184
16. Hanley SD, Gun MT, Osti O, Shanahan EM (1999) Radiology of intervertebral cages in spinal surgery. Clin Radiol 54:201–206
17. Hodgson AR, Stock FE et al (1994) The classic anterior spinal fusion: a preliminary communication on the radical treatment of Pott's disease and Pott's paraplegia. Clin Orthop Rel Res 300.16–23
18. Hutter CG (1983) Posterior intervertebral body fusion: a 25-year study. Clin Orthop 179:86–96
19. Janssen ME, Nguyen C et al (2000) Biological cages. Eur Spine J 9:S102–S109
20. Kozak JA, Heilman AE et al (1994) Anterior lumbar fusion options: techniques and graft materials. Clin Orthop Rel Res 300:45–51
21. Loguidice VA, Johnson RG, Guyer RD, Stith WJ et al (1988) Anterior lumbar interbody fusion. Spine 13: 366–369
22. Lorenz M, Zindrick M, Schwaegler P et al (1991) A comparison of single-level fusions with and without hardware. Spine 16:S455
23. Mankin HJ, Sell KW (eds) (1981) Osteochondral allografts: biology, banking, and clinical applications. Little Brown, New York
24. Mercer W (1936) Spondylolisthesis: with a description of a new method of operative treatment and of ten cases. Edinburgh Med J 43:545–527
25. Perry O (1957) Fracture of the vertebral endplate in the lumbar spine. Acta Orthop Scand [Suppl]
26. Postaccini F (1999) The lumbar spine in the 2000s. Spine (24)10:991–995
27. Schlegel J, Yuan HA, Fredrickson B (1991) Anterior interbody fixation devices. The adult spine: principals and practice. Raven, New York
28. West JL, Bradford DS, Ogilvie JW (1991) Results of spine arthrodesis with pedicle-screw fixation. J Bone Joint Surg [Am] 73:1179–1184
29. White AA, Panjabi MM (1990) Autogenic versus allogenic bone grafts in anterior lumbar interbody fusion. Clin Orthop 360:122–126
30. Younger EM, Chapman MW (1989) Morbidity at bone graft donor sites. J Orthop Trauma 3:192–195
31. Zindrick, MR, Selby, D: Lumbar spine fusion (1996) Different types and indications. In: Janssen ME, Larson A, Beckham R (eds) The lumbar spine, 2nd edn. Saunders, Philadelphia, pp 588–619

Sigurd Berven
Bobby K.B. Tay
Frank S. Kleinstueck
David S. Bradford

Clinical applications of bone graft substitutes in spine surgery: consideration of mineralized and demineralized preparations and growth factor supplementation

Abstract Bone graft substitutes may be broadly classified as mineralized and demineralized preparations. This article reviews the basic science and biology underlying each preparation. A review of the clinical and experimental applications of each preparation follows. The text concludes with a review of growth factors as biological supplements.

Keywords Allograft · Demineralized bone matrix · Ceramics · Growth factors · Spinal fusion

S. Berven (✉) · F.S. Kleinstueck
D.S. Bradford
Department of Orthopedic Surgery,
UC San Francisco,
500 Parnassus Avenue-MU320W,
San Francisco, CA 94143, USA
e-mail: bervens@orthosurg.ucsf.edu,
Tel.: +1-415-5142064,
Fax: +1-415-4761304

B.K.B. Tay
Division of Orthopedic Surgery,
San Francisco General Hospital and the
Veterans Administration Medical Center,
UCSF, San Francisco, CA 94143, USA

Introduction and background

Tissue and mineral grafts in the spine perform mechanical and biologic functions. Their capacity for each function is dependent upon the structural, cellular, and biochemical properties of the particular graft chosen. Autogenous bone offers an optimal balance of osteogenic, osteoinductive, and osteoconductive capacities, structural stability, and biocompatibility. However, the availability of autogenous bone graft is clearly limited, and the complications of autogenous harvest are well known [6, 16, 17, 19, 23, 29, 30, 36, 46, 78, 95]. In choosing bone graft substitutes for clinical application, the spine surgeon's decision generally involves a compromise of mechanical and biological functional considerations. This article will address the clinical applications of mineralized and demineralized bone graft preparations in spinal surgery, reviewing the basic science and clinical experience supporting the use of these substitutes.

A bone graft material is any implanted material that alone or in combination with other materials promotes a bone healing response by osteogenic, osteoconductive, or osteoinductive activity at a local site [56]. Graft material that is osteogenic contains viable cells at some stage of osteoblastic differentiation and is capable of forming new bone directly. Osteoinductive graft materials contain cytokines capable of inducing differentiation of host cells into bone forming cells. Osteoconductive graft materials provide a biocompatible matrix that supports new bone formation. Substitutes for autogenous bone graft may have variable capacities for each of these functions. In spinal surgery, the ideal bone graft substitute should be osteogenic, biocompatible, bioabsorbable, easy to use, and cost effective and should provide structural support. However, the success of a particular material in achieving these goals depends upon the material and biologic properties of the grafting material as well as the particular host environment in which it is placed.

Mineralized bone matrices

Bone is a composite tissue consisting of mineral and organic phases. While the mineral phase is primarily structural in function, the regulation of bone metabolism and turnover involves a complex interaction between these two phases. The inorganic component of bone is principally composed of a calcium phosphate mineral analogous to crystalline calcium hydroxyapatite [$Ca_{10}(PO_4)_6(OH)_2$]. Calcium hydroxyapatite exists as plate-like crystals approximately 20–80 nm long and 5 nm thick. The physical properties of apatite, including solubility and stiffness, are determined by its crystalline structure. Significant differences in the crystalline structure of mature bone, immature bone, and synthetic bone substitutes have been demonstrated by P^{32} MRI [94]. These differences, in turn, determine the biologic behavior of the material in the spinal fusion bed.

Mineralized bone matrices provide an osteoconductive matrix for new bone formation. In isolation, mineralized bone matrix has little osteoinductive or osteogenic potential. In situ, its osteoinductivity is dependent upon the biologic capacity of the host bed or the local environment [76]. The potential for osteogenesis relies on cellular and chemical contributions from the host bed. The principle determinants of host-graft union include stability of the construct, contact between host bone and graft, and vascularity of the graft bed. Factors that inhibit bone graft incorporation include histocompatibility mismatch and reduction of the biologic activity of the graft by processing.

The process of graft incorporation involves hemorrhage, inflammation, tissue revascularization, and substitution and remodeling of the graft with locally derived tissue. New bone formation occurs by a process of creeping substitution in which calcium phosphate cements are replaced by bone with normal organic and mineral phases. Resorption of the mineral component of the matrix may be variable. The resorption of implanted hydroxyapatite is dependent upon pore size, crystalline structure, and local host reaction [61]. Overall, mineralized bone matrices have the advantage of offering immediate structural support and, in unstable osseous defects, stabilization may contribute importantly to the creation of a microenvironment that promotes osteoneogenesis [3,86]. However, the mechanical strength and fatigue properties of the mineralized bone substitutes are generally inferior to those of cortical bone. Mineralized bone matrices used in spine surgery include allograft, corraline hydroxyapatite, and synthetic hydroxyapatite. The clinical use of each in spinal surgery will be reviewed below.

Allograft

Allograft is the most commonly used nonautogenous grafting material in spinal surgery, and 35% of all bone transplantations involve the use of human allograft tissues. Mineralized allograft is primarily osteoconductive, with weak osteoinductive capacity and no osteogenic potential because graft cells do not survive processing and transplantation. Allograft used for orthopedic applications is fresh-frozen, freeze-dried, or demineralized. The method of preparation has significant effects on graft strength, immunogenicity, capacity for incorporation, and potential for disease transmission. Fresh-frozen allografts retain much of their original mechanical strength, while freeze-drying can reduce graft strength up to 50% [37,66]. The freezing process also reduces immunogenicity of allografts [39,76].

The effect of immunogenicity in compromising graft incorporation may be significant [73, 72, 75,77]. Transmission of disease from donor to recipient is a problem with human allografts. The principle pathogens involved are human immunodeficiency virus (HIV) and hepatitis viruses B and C. The risk of disease transmission is determined by the rigor of screening procedures for donors and tissue, and the only cases of disease transmission in musculoskeletal allografts from the method of graft preparation to date have involved frozen, unprocessed grafts [82]. Tissue processing techniques include high pressure lavage to clear out marrow elements and donor cells and chemical treatments to eliminate viruses and reduce immunogenicity of the graft. The combination of donor screening, tissue testing, and tissue processing reduces the risk of viral transmission to less than one event per million grafts [5].

Allograft is available in many preparations. However, the majority are composed of primarily cancellous or cortical bone. Cortical allografts provide significant mechanical stability and structural support, while cancellous bone lends little mechanical stabilization on implantation but has a faster rate of incorporation. Cancellous allograft and particulate allograft preparations (cancellous or cortical) incorporate with new bone forming on the surfaces of trabeculae, with a large surface area available for new bone formation [7,74]. In contrast, cortical incorporation occurs slowly via a process of periosteal new bone formation around the allograft as an external callus derived from the host bone [28].

Particulate and structural grafts demonstrate significant differences in the histology of incorporation. Particulate grafts demonstrate more rapid and complete revascularization than structural grafts. Particulate bone remodels completely with time, while cortical bone remains a mixture of necrotic and viable bone. The process of creeping substitution is also differs significantly between these forms of allograft, with new bone formation occurring appositionally followed by resorption in cancellous bone, which process is reversed in cortical allografts [11]. These differences in biologic capacity between graft types lead to significant differences in optimal clinical applications.

The use of bone allografts in the spine has been reviewed previously by the senior author [12]. Structural cortical allografts are most useful in interbody arthrodesis of the lumbar and cervical spine, with low rates of graft subsidence or resorption. In revision lumbar surgery, tricortical allograft may be as effective as iliac crest in promoting anterior arthrodesis of the spine [13]. Crushed cortical or cancellous allograft may be useful as an autograft extender in posterior spinal fusion. In thoracolumbar deformity, cancellous allograft with instrumentation may give satisfactory results in the pediatric population but yields inferior results in adults. The conclusion from the senior author's experience is that successful use of allograft bone in the spine is dependent on the type of allograft bone used, the anatomic site of fusion, and patient age.

A review of other clinical applications of allograft compared with autogenous bone in spinal surgery is useful. In cervical spine, the use of allograft vs autograft has been debated since the first anterior discectomies and interbody fusions. Smith and Robinson used autogenous iliac crest graft and reported radiographic union in 18/21 patients [71]. Concurrently, Cloward reported resorption of only 3/46 grafts using his dowel technique with fresh-frozen allograft [18]. More recent reviews demonstrated similar fusion rates using autogenous and allogenous grafts in single level cervical surgery but significant differences in multilevel cervical fusions [38, 96,98].

In posterolateral arthrodesis of the lumbar spine, differences in function between allograft and autograft are more significant. In a prospective comparison of autograft and allograft preparations in posterolateral arthrodesis of the spine, differences in fusion mass were radiographically clearly apparent, reliable arthrodesis being achieved with autograft, followed by mixed autograft and allograft, and frozen allograft, and the least reliable graft material was freeze-dried allograft [1]. Similarly, a prospective evaluation of mineralized and demineralized allograft mixed with autogenous bone radiographically demonstrated fusion inferior to that from posterolateral arthrodesis with iliac autograft [44].

In summary, cortical allografts provide a useful structural matrix that is osteoconductive and has limited osteoinductivity. Cortical allografts are less likely than cancellous allograft to incorporate with adjacent host bone, but outcome and fusion rates in anterior lumbar and single level cervical applications are comparable to those with autogenous graft. Cancellous bone is useful as a graft extender in posterolateral arthrodesis of the spine but is an unreliable substitute in instrumented thoracolumbar deformity, especially in adults.

Ceramic matrices

Ceramic matrices include inorganic, ionically bonded preparations that mimic the mineral phase of bone [80]. Ceramic preparations that have been used in spinal reconstructive surgery include hydroxyapatite, tricalcium phosphate (TCP), and combinations of the two. Early formulations of hydroxyapatite used as bone void fillers were sintered by heating the precipitate at temperatures reaching or exceeding 1100°C. Products such as Pro-Osteon and Interpore are hydroxyapatite lattices created from a coralline scaffold. They are created by heating the calcium carbonate skeleton of coral in the presence of an aqueous phosphate solution that drives the exchange of the calcium carbonate of the coral with a calcium phosphate replica. The coral species *Porites astreoides* was chosen because of its theoretically ideal pore size for the ingrowth of bone. On electron microscopic examination, the average pore size of *Porites astreoides* was found to be 153.95±25.36 μm [61,62].

Ceramic matrices provide a biocompatible osteoconductive surface for bone regeneration and may contribute limited structural support [14,43]. Advantages of ceramic matrices include low immunogenicity and toxicity, stability at physiologic pH levels, and the ability to withstand sterilization procedures without losing structural integrity. While the organic phase of bone confers bone stiffness and compressive strength, ceramics are inherently brittle and susceptible to fracture, with elasticity moduli significantly higher than those of cortical and cancellous bone, and with low tensile strength. Bone mineral is distinct from the synthetic or geologic mineral hydroxyapatite. Although the overall crystal structure and composition of bone apatite is similar to that of hydroxyapatite [$Ca_{10}(PO_4)_6(OH)_2$], the former displays highly significant functional differences concerning crystal size, short-range order, and the presence of carbonate (CO_3^{-2}) and acid phosphate (HPO_4^{-2}) [93]. This may explain differences observed in remodeling and resorption of synthetic apatite matrices used in spinal arthrodesis. Overall, more crystallization and higher mineral density yield greater mechanical strength and lasting stability. In contrast, an amorphous, simple preparation of calcium phosphate and calcium sulfate may also provide an osteoconductive matrix useful as a bone graft extender in spinal fusion while retaining a rate of resorption that equals the rate of formation. Optimal remodeling of the spinal fusion mass is dependent upon biodegradability of the ceramic, which, depending on the crystalline structure and composition, may take from several months to several years.

There are several currently used preparations of ceramic matrices that differ in biological and mechanical characteristics. Calcium sulfate and calcium phosphate are purely osteoconductive, with resorption profiles closely matching the rate at which new bone is deposited. These materials are replaced by host bone through a process of creeping substitution. These materials exist in many different preparations including powders, pellets, putty, and injectable cements. Tricalcium phosphate [$Ca_3(PO_4)_2$] (TCP) has been used as a bone void filler. It has advantages similar to those of hydroxyapatite since it is biocompatible and bioabsorbable [25,31]. However, it is brittle, with very low impact resistance. Porous TCP contains micropores 3–5 nm in diameter and has compressive and tensile

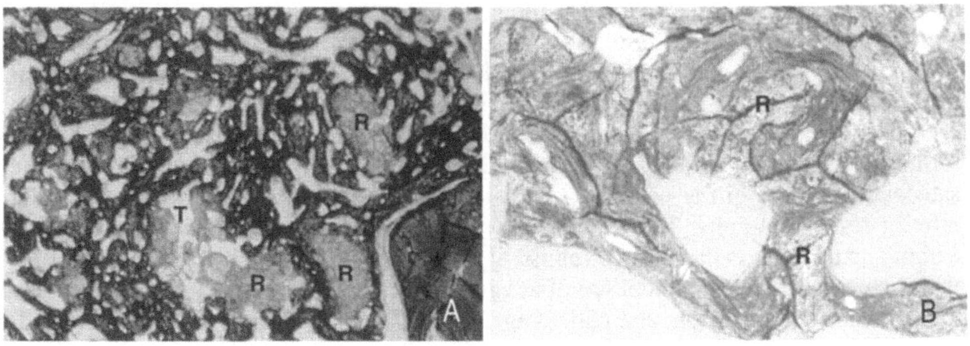

Fig. 1A, B Low (**A**) and high magnification (**B**) histologic sections of femoral slot defects filled with alpha-BSM (courtesy of ETEX)

strengths similar to but lower than those of cancellous bone [43]. It also dissolves more rapidly than hydroxyapatite, especially in an acidic milieu. Collagraft (Zimmer, Warsaw, Ind., USA) is a combination of TCP with hydroxyapatite and type 1 collagen.

Calcium phosphate cements that set in situ are now commercially available or in the final stages of U.S. Federal Drug Administration approval. These include SRS skeletal repair system (Norian, Cupertino, Calif., USA) and alpha-BSM (ETEX, Cambridge, Mass., USA). These calcium phosphate preparations have the advantage of excellent biocompatibility as well as in situ setting without shrinkage or generation of heat. The endothermic setting of these cements makes them ideal carriers for growth factors and cytokines.

The Norian SRS is a biocompatible and resorbable calcium phosphate cement combined from monocalcium phosphate, TCP, calcium carbonate, and a sodium phosphate solution mixed into an injectable paste. Under physiologic conditions, the material hardens within minutes into a dahllite (carbonated hydroxyapatite) in a nonexothermic reaction. It reaches 85–95% of completion within 12 h and has a final compressive strength of 55 MPa [42]. This material appears to offer significant mechanical integrity for the augmentation of fixation devices such as pedicle screws.

Alpha-BSM provides poorly crystalline calcium phosphate apatite with favorable absorption characteristics and easy intraoperative handling characteristics. It is composed of a calcium phosphate material that can be hydrated with saline to form a workable paste. This paste remains formable for hours at room temperature but hardens within 20 min at physiologic body temperature (37°C) and can be prepared to harden to a variety of compressive strengths (5–40 MPa). However, it is still significantly weaker than cortical bone. The poorly crystalline nature of the cement also closely mimics the mineral phase of bone, thus providing an excellent osteoconductive scaffold for cell-mediated absorption and remodeling into natural host bone (Fig. 1).

Clinical applications of ceramics in spinal surgery include animal and human studies. The application of ceramic matrices in animal models of spine fusion has demonstrated mixed results. In lumbar fusion in sheep, a ceramic composite containing 65% hydroxyapatite, 35% tricalcium phosphate, and type 1 bovine dermal collagen (Collagraft, Zimmer) demonstrated radiographic and histologic evidence of better fusion as a bone graft substitute than autogenous bone [88]. However, in a study on dogs, a similar preparation demonstrated union inferior to that of an equal volume of autogenous cancellous bone. In addition, the combination of collagen ceramic composite with autogenous cancellous bone graft significantly reduced the effectiveness of the autogenous bone graft [57]. Studies using arthrodesis in dogs demonstrate the importance of the local environment in promoting incorporation of ceramic matrices in spinal fusion. In one study with a biphasic material composed of 60% hydroxyapatite and 40% TCP, the biomechanical properties of the posterolateral fusion were equal to those with autograft and ceramic grafts, and the amount of new bone formation was related to contact area with bone and decortication of the host graft site [27]. In a study of anterior interbody arthrodesis in the canine thoracic spine, calcium carbonate graft led to arthrodesis that was significantly weaker biomechanically and histologically than with autograft. Internal fixation of the fused segment did, however, significantly improve revascularization and remodeling in both autograft and ceramic graft specimens [34].

In rabbits, the effectiveness of ceramic matrix grafts in promoting spinal arthrodesis was limited. A comparison of natural coral with autogenous bone in rabbit anterior interbody fusion demonstrated no signs of integration of the natural coral, with no evidence of fusion at 3 months. In contrast, autogenous graft promoted reliable arthrodesis [81]. In posterolateral arthrodesis in rabbits, coralline hydroxyapatite as an isolated graft material led to unreliable arthrodesis compared with autograft (Fig. 2). However, supplementation of the ceramic matrix with osteoinductive bone protein extract or with direct current electrical stimulation led to reliable spinal arthrodesis [8, 10, 79].

Although a recent study reported the utility of ceramics in spinal arthrodesis in adolescent idiopathic scoliosis, its efficacy in this situation is still a subject of controversy. In a prospective trial comparing ceramic matrix (porous biphasic calcium phosphate ceramic blocks comprised of

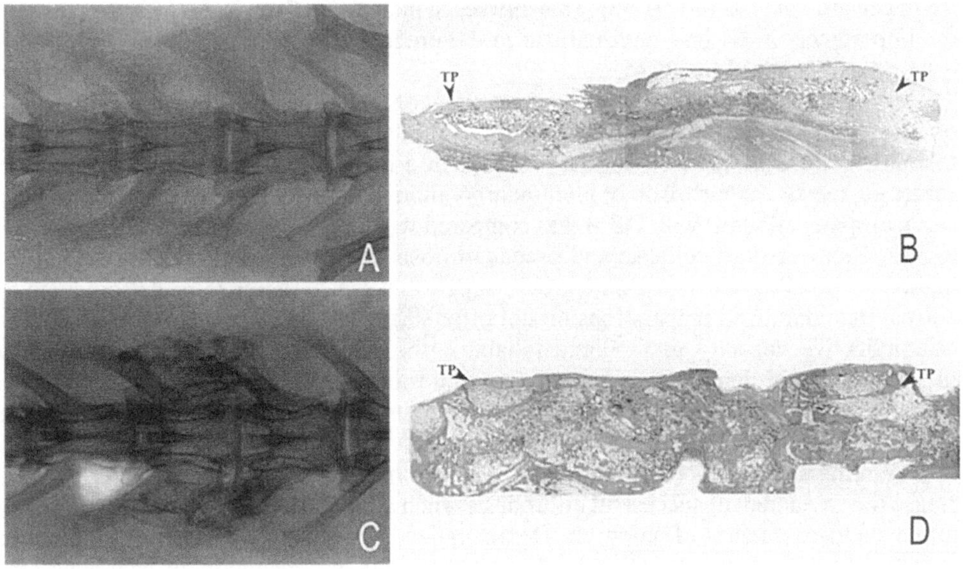

Fig. 2A–D The use of hydroxyapatite matrices in rabbit spinal fusion. **A** Commercially available collagen hydroxyapatite matrix placed in the intertransverse area of a rabbit spine showing no bony fusion at 8 weeks. **B** Sagittal histological cross-section with hematoxylin-eosin staining showing fibrous tissue interposition between the decorticated transverse processes and no evidence of fusion. **C** Autogenous iliac crest graft placed in the intertransverse area showing solid fusion at 8 weeks. **D** Sagittal histological cross-section of the fusion area with hematoxylin-eosin showing a mature cortical rim

hydroxyapatite and TCP) with autograft alone, fusion rates were similar at 1 year, and donor site morbidity and blood loss were lower in the ceramic group [27]. However, these results must be interpreted with caution. In the cases of adolescent scoliosis treated with spinal fusion, the ceramic was used as a bone graft extender to supplement the local bone used for graft materials. In addition, the patient population studied in this trial has a high propensity to healing, even without the addition of bone grafts. As thoracoplasty is used more routinely for correcting the rib hump deformity in children with scoliosis, sufficient bone can be obtained from the resected ribs to eliminate the need for iliac crest bone. This virtually eliminates the morbidity associated with graft harvest from that site. Thus, the utility of ceramics as bone graft extenders in the surgical treatment of children with adolescent idiopathic scoliosis is questionable.

The variability of clinical results for arthrodesis may be related to variance in local environment (segmental stability, exposed bone) and to the significant variation in biological properties (pore size, osteophilicity, resorbability) of the different ceramic preparations. The tissue surrounding the ceramic matrix is the most important determinant of the kinetics of graft incorporation, as this material has weak osteophilic properties and lacks the capacity for osteoinduction [26]. Enhancement of the local environment for osteoneogenesis, including segmental stabilization, optimizing the supply of osteogenic cells, providing osteoinductive material, and possibly adding electrical stimulation, enhances the effectiveness of ceramic matrices in promoting spinal arthrodesis. It is clear that both host and donor cells contribute to the formation of the final fusion mass [35]. Despite the presence of an adequate osteoinductive and osteoconductive environment, the lack of sufficient numbers of osteoprogenitor cells will adversely affect formation of the fusion mass. Further work is needed to determine the optimal biologic characteristics of ceramic matrices with regard to mechanical stability and resorbability [69]. Ceramic composites consisting of an osteoconductive ceramic matrix and an osteoinductive substance (autograft, DBM, growth factors, electrical current) may offer the most effective graft material for promoting arthrodesis [9].

Demineralized bone matrices

The osteoinductive factors of bone are contained within the organic phase. While mineralized matrices have minimal osteoinductive activity, demineralized preparations have demonstrated a potent effect on the differentiation of osteoprogenitor cells into osteoblasts. Marshall Urist first identified a bone morphogenetic substance in his pioneering work using soluble extracts from demineralized bone [84]. The demonstration of osteoneogenesis in response to ectopic submuscular implants of demineralized bone was pivotal in further identification and cloning of the identified bone morphogenetic proteins [93]. De novo bone formation in ectopic, submuscular sites has become the standard means of assessing molecules with bone morphogenetic activity. The capacity of demineralized bone matrix (DBM) to induce new bone formation is well established [83,85]. The primary osteoinductive component of DBM consists of small amounts of glycoproteins in the organic phase of bone, the most important of which are the bone morphogenetic proteins. The major pathway of osteoneogenesis induced by DBM is endochondral in subcutaneous and submuscular implants and by direct induction of resident mesenchymal stem cells to osteoblasts and direct formation of bone without a cartilaginous intermediate in calvarial defects [90, 91,92]. This difference indicates the importance of the host environment in the process of osteogenesis induced by DBM.

Despite animal data suggesting a positive effect of DBM on spinal fusions, the clinical utilization of DBM in spinal fusion has not demonstrated similar efficacy. In a multicenter prospective comparison of graft incorporation in the cervical spine, allograft with DBM was compared with autograft. Rates of graft collapse and pseudoarthrosis were higher in the allograft with DBM group, suggesting that current demineralized preparations do not offer sufficient osteoinductive capacity to facilitate reliable arthrodesis [2]. The utility of demineralized matrix gel in posterolateral lumbar spinal fusion was demonstrated in rabbits. The DBM appeared more effective than frozen allograft alone in promoting arthrodesis [58]. However, DBM did not increase the frequency of successful arthrodesis when added to the standard amount of autograft. Demineralized bone matrix preparations may be effective as graft extenders in the setting of limited autograft [53] and as graft enhancers when comparing fusion quality to that with autograft alone [50]. A role for DBM as a graft extender was further supported by results of a dog study [33]. In other studies on dogs, DBM has not been shown useful in promoting spinal arthrodesis. Cook et al. demonstrated that DBM alone or in combination with allograft did not produce reliable spinal arthrodesis [22] and may have an inhibitory effect on arthrodesis of the spine compared with autogenous bone alone and with recombinant osteogenic protein (rhOP-1) [20,40]. The differing efficacy of DBM in spinal fusion demonstrated in these studies is likely a result of the different DBM preparations used. It is important to note that the osteogenic activity of a DBM preparation is highly dependent upon the type and specific preparation of bone used. In addition, the carrier with which the DBM is mixed may affect its osteoinductivity. Current preparations of DBM which are mixed with a glycerol carrier (Grafton, Osteotech, Eatontown, N.J., USA) are very acidic. The low pH may have detrimental effects on host cells if it is used in large quantities. Other preparations containing hyaluronic acid (DBX, Synthes) have a more neutral pH and thus may be less harmful to host tissues. In hosts with compromised osteogenic capacity, such as smokers, DBM may be useful as a supplement to autogenous bone graft [70].

In summary, despite good evidence for osteogenic activity in DBM, there is little evidence suggesting its effectiveness as a substitute for autogenous bone graft. There is tremendous variability in the osteoinductive capacity of different commercial demineralized bone graft preparations as assessed by submuscular assay [68], and this may contribute to variability in clinical experience. Demineralized bone matrix offers no structural or mechanical stability independently of its carrier and does not appear to be a reliable substitute for autogenous bone graft. The material may have a role as a graft extender or as a supplement in hosts with compromised bone forming capacity.

Growth factors and composite grafts

Recent advances in cellular and molecular biology led to the identification of specific cytokines that are active in mediating cellular activities including mitogenesis, anabolic activity, and differentiation. The ability to control cellular activity is a potentially powerful tool in the management of orthopedic disorders and surgical reconstructions. Many growth factors and other cytokines have been shown to be osteoinductive in animal models. The growth factors that may enhance bone formation in vitro include insulin-like growth factor (IGF-1), fibroblast growth factor (aFGF, bFGF), platelet-derived growth factor (PDGF), and transforming growth factor beta (TGF-ß) [4, 15, 45, 48, 51, 54,55]. Bone morphogenetic proteins are a subset of the TGF-ß superfamily and are the only cytokines that demonstrated a capacity to induce new bone formation in vivo [87]. Bone morphogenetic proteins are important mediators of new bone formation and repair in all stages of life from embryonic development to adulthood [41,63]. Recent developments in recombinant techniques permit isolation of BMP in pharmacologic quantities, in contrast to isolation through demineralization, in which less than 20 µg of osteoinductive material could be extracted from 10 kg of bovine cortical bone [89]. Clinical experience with bone morphogenetic proteins in spinal fusion studies suggest a valuable role as bone graft supplements or substitutes [9, 21, 24, 32, 49, 59, 64, 65, 67,97].

Composite grafts permit combination of the osteoinductive and osteogenic capacities of growth factors or autogenous bone with the structural capacity of mineralized matrices [9]. The optimal carrier for bone growth morphogenetic proteins has not been determined but would have a reversible affinity to the glycoprotein, structural characteristics possibly including malleability or mechanical rigidity, limited immunogenicity and toxicity, and resorbability to permit complete replacement by bone. Inorganic carriers of BMP that have demonstrated efficacy in promoting spinal arthrodesis include true bone ceramic (TBC) derived from sintered bovine bone, and hydroxyapatite-TCP [52]. Organic carriers include polylactic acid polymers (PLA), collagen and noncollagenous protein carriers, mineralized or demineralized bone matrix, and autograft [47,60]. Advantages of organic carriers include the capacity for chemical bonding to growth factors and the provision of a biodegradable environment for new bone formation and graft incorporation. However, many organic carriers are weakly immunogenic and lack the osteoconductive function of inorganic bone cements. The structural capacity of inorganic cements is a further advantage of this carrier. Composite grafts offer potential for the design of bone graft substitutes that are specific for the structural and biologic demands of the host, and it is likely that very different composites will be used for anterior interbody arthrodesis than for long-instrumented posterior fusion.

Conclusions

Effective clinical application of mineralized and demineralized bone matrix substitutes requires an understanding of their biologic and structural characteristics. Existing preparations have clear limitations in clinical efficacy. Experience to date suggests that grafting materials and composites will continue to evolve for specific applications, and the choice of bone graft materials will be determined by the properties of the local host environment, including anticipated loading and vascular and soft tissue envelope. The development of growth factors and other cytokines that function as potent induction agents for osteoneogenesis offers tremendous potential for the design of composite materials providing osteoinductive, osteoconductive, and structural functions. New techniques in tissue engineering and gene therapy will add a further osteogenic capacity to future bone graft substitutes.

References

1. An HS, Lynch K, Toth J (1995) Prospective comparison of autograft vs allograft for adult posterolateral lumbar spine fusion: differences among freeze-dried, frozen, and mixed grafts. J Spinal Disord 8:131–135
2. An HS, Simpson JM, Glover JM, Stephany J (1995) Comparison between allograft plus demineralized bone matrix versus autograft in anterior cervical fusion. A prospective multicenter study. Spine 20:2211–2216
3. Aronson J, Harrison BH, Stewart CL, Harp JH Jr (1989) The histology of distraction osteogenesis using different external fixators. Clin Orthop 241:106–116
4. Aspenberg P, Albrektsson T, Thorngren K (1989) Local application of IGF-1 to healing bone. Acta Orthop Scan 60:607
5. Asselmeier MA, Casperi RB, Bottenfeld S (1993) A review of allograft processing and sterilization techniques and their role in transmission of the human immunodeficiency virus. Am J Sports Med 21:170–175
6. Banwart JC, Asher MA, Hassanein RS (1994) Iliac crest bone graft harvest donor site morbidity: a statistical evaluation. Spine 20:1055–1060
7. Bauer TW, Muschler GF (2000) Bone graft materials. An overview of the basic science. Clin Orthop 371:10–27
8. Boden SD, Martin GJ, Morone M, Ugbo JL, Hutton WC (1999) The use of coralline hydroxyapatite with bone marrow, autogenous bone graft, or osteoinductive bone protein extract for posterolateral lumbar spine fusion. Spine 24:320–327
9. Boden SD, Martin GJ, Morone MA, Ugbo JL, Moskovitz PA (1999) Posterolateral lumbar intertransverse process spine arthrodesis with recombinant human bone morphogenetic protein 2/hydroxyapatite-tricalcium phosphate after laminectomy in the nonhuman primate. Spine 24:1179–1185
10. Bozic KJ, Glazer PA, Zurakowski D, Simon BJ, Lipson SJ, Hayes WC (1999) In vivo evaluation of coralline hydroxyapatite and direct current electrical stimulation in lumbar spine fusion. Spine 24:2127–2133
11. Burchardt H (1983) The biology of bone graft repair. Clin Orthop 174:28–42
12. Butterman GR, Glazer PA, Bradford DS (1996) The use of bone allografts in the spine. Clin Orthop 324:75–85
13. Buttermann GR, Glazer PA, Hu SS, Bradford DS (1997) Revision of failed lumbar fusions. A comparison of anterior autograft and allograft. Spine 22: 2748–2755
14. Cameron HV, Macnab I, Pillar RM (1977) Evaluation of a biodegradable ceramic. J Biomed Mater Res 11:179–186
15. Canalis E, McCarthy T, Centrella M (1988) Growth factors in the regulation of bone remodeling. J Clin Invest 81: 277
16. Catinella FP, Delaria GA, De Wald RL (1990) False aneurysm of the superior gluteal artery – a complication of iliac crest bone grafting. Spine 15:1360–1362
17. Challis JH, Lyttle JA, Stuart AE (1975) Strangulated lumbar hernia and volvulus following removal of iliac crest bone graft. Acta Orthop Scan 46:230–233
18. Cloward RB (1958) The anterior approach for removal of ruptured discs. J Neurosurg 15:602
19. Cockin J (1971) Autogenous bone graft complications and the donor site. J Bone Joint Surg Br 53:153
20. Cook SD, Dalton JE, Tan EH, Whitecloud TS, Rueger DC (1994) In vivo evaluation of recombinant human osteogenic protein (rhOP-1) implants as a bone graft substitute for spine fusions. Spine 19:1655–1664
21. Cook SD, Rueger DC (1996) Osteogenic protein-1. Biology and applications. Clin Orthop 324:29–38
22. Cook SD, Dalton JE, Prewett AB, Whitecloud TS 3rd (1995) In vivo evaluation of demineralized bone matrix as a bone graft substitute for posterior spinal fusion. Spine 20:877–886
23. Coventry MB, Tapper EM (1972) Pelvic instability – a consequence of removing iliac crest for bone grafting. J Bone Joint Surg Am 54:83–101
24. Cunningham BW, Kanayama M, Parker LM, Weis JC, Sefter JC, Fedder IL, McAfee PC (1999) Osteogenic protein versus autologous interbody arthrodesis in the sheep thoracic spine. A comparative endoscopic study using the Bagba and Kuslich interbody fusion device. Spine 24:509–518
25. Cutright DE, Bhaskar SN, Brady JM et al (1972) Reaction of bone to tricalcium phosphate ceramic pellets. Oral Surg Oral Med Oral Pathol 33:850–856
26. Delecrin J, Aguado E, Nguyen JM, Pyre D, Royer J, Passuti N (1997) Influence of local environment on incorporation of ceramic for lumbar fusion. A comparison of laminar and intertransverse sites in a canine model. Spine 22:1683–1689
27. Delecrin J, Takahashi S, Gouin F, Passuti N (2000) A synthetic porous ceramic as a bone graft substitute in the surgical management of scoliosis: a prospective, randomized study. Spine 25:563–569
28. Enneking WF, Mindell ER (1991) Observations on massive retrieved human allografts. J Bone Joint Surg Am 73: 1123–1142
29. Escales F, De Wald RL (1977) Combined traumatic arteriovenous fistula and ureteral injury: a complication of bone grafting. J Bone Joint Surg Am 59:270–271
30. Fernyhough JC, Schimandle JJ, Weigel MC et al (1992) Chronic donor site pain complicating bone graft harvest from the posterior iliac crest for spinal fusion. Spine 17:1474–1480

31. Ferraro JW (1979) Experimental evaluation of ceramic calcium phosphate as a substitute for bone grafts. Plast Reconstr Surg 63:634–640
32. Fischgrund JS, James SB, Chabot MC, Hankin R, Herkowitz HN, Wozney JM, Shirkhode A (1997) Augmentation of autograft using reBMP-2 and different carrier media in the canine spine fusion model. J Spinal Disord 10:467–472
33. Frenkel SR, Moskovich R, Spivak J, Zhang ZH, Prewett AB (1993) Demineralized bone matrix. Enhancement of spinal fusion. Spine 18:1634–1639
34. Fuller D, Stevenson S, Emery SE (1996) The effects of internal fixation on calcium carbonate. Ceramic anterior spinal fusion in dogs. Spine 21:2131–2136
35. Gould S, Rhee J, Tay BK: Cellular contribution of bone graft to fusion. J Orthop Res (in press)
36. Goulet JA, Senunas LE, DeSilva GL, Greengield MLVH (1997) Autogenous iliac crest bone graft. Complications and functional assessment. Clin Orthop 339:76–81
37. Hamer AJ, Strachan JR, Black MM, Ibbotson CJ, Stockley I, Elson RA (1996) Biomechanical properties of cortical allograft bone using a new method of bone strength measurement: a comparison of fresh, fresh-frozen, and irradiated bone. J Bone Joint Surg Br 78:363–368
38. Hanley EN, Harvell JC, Shaparo DE (1989) The use of allograft bone in cervical spine surgery. Semin Spine Surg 1:262
39. Heiple KG, Chase SW, Herndon CH (1963) A comparative study of the healing process following different types of bone transplantation. J Bone Joint Surg Am 45:1593–1616
40. Helm GA, Sheehan JM, Sheehan JP, Jane JA Jr, diPierro CG, Simmons NE, Gillies GT, Kallmes DF, Sweeney TM (1997) Utilization of type I collagen gel, demineralized bone matrix, and bone morphogenetic protein-2 to enhance autologous bone lumbar spinal fusion. J Neurosurg 86:93–100
41. Hogan B (1996) Bone morphogenetic proteins. Multifunctional regulators of vertebral development. Genes Dev 10: 1580–1594
42. Ison I FB, Barr B, Constantz B (1994) Synthesis of dahllite: the mineral phase of bone. CRC Press, Boca Raton
43. Jarcho M (1981) Calcium phosphate ceramics as hard tissue prosthetics. Clin Orthop 157:259–278
44. Jorgenson SS, Lowe TG, France J, Sabin J (1994) A prospective analysis of autograft versus allograft in posterolateral lumbar fusion in the same patient. A minimum of 1-year follow-up in 144 patients. Spine 19:2048–2053
45. Jungushi S, Heydemann A, Kana SK, Macey LR, Bolander M (1990) aFGF injection stimulates cartilage enlargement and inhibits collagen gene expression in a rat fracture healing model. J Orthop Res 8:364
46. Kuhn DA, Moreland MS (1986) Complications following iliac crest bone grafting. Clin Orthop 209:224–226
47. Lindholm TS, Gao TJ (1993) Functional carriers for bone morphogenetic proteins. Ann Chir Gynaecol 82:3–12
48. Linkhart TA, Mohan S, Baylink DJ (1996) Growth factors for bone growth and repair: IGF, TGF-B, BMP. Bone 19:1S–12S
49. Martin GJ, Boden SD, Morone MA, Moskovitz PA (1999) Posterolateral intertransverse process spinal arthrodesis with rhBMP-2 in a nonhuman primate: important lessons learned regarding dose, carrier, and safety. J Spinal Disord 12:179–186
50. Martin GJ, Boden SD, Titus L, Scarborough NL (1999) New formulations of demineralized bone matrix as a more effective graft alternative in experimental posterolateral lumbar spine arthrodesis. Spine 24:637–645
51. Massague J (1990) The TGF-B family. Annu Rev Cell Biol 6:597
52. Minamide A, Tamaki T, Kawakami M, Hashizume H, Yoshida M, Sakata R (1999) Experimental spinal fusion using sintered bovine bone coated with type I collagen and recombinant human BMP-2. Spine 24:1863–1872
53. Morone MN, Boden SD (1998) Experimental posterolateral lumbar spinal fusion with a demineralized bone matrix gel. Spine 23:159–167
54. Muller R, Bravo R, Burckhardt J, Currant T (1984) Induction of c-fos gene and protein by growth factors precedes activation of c-myc. Nature 312:716
55. Mundy GR (1996) Regulation of bone formation by bone morphogenetic proteins and other growth factors. Clin Orthop Rel Res 324:24–8
56. Muschler GF, Lane JM (1992) Orthopaedic surgery. In: Habal MB, Reddi AH (eds) Bone grafts and bone substitutes. Saunders, Philadelphia, pp 375–407
57. Muschler GF, Negami S, Hyodo A et al (1996) Evaluation of collagen ceramic composite graft materials in a spinal fusion model. Clin Orthop 328: 250–60
58. Oikarinen J (1982) Experimental spinal fusion with decalcified bone matrix and deep-frozen allogeneic bone in rabbits. Clinical Orthop Rel Res 162: 210–218
59. Riley EH, Lane JM, Urist MR, Lyons KM, Lieberman JR (1996) Bone morphogenetic protein-2. Biology and applications. Clin Orthop 324:39–46
60. Ripamonti U (1993) Delivery systems for bone morphogenetic proteins. A summary of experimental studies in primate models. Ann Chir Gynaecol 82:13–25
61. Roudier M, Bouchon C, Rouvillain JL et al (1995) The resorption of bone-implanted corals varies with porosity but also with the host reaction. J Biomed Mater Res 29:909–915
62. Roy DM, Linnehan SK (1974) Hydroxyapatite formed from coral skeletal carbonate by hydrothermal exchange. Nature 247:220–222
63. Sandberg M, Aro HT, Vuorio EI (1993) Gene expression during bone repair. Clin Orthop 289:292–312
64. Sandhu HS (2000) Anterior lumbar interbody fusion with osteoinductive growth factors. Clin Orthop 371:55–60
65. Sandhu HS, Kanim LE, Toth JM, Kabo JM, Liu D, Delamarter RB, Dawson EG (1997) Experimental spinal fusion with recombinant human bone morphogenetic protein-2 without decortication of the osseous elements. Spine 22: 1171–1180
66. Sandhu HS, Grewal HS, Parvataneni H (1999) Bone grafting for spine fusion. Orthop Clin North Am 30:685–698
67. Schimandle JH, Boden SD, Hutton WC (1995) Experimental spinal fusion with recombinant human bone morphogenetic protein-2. Spine 20:1326–1337
68. Schwartz Z, Mellonig JT, Carnes DL Jr, de la Fontaine J, Cochran DL, Dean DD, Boyan BD (1996) Ability of commercial demineralized freeze-dried bone allograft to induce new bone formation. J Periodontol 67:918–926
69. Shimazaki K, Mooney V (1985) Comparative study of porous hydroxyapatite and tricalcium phosphate as bone substitutes. J Orthop Res 3:301–310
70. Silcox DH 3rd, Boden SD, Schimandle JH, Johnson P, Whitesides TE, Hutton WC (1998) Reversing the inhibitory effect of nicotine on spinal fusion using an osteoinductive protein extract. Spine 23:291–297
71. Smith GW, Robinson RA (1958) The treatment of certain cervical spine disorders by anterior removal of the intervertebral disc and interbody fusion. J Bone Joint Surg Am 40:607–624

72. Stevenson S (1987) The immune response to osteochondral allografts in dogs. J Bone Joint Surg Am 69:573–582
73. Stevenson S, Horowitz M (1992) The response to bone allografts. J Bone Joint Surg Am 74:939–950
74. Stevenson S, Horowitz M (1992) The response to bone allografts: curent concepts review. J Bone Joint Surg Am 74:939–949
75. Stevenson S, Li XQ, Martin B (1991) The fate of cancellous and cortical bone after transplantation of fresh and frozen tissue-antigen-matched and mismatched osteochondral allografts in dogs. J Bone Joint Surg Am 73:1143–1156
76. Stevenson S, Emery SE, Goldberg VM (1996) Factors affecting bone graft incorporation. Clin Orthop 324:66–74
77. Strong DM, Friedlaender HE, Tomford WW et al (1996) Immunlogic responses in human recipients of osseous and osteochondral allografts. Clin Orthop 326:107–114
78. Summers BN, Eisenstein SM (1989) Donor site pain from the ilium: a complication of lumbar spine fusion. J Bone Joint Surg Br 71:677–680
79. Tay BK, Le AX, Heilman M, Lotz J, Bradford DS (1998) Use of a collagen-hydroxyapatite matrix in spinal fusion. A rabbit model. Spine 23:2276–2281
80. Tay BK, Patel VV, Bradford DS (1999) Calcium sulfate and calcium phosphate-based bone substitutes. Mimickry of the moneral phase of bone. Orthop Clin North Am 30:615–623
81. Tho KS, Krishnamoorthy S (1996) Use of coral grafts in anterior interbody fusion of the rabbit spine. Ann Acad Med Singapore 25:824–827
82. Tomford WW (1995) Transmission of disease through transplantation of musculoskeletal allografts. J Bone Joint Surg Am 77:1742–1754
83. Tuli SM, Singh AD (1978) The osteoinductive property of decalcified bone matrix: an experimental study. J Bone Joint Surg Br 60:116–123
84. Urist MR (1965) Bone formation by autoinduction. Science 150:893–899
85. Urist MR, Silverman BF, Buring K, Dubuc FL, Rosenberg JM (1987) The bone induction principle. Clin Orthop 53:243–283
86. VanderGriend RA (1994) The effect of internal fixation on the healing of very large allografts. J Bone Joint Surg Am 76:657–663
87. Vukicevic S, Stanljenic A, Pecina M (1995) Discovery and clinical applications of bone morphogenetic proteins. Eur J Clin Chem Clin Biochem 33: 661–671
88. Walsh WR, Harrison J, Loefler A, Martin T, Van Sickle D, Brown MKC, Sonnabend DH (2000) Mechanical and histologic evaluation of collagraft in an ovine lumbar fusion model. Clin Orthop 375:258–266
89. Wang EA, Rosen V, Cordes P, Hewick RM, Kriz MJ, Luxenberg DP, Sibley BS, Wozney JM (1988) Purification and characterization of other distinct bone-inducing factors. Proc Natl Acad Sci U S A 85:9484–9488
90. Wang J, Glimcher MJ (1999) Characterization of demineralized bone matrix-induced osteogenesis in rat calvarial bone defects: I. Origins of bone forming cells. Calcif Tissue Int 65: 486–493
91. Wang J, Glimcher MJ (1999) Characterization of matrix-induced osteogenesis in a rat calvarial bone defect: I. Differences in the cellular response to demineralized bone matrix implanted in calvarial defects and subcutaneous sites. Calcif Tissue Int 65:156–165
92. Wang J, Yang R, Gerstenfeld LC, Glimcher MJ (2000) Characterization of demineralized bone matrix-induced osteogenesis in rat calvarial bone defects: III. Gene and protein expression. Calcif Tissue Int 67:314–20
93. Wozney JM, Rosen V, Celeste AJ (1988) Novel regulators of bone formation: molecular clones and activities. Science 242:1528–1534
94. Wu Y, Chellser DA, Glimcher MJ, Garrido L, Wang J, Jiang HJ, Ackerman JL (1999) Multinuclear solid-state three-dimensional MRI of bone and synthetic calcium phosphates. Proc Natl Acad Sci U S A 96:1574–1578
95. Younger EM, Chapman MW (1989) Morbidity at bone graft donor sites. J Orthop Trauma 3:192–195
96. Zdeblick TA (1993) A prospective randomized study of lumbar fusion: preliminary results. Spine 18:983–991
97. Zdeblick TA, Ghanayem AJ, Rapoff AJ, Swain C, Bassett T, Cooke ME, Markel M (1998) Cervical interbody fusion cages. An animal model with and without morphogenetic protein. Spine 23:758–765
98. Zhang ZH, Yin H, Yang K et al (1983) Anterior intervertebral disc excision and bone grafting in cervical spondylitic myelopathy. Spine 8:16

Michael Muschik
Ralph Ludwig
Silke Halbhübner
Kathrin Bursche
Thierry Stoll

β-tricalcium phosphate as a bone substitute for dorsal spinal fusion in adolescent idiopathic scoliosis: preliminary results of a prospective clinical study

Dedicated to Prof. Hartmut Zippel, MD, Head of the Orthopedic Clinic in the Charité Hospital, where all the surgery was done

M. Muschik (✉)
Seehospital Sahlenburg
der Nordheimstiftung, Norddeutsches Wirbelsäulenzentrum,
Nordheimstrasse 201,
27476 Cuxhaven, Germany
e-mail: Muschik@seehospital-sahlenburg.de,
Tel.: +49-4721-604211,
Fax: +49-4721-205317

R. Ludwig · S. Halbhübner
Orthopädische Klinik der Charité,
Humboldt-Universität, Berlin, Germany

K. Bursche
Spine Group – Zentrum für Wirbelsäulenerkrankungen GmbH,
Berlin, Germany

T. Stoll
Mathys Medical Ltd., Bettlach, Germany

Abstract The aim of this study is to evaluate the ability of β-tricalcium phosphate (TCP) in granular form to achieve dorsal spondylodesis in adolescent idiopathic scoliosis (AIS). Twenty-eight patients underwent surgical correction and were followed up for 13±8 (range 6–33) months. Posterolateral grafting was performed, using either autograft bone mixed with allograft bone (n=19; "bone group") or autograft bone mixed with 25 g TCP (n=9; "TCP group"). Patients were followed by clinical examination, X-rays and computed tomographic (CT) scans to measure bone mineral density. Fusion involved 12±1 (range 10–14) vertebrae. The segments were fused after 6±1 months in both groups according to the radiographs. No pseudarthrosis was observed. Bone mineral density was 430±111 (range 273–629) mg/cm^3 in the TCP group versus 337±134 (range 130–669) mg/cm^3 in the bone group. Resorption of TCP was complete on the radiographs after 8±2 (range 6–10) months. Based upon the results of this small preliminary study, the use of TCP appears to be a valuable alternative to allografts for application in the spine, even when large amounts of bone are needed.

Keywords Scoliosis · Spinal fusion · Bone substitutes · Bone regeneration

Introduction

Despite modern fixation techniques, pseudarthrosis is a major cause of failure in the surgical treatment of idiopathic scoliosis. To avoid this, dorsal spondylodesis requires the use of large quantities of bone graft. Autologous bone graft from spinal process and iliac crest often provides insufficient quantities. In addition, morbidity after harvesting bone from the pelvis is considerable [1, 7]. Allograft bone from bone banks carries known risks of bacterial contamination and viral transmission [2, 5].

Because of these problems, there is an increasing interest in biodegradable osteoconductive ceramic bone graft substitutes. These materials must fulfil certain properties [1, 13]: compatibility with surrounding tissues, chemical stability in body fluids, compatibility of mechanical and physical properties, ability to be produced in functional shapes and to withstand the sterilization process, reasonable cost of manufacture and reliable quality control.

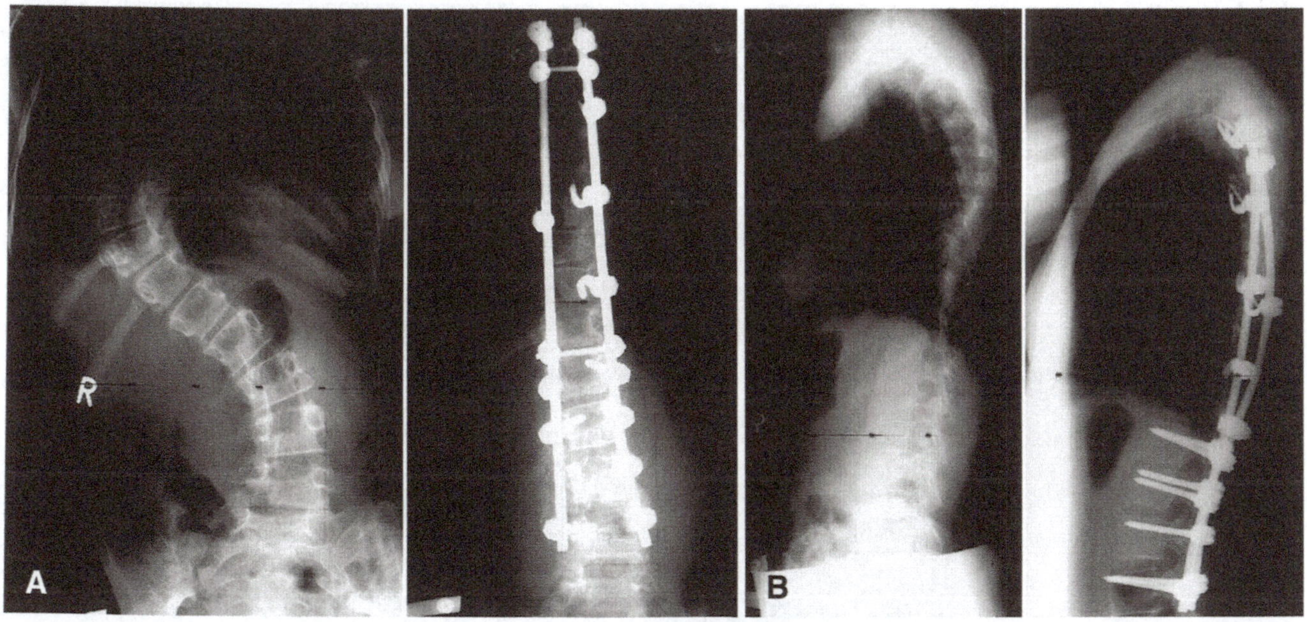

Fig. 1 **A** Posteroanterior and **B** lateral radiograph of an idiopathic adolescent scoliosis ("bone group"), before and after surgery

Calcium phosphate ceramics, whose composition is similar to that of mineral bone, are known to be safe and non-allergenic, with good bone bonding capacity. They have been explored and used as substitutes for bone graft in orthopaedic, maxillofacial and dental operations over the last 30 years. Hydroxyapatite (HA) is generally considered to be only slightly resorbable, while tricalcium phosphate (TCP) is resorbed by a cellular pathway, leaving newly formed bone tissue [3, 19]. When used for spinal arthrodesis, the quality of grafts obtained has been found to be satisfactory in animal models and in human spinal fusion [4, 8, 9, 12, 14, 15].

In previous studies of treatment of idiopathic scoliosis with synthetic bone substitutes, blocks or sticks of TCP composites were used (biphasic ceramic TCP/HA [15, 17], composite collagen/TCP [11]). The aim of this prospective study is to evaluate the performance of TCP in granular form in human dorsal spine fusion and to assess the quality of bone fusion obtained in the treatment of adolescent idiopathic scoliosis.

Materials and methods

Between October 1998 and April 1999, 28 patients with idiopathic adolescent scoliosis were operated. There were 22 female and 6 male patients with an average age of 14.5±1.6 (range 10–17) years. The hospital stay was 14±3 (range 10–23) days. We carried out a dorsal spondylodesis with USS-titanium implants (Mathys Medical, Ltd) (Fig. 1). The surgical procedure for operative correction of the scoliosis was performed analogously to the rod rotation procedure of Cotrel and Dubousset. All operations were performed by one surgeon (M. M.). No anterior release or anterior fusion was considered to be necessary. Convex side rib hump resection was added in 24 patients during the operation. Posterolateral grafting was performed with two sorts of graft: autograft bone mixed with allograft bone (*n*=19; "bone group") and autograft bone mixed with 25 g TCP (chronOS, Mathys Medical, Ltd) (*n*=9; "TCP group") (Fig. 2, Fig. 3).

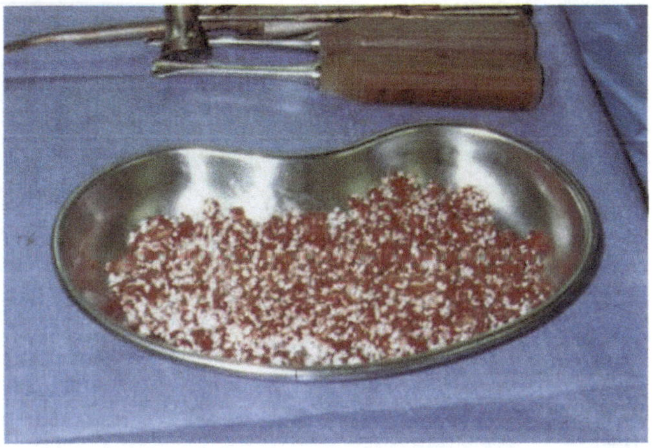

Fig. 2 Mixture of β-tricalcium phosphate (TCP) and morcellised autologous bone

In both patient groups, perioperative antibiotics were given. The patients were mobilized without corset, starting on the 2nd postoperative day.

Patients were followed up for 13±8 (6–33) months. Clinical examination and posteroanterior and lateral radiographs of the spine in standing position were carried out preoperatively and postoperatively at 3 months, 6 months, 1 year and 2 years.

The evaluation of the patient records and radiographic measurements were performed by an independent observer (S.H.). For each patient, the intraoperative blood loss, the duration of surgery and complications were recorded. From the posteroanterior view we measured not only the Cobb angles of the thoracic major curve and the lumbar secondary curve, but also the rotation of the apex and the sagittal profile (kyphosis T4–12 and lordosis L1–5) according to Pedriolle [16]. To measure bone mineral density, all patients underwent one computed tomographic (CT) scan at 11±8

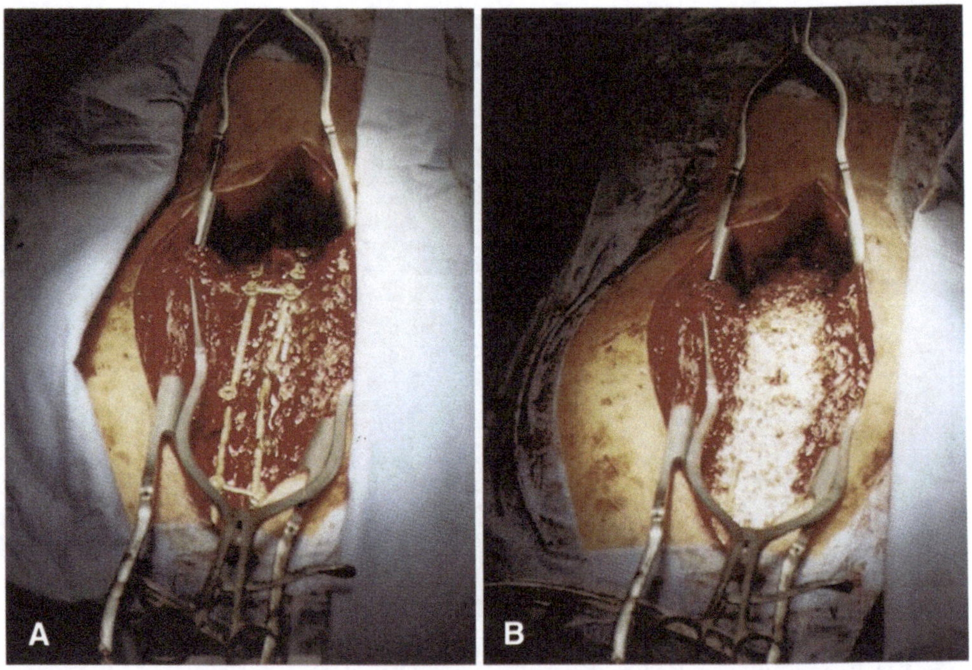

Fig. 3 Idiopathic adolescent scoliosis, instrumented with USS, before (**A**) and after (**B**) augmentation with autologous bone and β-tricalcium phosphate (TCP)

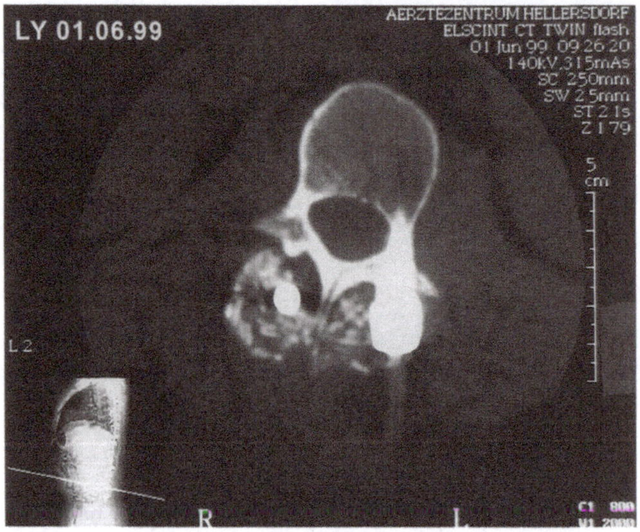

Fig. 4 Computed tomographic (CT) scan 3 months after dorsal instrumented spondylodesis with good coverage of the metal implants with autologous bone/β-tricalcium phosphate (CP)

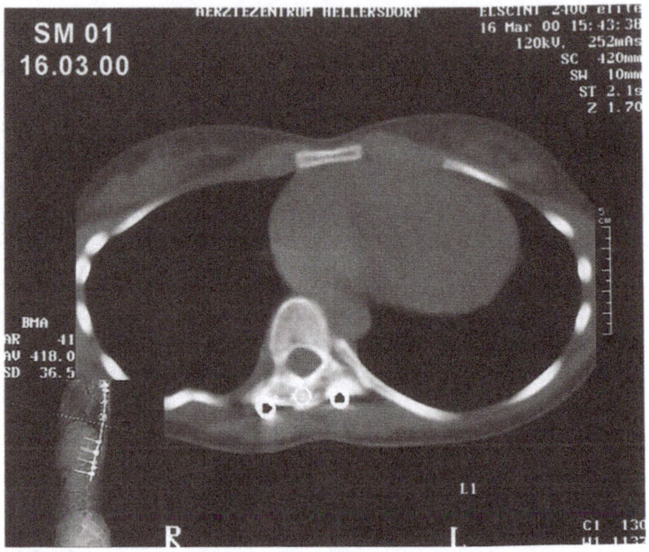

Fig. 5 CT scan 8 months after dorsal instrumented spondylodesis ("TCP group") shows homogeneous bone formation between the transverse process and the measurement results of the bone mineral density (418 mg/cm^3)

(range 3–33) months (Fig. 4, Fig. 5). The CT scans were carried out by one radiologist (K.B.), who was not informed of the aim of the study. To reduce the radiation exposure of the patients, only one vertebral level was scanned. It was agreed to use the setting of the instrumentation resulting in darker images (setting C1=800, W1=2000), thus reducing the artifacts and emphasising bone.

Results

The distribution of age, gender, type of scoliosis according to King as well as the stay in the hospital were similar in the two groups (Table 1). Significant correction of the spine was achieved by surgery in both groups. No differ-

Table 1 Comparison of the bone and β-tricalcium phosphate (*TCP*) group according to patient age (mean ±SD with range in parentheses), gender, type of scoliosis (King classification) and stay in hospital

	Bone group	TCP group
Age (years)	14.3±1.7 (10–17)	14.8±1.5 (12–17)
Gender	14 girls, 5 boys	8 girls, 1 boy
King type 2	10	5
King type 3	7	2
King type 4	2	2
Days in hospital	14.1±3.1 (10–21)	13.9±4.0 (10–23)

Table 2 Comparison of preoperative and follow-up measurements of the thoracic major curvature, the lumbar secondary curvature, the thoracic and lumbar rotation at the apex of the curvature, and the thoracic kyphosis and lumbar lordosis between the β-tricalcium phosphate (*TCP*) and the bone group (all measurements expressed in degrees with mean± SD, and minimum and maximum values in parentheses)

	Bone group	TCP group	Significance
Preoperative values			
Thoracic major curvature	53±8 (36–66)	54±10 (46–72)	*P*=0.87 (n.s.)
Lumbar secondary curvature	31±11 (0–45)	35±8 (19–43)	*P*=0.38 (n.s.)
Thoracic rotation (apex)	25±8 (5–35)	18±4 (10–25)	*P*=0.02
Lumbar rotation (apex)	7±6 (0–20)	6±5 (0–15)	*P*=0.38 (n.s.)
Thoracic kyphosis (T4–12)	29±13 (9–48)	17±14 (2–43)	*P*=0.03
Lumbar lordosis (L1–5)	37±16 (5–45)	38±14 (21–60)	*P*=0.87 (n.s.)
Follow-up values			
Thoracic major curvature	17±6 (8–30)*	16±6 (7–23)*	*P*=0.73 (n.s.)
Lumbar secondary curvature	8±7 (0–22)*	7±6 (0–16) *	*P*=0.73 (n.s.)
Thoracic rotation (apex)	16±10 (0–30)*	11±4 (5–15)**	*P*=0.27 (n.s.)
Lumbar rotation (apex)	2±5 (0–15)**	6±6 (0–15) $n.s._{pre}$	*P*=0.15 (n.s.)
Thoracic kyphosis (T4–12)	22±9 (6–34) $n.s._{pre}$	22±8 (8–32) $n.s._{pre}$	*P*=0.99 (n.s.)
Lumbar lordosis (L1–5)	37±10 (19–50) $n.s._{pre}$	28±6 (21–36) $n.s._{pre}$	*P*=0.08 (n.s.)

**P*<0.01; ***P*<0.05; $n.s._{pre}$ (not significant): all compared with preoperative values

Table 3 Comparison of patients' blood loss (intraoperative and postoperative; mean±SD with range in parentheses), number of patients who received blood transfusion (autologous and blood from blood bank) and operation time between the two groups

	Bone group (*n*=19)	TCP group (*n*=9)	Significance
Blood loss (ml)	1793±486 (900–2600)	1850±524 (1100–2400)	n.s.
Intraop. blood loss (ml)	1207±506 (400–2000)	1150±476 (700–1800)	n.s.
Postop. blood loss (ml)	612±209 (200–3000)	678±248 (200–1000)	n.s.
Blood transfusion (no. of patients)	16	6	n.s.
Only autologous blood	12	4	
Blood from bank	4	2	
Operation time (min)	181±29 (135–240)	186±46 (135–290)	n.s.

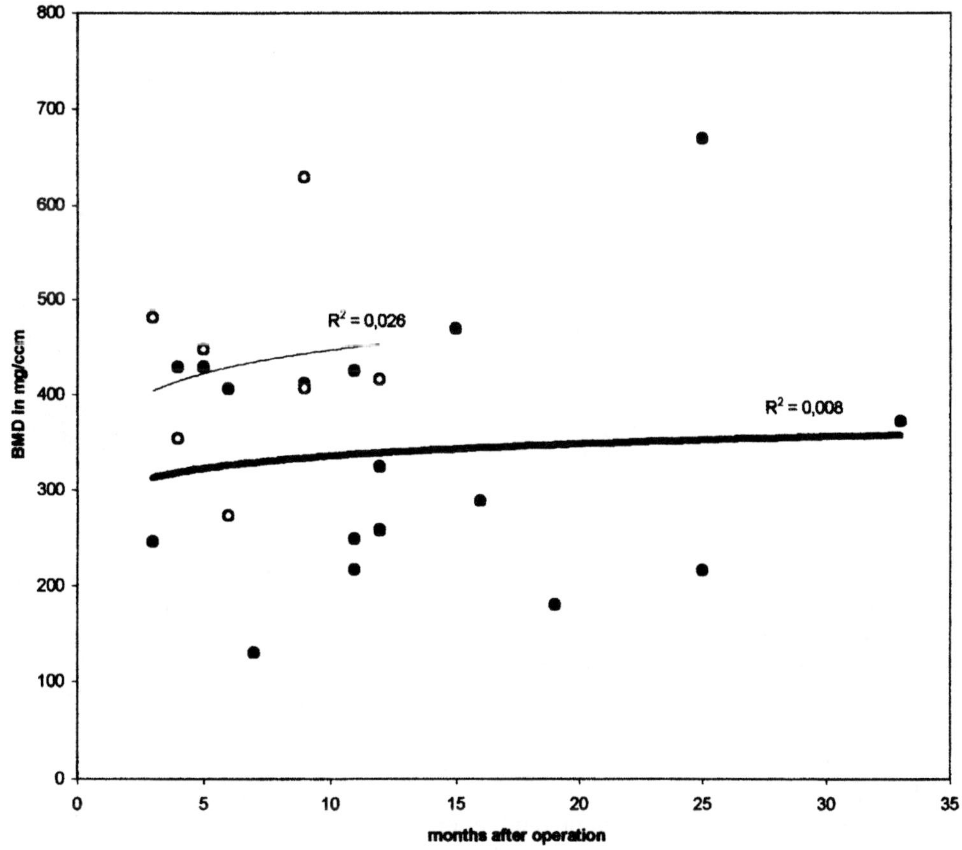

Fig. 6 Measurements of bone mineral density (BMD in mg/ccm) in the bone group and in the β-tricalcium phosphate (TCP) group, and logarithmic regression analysis of the values (*filled circles* bone group, *open circles* TCP group, *thick line* bone group trend line, *thin line* TCP group trend line)

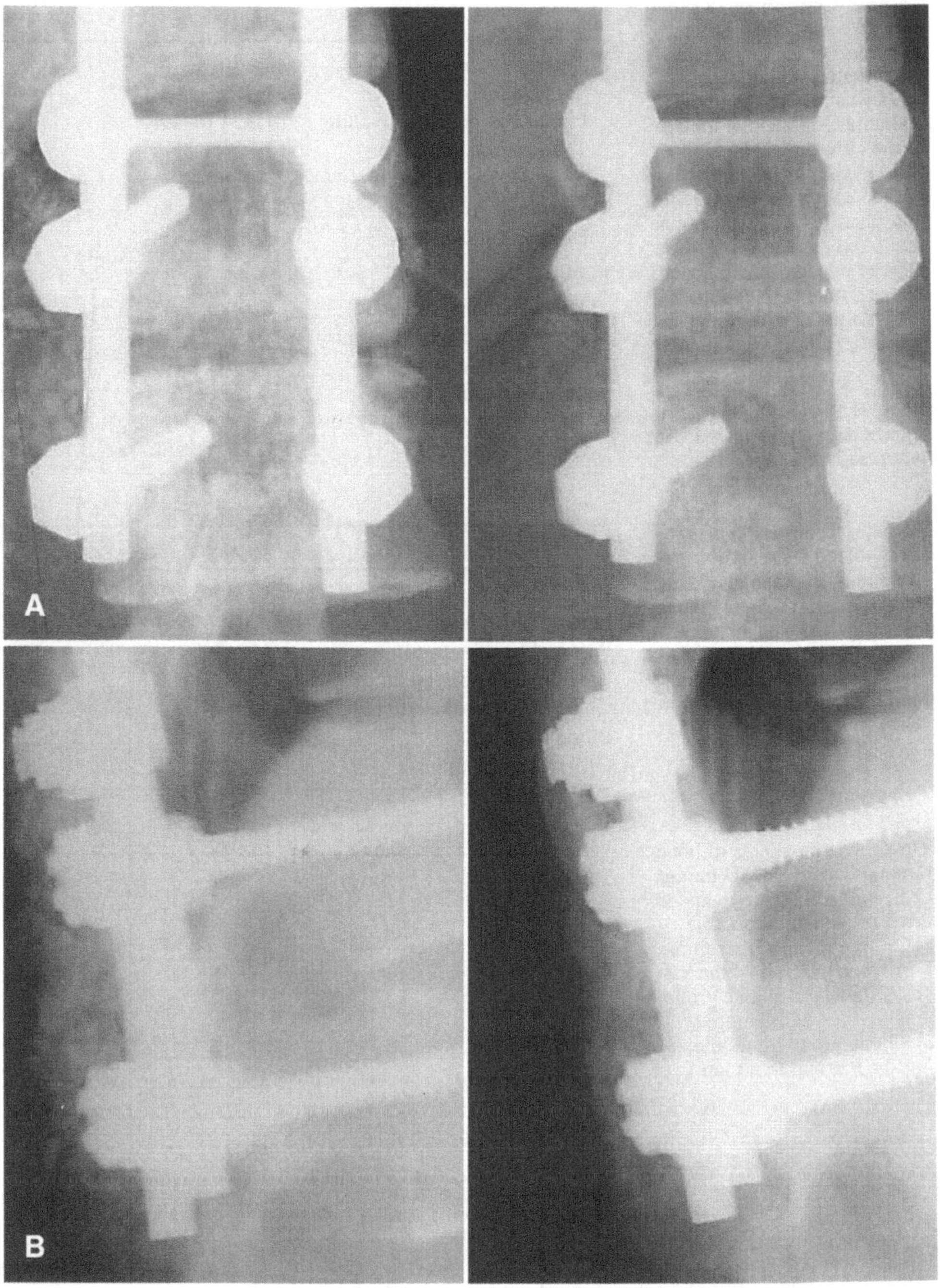

Fig. 7 **A** Anteroposterior and **B** lateral radiographs, immediately (*left*) and 6 months (*right*) after surgery, showing β-tricalcium phosphate granules resorption and formation of solid bone fusion

ence according to the amount of the correction of the thoracic major curve, the lumbar secondary curve, the thoracic rotation, the thoracic kyphosis or the lumbar lordosis was observed between the two patient groups (Table 2). Comparison of the preoperative and follow-up measurements of lumbar rotation demonstrated a significant correction in the bone group, but was not observed in the TCP group.

Blood loss during the operation and after surgery, transfusion of blood (autologous blood or blood from the bank) and the operation time were recorded (Table 3). No significant differences were seen between these parameters. Three of 19 patients (15%) in the bone group and 3 of 9 patients (33%) in the TCP group did not need any blood transfusion. We had one patient from the bone group with local pain at the iliac crest 6 months after surgery. However, pain disappeared without any therapy.

The CT scans to measure the bone mineral density were performed at 11±8 (range 3–33) months after surgery. Seven CT scans were available in the TCP group

Table 4 Complications and management of these complications. *TCP* β-tricalcium phosphate

Complication	Bone group (n=19)	TCP group (n=9)
Lumbar decompensation, no reoperation required	1	
Cast syndrome, infusion therapy		1
Puncture of a deep haematoma	1	
Late deep infection, hardware removal and anterior fusion (VDS according to Zielke)		1

and 17 in the bone group. The mean value of the bone mineral density was 430±111 (range 273–629) mg/cm^3 in the TCP group and 337±134 (range 130–669) mg/cm^3 in the bone group (P=0.16; n.s.). The results of the CT measurements relative to the bone density are summarised in Fig. 6.

No pseudarthrosis was observed. The time until the TCP granules disappeared on the plain X-ray films and were completely substituted by homogeneous bone was 8±2 (range 6–10) months (Fig. 7).

Complications were seen in four patients (14%; Table 4), but these complications were not related to the bone graft or the bone substitute.

Discussion

The efficacy of different ceramics in obtaining spinal arthrodesis has been studied both in animal models and in selective clinical studies [13]. In animal models the fusion has been analysed mainly in sheep [8, 9]. Some authors demonstrated better results with autologous bone, others found similar results, in term of fusion rate, when using a mixture of hydroxyapatite and TCP or coralline hydroxyapatite [13, 18].

Clinical data on the use of ceramics as graft extenders for autologous bone fusion of deformities have been presented by Delecrin et al., Heise et al., Le Huec et al., Passuti et al. and Ransford et al. [6, 10, 12, 15, 17].

Delecrin et al. operated on 58 patients with idiopathic scoliosis using Cotrel Dubousset (CD) instrumentation [6]. Posterior spinal fusion was performed using autologous bone in 30 patients using local bone combined with blocks containing both hydroxyapatite and β-tricalcium phosphate in 28 patients. They observed less blood loss in the patient group with ceramic blocks. The satisfactory correction of the deformity was maintained to a similar degree in the two groups. They concluded that harvesting iliac bone is no longer necessary for such surgeries.

Le Huec et al. presented a study of 54 patients who underwent dorsal spondylodesis for idiopathic scoliosis [12]. Twenty-four patients underwent grafting with a mixture of autologous cortico-cancellous bone and TCP sticks, while 30 patients received a graft consisting of a mixture of autologous and allogenic bone frozen at −80°C, as in our study. The authors found TCP resorption after 2 years, which is clearly a longer time period than the one we found in our study using TCP granules. Loss of correction was 8% in the autograft/allograft group, but only 2% in the TCP group.

Passuti et al. [15] used calcium phosphate blocks in 12 patients with scoliosis for whom sufficient bone graft was difficult to obtain (neurologic scoliosis and osteogenesis imperfecta). They found normal clinical and radiologic outcome with histologic evaluation, as performed in two patients, demonstrating both the bioactivity and the osteoconduction of this material.

In a prospective randomised study at five hospitals in the UK and France, Ransford et al. investigated 341 patients with idiopathic scoliosis. The patients were grafted with autologous bone (n=171) or synthetic porous ceramic (n=170) [17]. They also found a loss of correction of 8% in the autograft group versus 3% in ceramic group. Fifteen autograft patients had pain at the donor site at 3 months. They found normal haematological and serum biochemistry results and no adverse events related to the graft material or evidence of allergenicity.

We found comparable results in our study when compared with the literature. However, it was difficult to assess whether a solid fusion had occurred. It is critical to use bone mineral density as a way to assess the bone quality or the rate of spinal arthrodesis. Further research is needed to investigate this problem in more detail.

Conclusion

Based on the results of this small study, we consider β-tricalcium phosphate to be a good bone substitute for dorsal spinal fusion in adolescent idiopathic scoliosis. According to clinical and radiological parameters, together with the bone mineral density results, β-tricalcium phosphate in granular form has similar fusion rates to autologous bone.

References

1. Banwart JC, Asher MA, Hassanein RS (1995) Iliac crest bone graft harvest donor site morbidity. A statistical evaluation. Spine 20:1055–1060
2. Centers for Disease Control (1988) Transmission of HIV through bone transplantation: case report and public health recommendations. JAMA 260: 2487–2488
3. Daculsi G, LeGeros R, Nery E, Lynch K, Kerebel B (1989) Transformation of biphasic calcium phosphate ceramics in vivo: ultrastructural and physicochemical characterisation. J Biomed Mater Res 23:883–894

4. Daculsi G, Passuti N, Martin S, Le Nihouannen JC (1989) Etude comparative de céramiques bioactives en phosphate de calcium après l'implantation en site osseux spongieux chez le chien. Rev Chir Orthop 75:65–71
5. Deijkers RLM, Bloem RM, Petit PLC, Brand R, Vehmeyer SBW, Veen MR (1997) Contamination of bone allografts. Analysis of incidence and predisposing factors. J Bone Joint Surg Br 79:161–166
6. Delecrin J, Takahashi S, Gouin F, Passuti N (2000) A synthetic porous ceramic as a bone graft substitute in the surgical managment of scoliosis: a prospectiv, randomized study. Spine 25: 563–569
7. Fernyhough J, Schimandle J, Weigel M, Edwards C, Levine A (1992) Chronic donor-site pain complicating graft harvesting from the posterior iliac crest for spinal fusion. Spine 17:1474–1480
8. Guigui P, Plais PY, Flautre B, Viguier E, Blary MC, Sales De Gauzy J, Chopin D, Lavaste F, Hardouin P (1994) Experimental model of posterolateral spinal arthrodesis in sheep. 1. Experimental procedures and results with autologous bone graft. Spine 19: 2791–2797
9. Guigui P, Plais PY, Flautre B, Viguier E, Blary MC, Chopin D, Lavaste F, Hardouin P (1994) Experimental model of posterolateral spinal arthrodesis in sheep. 2. Application of the model: evaluation of vertebral fusion obtained with coral (Porites) or with a biphasic ceramic (Triosite). Spine 19: 2798–2803
10. Heise U, Osborn J, Duwe F (1990) Hydroxyapatite ceramic as a bone substitute. Int Orthop 14:329–338
11. Husson JL, Poncer R, Chateller P, Morel G (1995) Phosphates tricalciques et arthrodèses lombaires: résultats cliniques, radiographiques at histologiques. Rev Chir Orthop 158 [Suppl II]:158
12. Le Huec JC, Lesprit E, Delavigne C, Clement D, Chauveaux D, Le Rebeller A (1997) Tri-calcium phosphate ceramics and allografts as bone substitutes for spinal fusion in idiopathic scoliosis: comparative clinical results at four years. Acta Orthop Belg 63: 202–211
13. Marchesi DG (2000) Spinal fusion: bone and bone substitutes. Eur Spine J 9:372–378
14. Nasca RJ, Lemons JE, Montgomery R (1991) Evaluation of cryopreserved bone and synthetic biomaterials in promoting spinal fusion. Spine 16 [8 Suppl]: 330–333
15. Passuti N, Daculsi G, Rogez JM, Martin S, Bainvel JV (1989) Macroporous calcium phosphate ceramic performance in human spine fusion. Clin Orthop 248:169–176
16. Pedriolle R, Vidal J (1987) Morphology of scoliosis: three-dimensional evolution. Orthopedics 10:909–915
17. Ransford AO, Morley T, Edgar MA, Webb P, Passuti N, Chopin D, Morin C, Michel F, Garin C, Pries D (1998) Synthetic porous ceramic compared with autograft in scoliosis surgery. J Bone Joint Surg Br 80:13–18
18. Steffen T, Marchesi D, Aebi M (2000) Posterolateral and anterior interbody spinal fusion models in the sheep. Clin Orthop 371:28–37
19. Zerwekh J, Kourosh S, Scheinberg R (1992) Fibrillar collagen: biphasic calcium phosphate composite as a bone graft substitute for spinal fusion. J Orthop Res 10:562–572

Akihito Minamide
Tetsuya Tamaki
Munehito Yoshida
Hiroshi Hashizume
Yukihiro Nakagawa

The use of sintered bone in spinal surgery

Abstract The sintered bovine bone True Bone Ceramics (TBC) is one of the biomaterials based on calcium phosphate, an organized crystal of bone mineral and a biomaterial possessing a natural trabecular structure. We examined whether the sintered bovine bone can integrate with recipient bone and adjust to the strength of recipient bone for anterior spinal fusion in an animal model. Based on radiographic evaluation, manual palpation, biomechanical testing, and histological examination, spinal fusion with TBC resulted in a composition and structure similar to that of autograft (and to no implantation). TBC, with its moderate strength, tended to adjust to the bone stiffness of the host bone in the respective specimens as new bone growth developed. Our observations warrant further clinical investigation of the use of sintered bone as an effective spinal arthrodesis, especially in patients who have fragile vertebrae, as in osteoporosis.

Keywords Animal model · Biomaterials · Biomechanics · Sintered bone · Spinal fusion

A. Minamide (✉) · T. Tamaki
M. Yoshida · H. Hashizume · Y. Nakagawa
Department of Orthopaedic Surgery,
Wakayama Medical College,
811–1 Kimiidera, Wakayama City,
Wakayama 641-8157, Japan
e-mail: aminami@emory.edu,
Tel.: +81-73-441-0645,
Fax: +81-73-448-3008

Introduction

Vertebral body destruction sometimes results in spinal instability or neural compression. Such conditions include osteoporosis, traumatic spinal injury, spinal tumors, and infectious diseases of the spine. Several reports of neurological compromise caused by delayed vertebral collapse after osteoporotic compression fracture have been recently published [11]. Anterior decompression of the vertebral body or vertebral corpectomy is indicated to relieve stress on the neural tissues, and to permit reconstruction of the destabilized spine. In reconstruction, autologous bone grafting has been the standard way to obtain bone fusion. However, the use of autografting is subject to limitations on suitable location and volume, and the harvesting of autologous bone grafts is responsible for significant morbid complications in as many as 30% of patients [5]. To avoid the disadvantages of autologous bone graft, considerable attention has been directed toward development of suitable biosynthetic bone graft substitutes. Synthetic biomaterials provide attractive alternatives for use in spinal fusion. However, such biomaterials have proved problematic, and reliable methods have not been established to apply these relatively stiff materials to patients who have fragile vertebrae, as in the case of osteoporosis. Implanted biomaterials have been reported to sink into the vertebra above or below the implantation site because of comparative differences in strength between recipient bone and the biomaterial [1]. As artificial substitutes designed to repair lost bone tissue morphologically, these materials must be fully biocompatible. They must also be able to provide for the rapid penetration of osteogenesis from the host bone bed to the center of the implant. The optimal substitute is one with a composition and a structure similar to that of human bone tissue, and one that has the biological ability to adjust to the unique bone stiffness of each recipient. For the biomaterial that can integrate with recipient bone and adjust to the stiffness of the recipient bone, the sintered bone, which is one of the natural biomaterials based on the calcium phosphate system, may be thought to be a candidate. The moderate mechanical strength and struc-

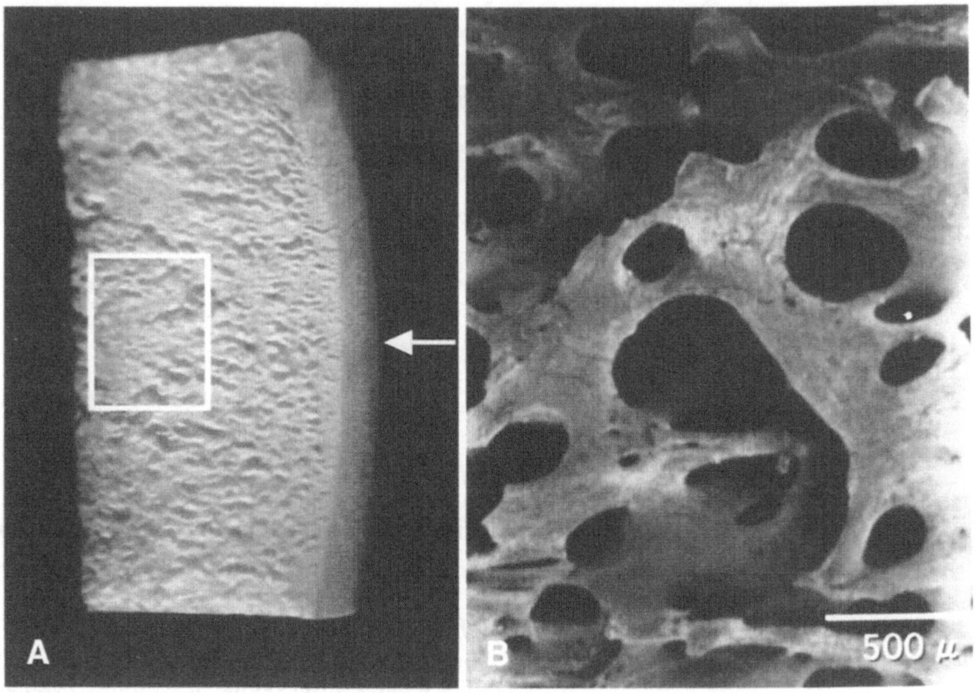

Fig. 1 **A** Micrograph of a True Bone Ceramics (TBC) block reveals a structure of both monocortical (*arrow*) and cancellous bone. **B** A higher magnification view of the TBC block. Scanning electron microscopy shows preservation of the microskeletal structure and interconnecting pores of cancellous TBC

ture of sintered bone may permit it to be used for spinal fusion in ageing patients.

We selected sintered bovine bone, True Bone Ceramics (TBC: Koken, Tokyo, Japan), developed by Ueno et al. [12, 13] in 1983, for the implanted biomaterial in spinal fusion. TBC is made by sintering bovine bone at high temperatures (initially 600°C, secondly 1450°C), and is one of the natural biomaterials, consisting mainly of calcium phosphate and an organized crystal of bone mineral that possesses moderate mechanical strength (mean compressive strength: 9.2±1.9 MPa). TBC is a biomaterial that possesses a natural trabecular structure with interstices connecting to the porous structure of natural bone (Fig. 1). It is thought that the natural bony structure of TBC facilitates the growth of vessels into the material and provides an ideal environment for bone formation [2, 4, 8, 12, 13]. TBC accelerates in vitro adhesion and calcification by osteoblasts more actively than does artificial hydroxyapatite [7].

Materials and methods

The purpose of the present study was to identify whether sintered bovine bone could integrate with recipient bone and adjust to the strength of recipient bone for anterior spinal fusion in an animal model. Seventeen mature pigs were used. A lumbar spinal body fusion was performed through an anterior retroperitoneal approach. The vertebral bodies of L2 and L3 were exposed and the single-level interbody fusion was performed. Either autologous iliac bone (autologous bone group) or sintered bovine bone (TBC group) was implanted for a spinal fusion. Some pigs underwent exposure of the spinal bodies without implantation (control group). The pigs were sacrificed 3 or 6 months after surgery. The lumbar spines were harvested en masse.

Results

Spinal fusion was confirmed by radiographic analysis, biomechanical testing, and histological examination. Fusion was successful in all pigs that received the sintered bovine bone or the autologous bone. Spinal fusion with TBC resulted in a composition and structure similar to that of the autograft (and of no implantation). The TBC, with its moderate strength, tended to adjust to the bone stiffness of the host bone in the specimens as new bone grew (Fig. 2). In the histological findings, trabeculae of regenerated bone were apposed directly to the TBC and there was no sign of intervening soft tissue between the bone and the implant. The new bony matrix was growing into pores located in the deeper regions of the TBC, so that all pores of TBC gradually filled up.

Augmentation to clinical study using sintered bone

Bioactive materials that possess excellent strength in themselves, such as titanium cage and Apatite and Wollastonite coating glass ceramics (A-W glass ceramics), have been applied clinically to reconstructive spinal stabilization [1, 3, 6, 10]. However, there are doubts about whether spinal reconstruction requires biomaterials that

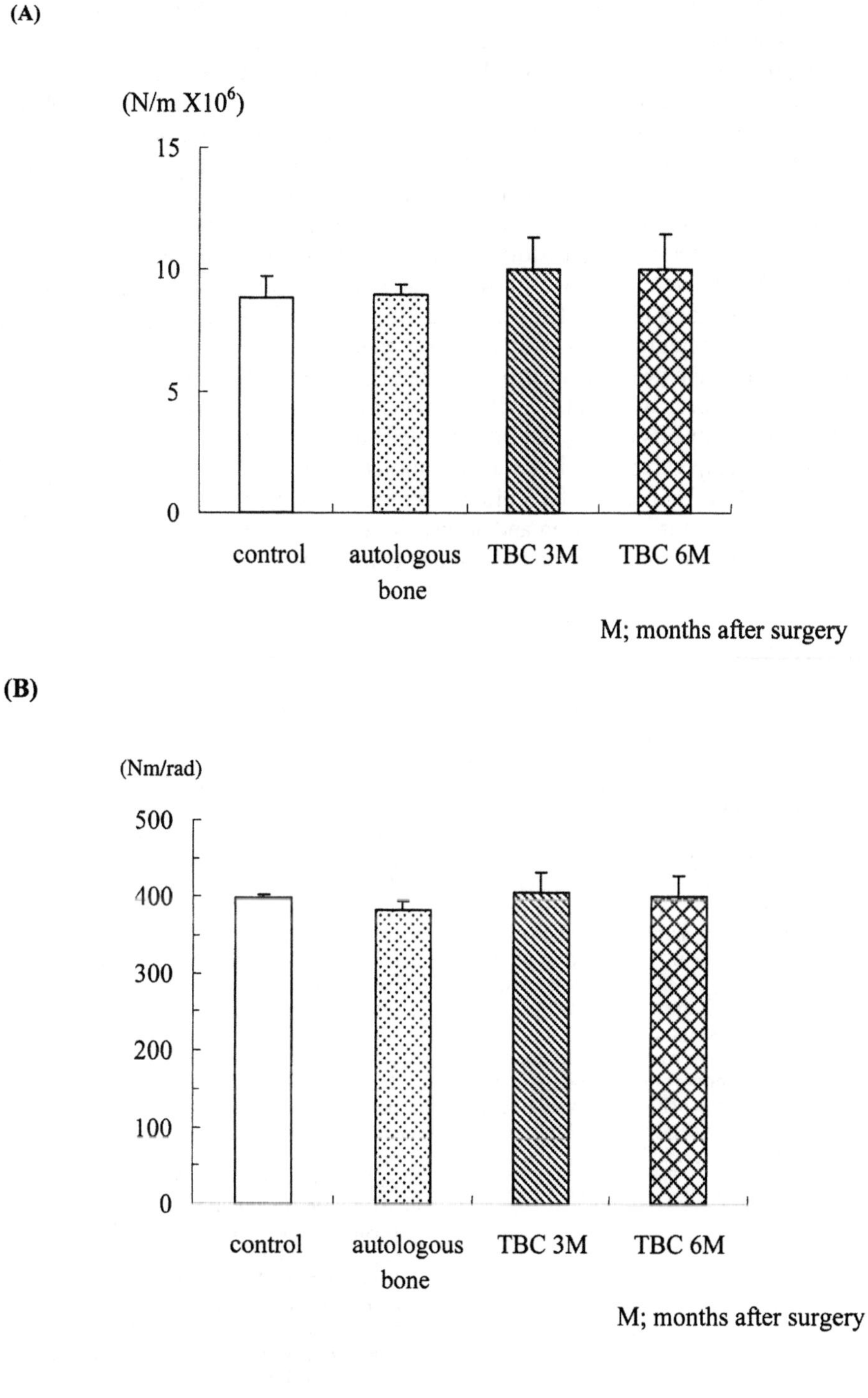

Fig. 2 Graphs showing the axial compressive (**A**) and torsional (**B**) stiffness of each construct. There were no significant differences in the stiffness of each loading method among samples from each group. The unfused L2-L3 motion segments in the control group were separated at the level of the L2-L3 disk. The L2 or L3 segments were tested biomechanically in an identical manner to obtain an internal control and to determine the strength of vertebra itself to minimize the effect of biological variation among different animals

are much harder than the recipient bone. In some studies, implanted biomaterials affected the adjacent vertebrae because of relative differences in strength between recipient bone and the implanted material [1, 6]. One phenomenon is that the implanted material may sink into the vertebra superior or inferior to the implant in patients who have fragile vertebrae, such as those with osteoporosis. Vertebrae in the ageing spine fail because they cannot support the internal stresses and strains that result from loads applied to the spine. With ageing and osteoporosis, the strength of the trabecular bone and the structural capacity of the vertebrae are compromised. Reductions in the apparent density and the bone mineral density of trabecular bone typify ageing and osteoporosis. In many experimental studies, the maximum force during compression of vertebral specimens has been assessed, and the failure force has been related to the apparent density and geometric properties of the vertebrae [9]. Measurements have shown that much lower failure force accompanies ageing and severe osteoporosis.

Therefore, the moderate mechanical strength of sintered bone may permit it to be used for spinal fusion in ageing patients with osteoporosis. The basis for this claim is that the optimal substitute material would be one that has a composition and structure similar to that of human bone tissue and one that would biologically adjust to the bone stiffness of a particular patient while allowing the substitute material to serve as a site for new bone formation. In biomechanical and histological testing, our experimental results were similar to those of the autograft and to the group with no implanted vertebrae. Because the implanted TBC integrated so well with the recipient bone and permitted the progressive growth of new bone into its pores, the stiffness of the TBC, with its moderate mechanical strength, appears to have adjusted biologically to match that of the respective host bone at the implantation site. Therefore, TBC appears to be a bioactive material, which forms a permanent integration and adjusts to the recipient bone in a similar manner to an autologous bone graft.

Conclusion

TBC, which is one of the natural biomaterials based on the calcium phosphate system, attained biomechanical and histological equivalency with the autograft (and with no implantation). Most importantly, sintered bone, with its moderate strength, tended to adjust to the stiffness of the bone in the host bed. Although it may be necessary to perform more detailed experimental studies on these improvements to sintered bone and on the use of instrumentation as an adjunct, our observations warrant further clinical investigation of the use of sintered bone as an effective spinal arthrodesis, especially in patients who have fragile vertebrae, as in osteoporosis.

Acknowledgements This work was supported in part by grants from the Japan Ministry of Education, Science and Culture, grant-in-aid for scientific research no. 11557110, 1999.

References

1. Abumi K, Kaneda K, Satoh E, Takeda N, Taneichi H, Ito M (1998) Anterior reconstruction of the thoracic and lumbar spine using Kaneda anterior spinal system: indication and results in destructive spinal disorders (in Japanese). Rinsho Seikeigeka 33:495–503
2. Hashizume H, Tamaki T, Oura H, Minamide A (1998) Changes in the extracellular matrix on the surface of sintered bovine bone implanted in the femur of a rabbit: an immunohistochemical study. J Orthop Sci 3:42–53
3. Kaneda K, Asano S, Hashimoto T, Satoh S, Fujiya M (1992) The treatment of osteoporotic posttraumatic vertebral collapse using the Kaneda device and bioactive ceramic vertebral prosthesis. Spine 17:S295–303
4. Katoh T, Sato K, Kawamura M, Iwata H, Miura T (1993) Osteogenesis in sintered bone combined with bovine bone morphogenetic protein. Clin Orthop 287:266–275
5. Kurz L, Grafin SR, Booth RE (1989) Harvesting autogenous iliac bone graft. A review of complications and techniques. Spine 14:1324-1331
6. Leong JCY, Chow SP, Yau ACMC (1994) Titanium-mesh block replacement of the intervertebral disk. Clin Orthop 300:52–63
7. Matsumoto T, Kawakami M, Kuribayashi K, Takenaka T, Minamide A, Tamaki T (1999) Effects of sintered bovine bone on cell proliferation, collagen synthesis and osteoblastic expression in MC3T3-E1 osteoblast-like cells. J Orthop Res 17:586-592
8. Minamide A, Tamaki T, Yoshida M, Hashizume H, Nakagawa Y (2000) An experimental approach to spinal fusion using sintered bovine bone in a pig model. J Spinal Disord 13:156–164
9. Myers ER, Wilson SE (1997) Biomechanics of osteoporosis and vertebral fracture. Spine 22:S25-31
10. Nibu K, Panjabi MM, Oxland T, Cholewicki J (1997) Multidirectional stabilizing potential of BAK interbody spinal fusion system for anterior surgery. J Spinal Disord 10:357-362
11. Shikata J, Yamamuro T, Iida H, Shimizu K, Yoshikawa J (1990) Surgical treatment for paraplegia resulting from vertebral fractures in senile osteoporosis. Spine 15:485-489
12. Tamaki T, Sakurai K, Kasamatsu N (1994) Results of basic and clinical studies of true bone ceramics. In: Urist MR, O'Connor BT, Burwell RG (eds) Bone grafts, derivatives and substitutes. Butterworth-Heinemann, Oxford, pp 235-244
13. Ueno Y, Shima Y, Ueyoshi A, Harada M, Sakata Y, Maeda T, Akiyama T (1985) Experimental studies of sintered bone implantation (in Japanese). Bessatsu Seikeigeka [Orthopedic Surgery, Suppl] 8:85-88

Alexander G. Hadjipavlou
James W. Simmons
Michael N. Tzermiadianos
Pavlos G. Katonis
David J. Simmons

Plaster of Paris as bone substitute in spinal surgery

A.G. Hadjipavlou (✉)
M.N. Tzermiadianos · P.G. Katonis
Department of Orthopaedics,
University of Crete, Heraklion, Greece
e-mail: ahadjipa@med.uoc.gr

J.W. Simmons
Alamo Bone and Joint Clinic,
San Antonio, Texas, USA

D.J. Simmons
Department of Orthopaedics
and Rehabilitation,
University of Texas Medical Branch,
Galveston, Texas, USA

A.G. Hadjipavlou
Department of Orthopaedic Surgery
and Traumatology,
University of Crete Medical School,
Heraklion, Crete 71110, Greece

Abstract In order to assess the effectiveness of calcium sulphate (plaster of Paris; POP) as a substitute for autologous bone graft, we performed lumbar intervertebral fusion in mature sheep using POP and a variety of other graft materials, and reviewed the literature. The osteoconductivity of the POP grafts was compared to that of grafts carried out with autogenous iliac crest, frozen allogeneic bone, and ProOsteon 500 coralline bone. We also compared the osteogenicity of POP to admixtures of autogenous iliac crest bone with POP and coralline bone, and to an osteoinductive demineralized sheep bone preparation (DBM). The substrates were loaded into tubular titanium mesh, implanted into excavated disc spaces and recovered after a period of 4 months. Fusion mass segments tested in flexion and tension showed that POP was equal to autogenous bone and most other substrates. The POP fusions were significantly tougher than the DBM fusions, even though histomorphometry failed to reveal differences in the amount of trabecular bone. We conclude that POP can be used to achieve a biomechanically stable interbody lumbar vertebral fusion. In addition, our literature review indicated that POP can be used as a vehicle for local delivery of antibiotics in bone infections.

Keywords Osteoinduction · Osteoconduction · Plaster of Paris · Replamineform coralline · Intervertebral fusion

Introduction

Stabilization of the spinal column is crucial to the preservation of neurologic function, and bone grafting is a prerequisite to obtaining the solid arthrodesis imperative to spinal stability [16]. Bone grafting is also essential for reconstruction of spinal defects and offers a surgical procedure for filling the bone defects caused by infection and tumors.

Early attempts at bone grafting date back more than 500 years to the Arab, indigenous Peruvian, and Aztec cultures. In modern times, the first documented case of autogenous bone grafting was reported by Merem in 1810, and the first successful allografting case has been attributed to Macewn in 1881 [32].

Our present knowledge and scientific base for understanding the biology, banking, and widespread clinical applications of bone grafting is largely due to the work of Albee [1], Barth [2], Lexter [28], Phemister [37] and Seen [42], during the late 19th and early 20th centuries. These substantive scientific contributions have made bone grafting techniques common and relatively effective clinical procedures.

There are three biologic processes that impact the success or failure of bone graft: osteogenesis, osteoconduction, and osteoinduction [5].

Osteogenesis refers to the process whereby bone forms directly from living cells, such as the stem cells within autogenous bone. Osteoconduction describes the process in which bone grows into and along the surface of a biocompatible structure when placed in direct apposition to host bone through the process of intramembranous bone formation. The ability to osteoconduct is a passive characteristic of bone that allows it to act as platform on which vascular invasion, resorption, and new bone formation can occur [16]. Osteoinduction is an endochondral bone growth stimulated by specific growth factors (morphogens and/or mitogens) on pluripotential cells, such as mesenchymal stromal or stem cells. In particular, bone morphogenic protein (BMP), identified through the seminal work of Urist and colleagues [48], has demonstrated the capacity for inducing the differentiation of host perivascular mesenchymal cells into cartilage and bone [26].

In varying degrees, bone grafting source materials and techniques use these mechanisms of bioincorporation. Thus, the ideal bone graft should be capable of these processes and also be free of immunologic antigens and microbial pathogens. There are a variety of bone grafts to choose from, each presenting a unique set of advantages and disadvantages. Autograft, or autogenous bone, represents the bone graft source used in the majority of clinical applications.

Autografts, because they are harvested from host bone stock from one body site for transfer to another location in the same individual, offer the maximum biologic potential and histocompatibility. Immunologic considerations and disease transmission are obviated through the use of autogenous bone.

The possibilities of meeting the needs of size, shape, and quantity of bone for any given procedure, however, are limited in autografting. The potential for morbidity by harvesting autologous iliac bone graft is ever present [52], and can be caused by nerve injuries [4, 7, 8, 9], vascular injuries [14, 27], hernia through the iliac bone donor site [17, 29], bowel obstructions [6], and other noteworthy drawbacks. Operating room time is extended, as is the period under which the patient must remain under anesthesia. Any complications arising from these events, especially if compounded by the sequelae of donor site morbidity, may also increase the duration of hospitalization. Moreover, such a procedure often renders the bone donor site unacceptable for a subsequent operation.

Despite these disadvantages, what makes the autograft the gold standard for bone grafting is that it fulfils the three requirements necessary for bioincorporation: it is osteogenic, osteoconductive, and osteoinductive.

Allografts, usually obtained from cadaveric sources or incidental to operative procedures, offer satisfactory biologic potential and eliminate the chance of donor site morbidity. For same species to species transfer, allografts provide an abundant supply of bone tissue, but the use of allografts for spinal fusion has proven disappointing, especially for onlay intertransverse bone grafts [19, 21, 45]. Moreover, the use of allografts poses biohazards arising from their potential to act as conduits for disease transmission from donor to recipient and the triggering of immunologic reactions. Thus, strict adherence to bone banking methodology and sterilization procedures are essential to proper handling of allografts [44].

Xenograft, or cross-species bone tissue, although in abundant supply, has been found to be a less reliable graft material than autogenous and allogeneic bone. The emergence of such concerns as major histocompatibility difference leading to immune response provocation, the incompatibility of other species' anatomies with human anatomic parts, lessened biological activity, and the need for rigorous, meticulous processing and sterilization of bone derived from non-human species have largely reduced the opportunities for effective orthopaedic reconstructive use of xenograft bone.

The endeavor to transcend the numerous drawbacks associated with natural sources of bone tissue has given rise to the development and manufacture of bone substitutes in various osteoinductive and osteoconductive forms [5, 16].

Osteoconductive agents are: tricalcium phosphate ceramics (TCP), hydroxyapatites(Ht), coral-derived biomaterials, mineralized collagen matrix (Healos), some osteoactive polymers and calcium sulphate (plaster of Paris; POP). Materials with osteoinductive properties are: demineralized bone matrix, bovine osteogenic factors and bone derivatives such as BMP and osteogenin. Osteogenesis refers to the process whereby bone forms directly from living cells, such as the stem cells within autogenous bone.

For some applications, such as intervertebral fusions, biologically compatible materials are most suitable when they provide geometric spaces that invite the ingrowth and osteogenic differentiation of primitive mesenchymal cells. "Industry" has exploited this knowledge by providing porous calcium phosphate ceramics [10, 18, 25] and the orthopedic implants with porous metallic coating, which are now widely employed in hip and knee replacement surgeries. Suitable "biological space" was also found in coelenterate coral skeletons. Once it was discovered how to chemically convert $CaCO_3$ to bone-like hydroxyapatite, this material was marketed as bone ingrowth system under a number of trademarks (e.g., Interpore 200/400; proOsteon Implant 500). There is now a sizeable outcome literature reporting successful use of replamineform coral implants. (i.e., bony union) in the canine mandible [23], and tibial plateau [23], in a rabbit tibia [43, 46], as well as in various human long bones [24]. However, osseous integration, which is usually promoted by hydroxyapatite coating, failed to occur on artificial intervertebral disc in dogs. To date, there is a single report that plate-stabilized blocks

(0.5 cm) of coralline material produce new bone within cervical disc spaces [49].

BMP has been demonstrated to improve the spinal fusion rate [47], but its expense and limited availability are not likely to encourage its widespread use in the near future. An inexpensive, readily available bone grafting material that has a high fusion success rate would be greatly welcomed. POP may prove to be such a material since, in non-vertebral settings, it is well tolerated by human tissue. POP-filled defects in bone are gradually vascularized and replaced by bone tissue derived from the host [11, 30, 33, 34, 35, 36].

The goal of this paper is:

1. To determine whether POP implants in resected vertebral bone spaces in adult sheep are as effective as autologous bone, allogeneic bone, demineralized bone and Interpore-500 in achieving lumbar intervertebral fusions, and
2. To review the pertinent literature on POP as bone substitute

Table 1 Graft materials used to fill tubular titanium mesh implants

Osteoconductive grafts	Osteoinductive graft
1. Autogenous iliac crest cancellous bone	Demineralized bone
2. Frozen allogeneic cancellous iliac crest	
3. Coralline hydroxyapatite (pro-Osteon 500)	
4. Plaster of Paris	
5. 1:1 autogenous iliac crest bone with:	
a) Frozen allogeneic bone	
b) Replamineform coral	
c) Plaster of Paris	

Materials and methods

Animals

Fifteen adult female sheep (30–40 kg body wt) were purchased through the UTMB Animal Resources Center. They were penned in individual cages with free access to food and tap of water. The full-time animal care staff monitored the health of the animals pre- and postoperatively, and the animals were inspected three times a day, including weekends. All experimental procedures were carried out with the approval of the Institutional Animal Use and Care Committee (ACUC Protocol # 94–07–036)

Surgical procedures

The animals were intubated, and anesthetized by deep halothane inhalation (2–4%). The skin was sheared and shaved over the region of their lumbar vertebrae, and was sterilized with a betadine scrub. Using aseptic conditions, the intervertebral discs between L1-L2, L3-L4, and L5-L6 were excised by sharp dissection and the use of a pituitary forceps, and the cartilaginous and bony end plates were cut away to expose the subchondral bone. Each space was then implanted with a 1.0×1.5-cm-long tubular titanium cage (DePuy Motech, Warsaw, Ind.), which had been filled with one of a variety of osteoconductive or osteoinductive demineralized bone substrates (Table 1, Fig. 1), or left empty as a control implant. The autogenous iliac crest implants containing bone and marrow were morselized (1–2 mm) prior to loading and implantation. The osteoinductive substrate was donated by Osteotech Inc., whose technical staff prepared the material from powdered/sieved (size range=100–500 mm) allogeneic sheep cortical bone according to the general methods reported by the Edwards' group [12]. POP was obtained from the Galveston Shriners Burne Hospital's orthotic laboratory, and implanted as 2- to 4-mm^3 pellets. The implant of a commercially available porous apatitic coralline material (Pro-Osteon 500, Orthopaedics Inc., Irvine, Calif.) was coarsely granular. Implant usage was randomized by implanting two grafts of each type at the three different levels (*n*=6/group) (Table 2). The subcutaneous muscles were reapproximated and sutured with 2–0 chromic sutures. The skin incisions were closed with surgical staples.

Immediately after surgery, the animals were removed to the ovine intensive care unit, where they were closely monitored for

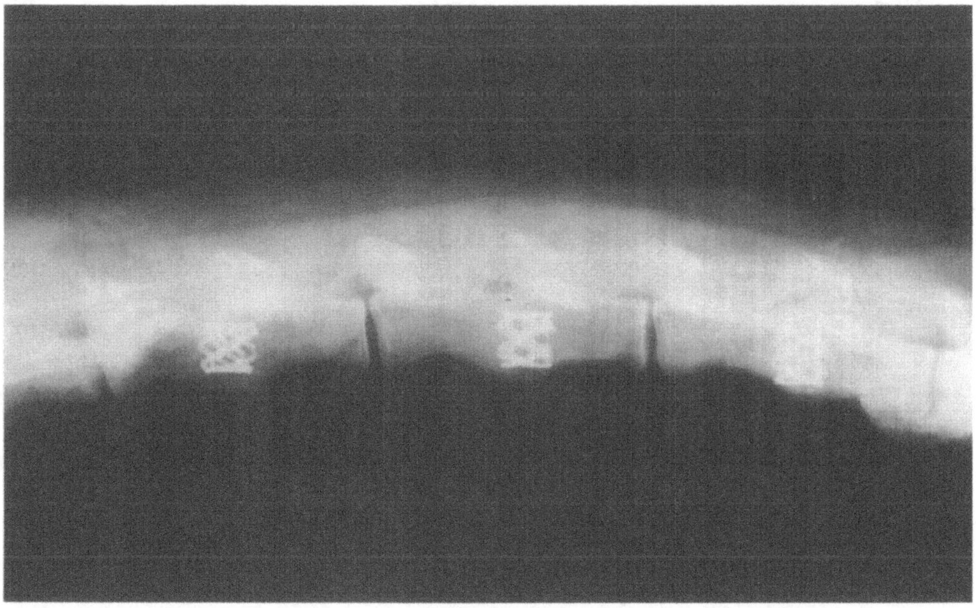

Fig. 1 Roentgenograph showing the positioning of titanium cages within excavated disc spaces in the lumbar spine of a sheep 4 months postoperatively. The interbody fusion masses represent the following graft types. *Top*: autogenous iliac crest bone/marrow; *middle*: demineralized allogeneic bone (DBM); *bottom*: 1:1 autograft:DBM. The roentgenograph is showing the interbody fusion masses within and around the titanium cages

Table 2 Example of distribution of graft types at three lumbar spinal levels in sheep (n=7/group)

Sheep no.	Disc space level	Graft material	Post-surgical radiology	Postop. time to sacrifice
1	L1–2	Autogenous iliac crest	48 h & 1,2,3,4 months	4 months
	L3–4	1:1 autogenous iliac crest and replamineform coral		
	L5–6	Replamineform coral		
2	L1–2	Autogenous iliac crest.	48 h & 1,2,3,4 months	4 months
	L3–4	1:1 autogenous iliac crest and plaster of Paris		
	L5–6	Plaster of Paris		

pain and discomfort, food and water consumption, and urinary output. Pain was managed by the subcutaneous administration of Buprenex (0.15 mg). All animals exhibited an unremarkable postoperative course, and were able to stand independently within 12–24 h. The animals were sacrificed 4 months postoperatively by an intravenous injection of Beuthenasia (1.0 ml/10lb body wt). At autopsy, the thoracolumbar vertebral columns were stripped of soft tissues and their posterior bony elements (facet joints), and frozen in saline for biomechanical and histomorphometric studies.

Biomechanical investigations

All testing was carried out using an MTS –858 Mini-Bionix machine (MTS Inc., Minneapolis, Minn.). Vertebrae were transected at their midlengths, so that the ends of individual segments, which included a single interbody graft, were mounted in methylmethacrylate. The stability of these segments was tested in two modes:

1. In torsional loading through a range of 5 N m (–2.5 to +2.5 N m) to establish rotational stability, and
2. In tensile loading to measure the tensile load to failure (N)

Longitudinal sections showed that the ±2.5 N m of torque applied to the normal vertebrae was insufficient to break trabecular bone structures (vide infra). Following the biomechanical extension test (which produced titanium-free bony cores), the tissues were recovered for histomorphometric investigations. In the protocol for (1), the loading rate was 0.1 Hz, and each sample was subjected to two complete cycles. In (2), the tensile loading was applied from a 0.05 N preload at a rate of 0.5 mm/s.

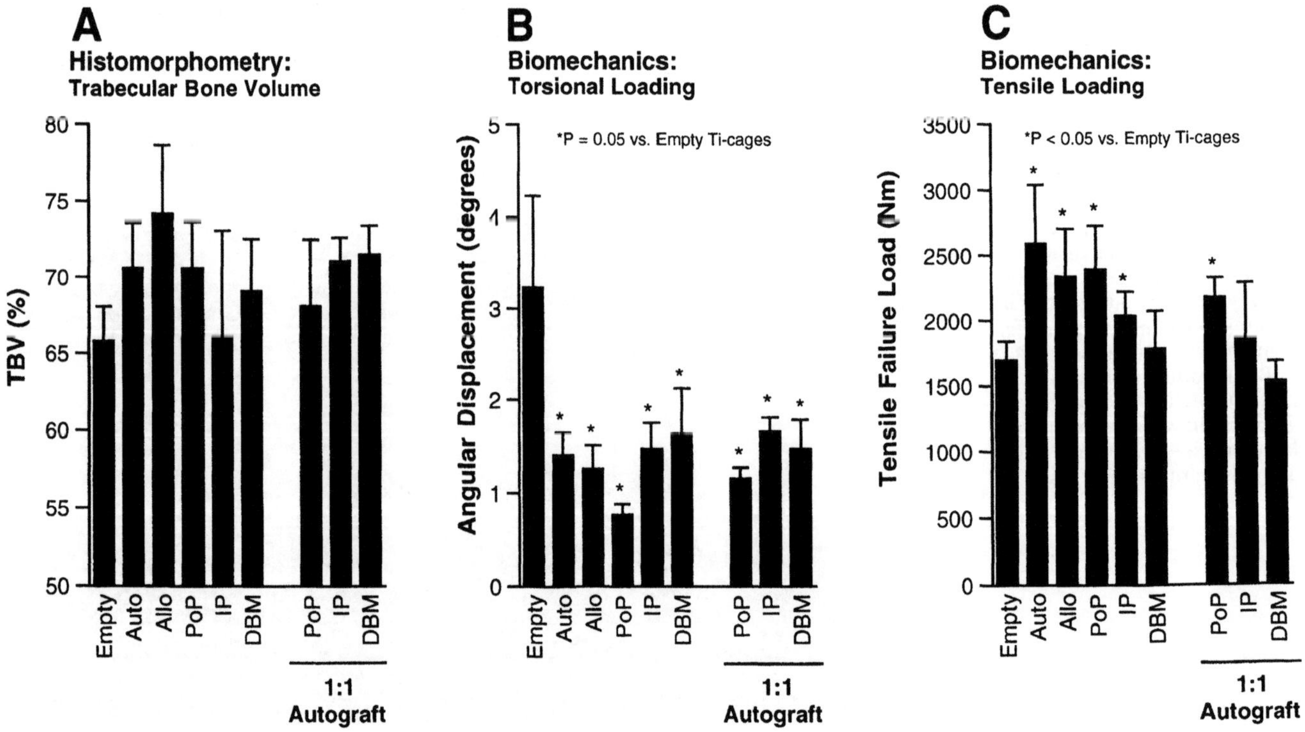

Fig. 2A–C Graphs showing the quantitative histomorphometric and biomechanical evaluations of the bone formed under the influence of osteoconductive and osteoinductive substrates implanted within excavated lumbar spine spaces. **A** Histomorphometry, **B** biomechanics – angular displacements between –2.5 and +2.5 N m loads, **C** biomechanics – tensile failure load. Implants of empty titanium cages served as the control group. Data represented by bars marked with an asterisk (*) were statistically different from the empty control data at the $P<0.05$ level of significance (*Auto* autograft, *Allo* frozen allografts, *PoP* plaster of Paris, *IP* replamineform coralline substrate, *BDM* demineralized allogeneic sheep bone)

Histomorphometric investigations

Interest focused on the relative volumes of bone that had formed within the titanium cages. The intact cores of bone with attached vertebrae were fixed in 95% ethyl alcohol, defatted in acetone, and embedded in methylmethacrylate, and serial longitudinal sections (100 μm thick) were obtained at midlength level using a low-speed Isomet saw (Buehler) equipped with a diamond blade. The sections were microradiographed on fine-grain 649–0 spectroscopic film (10 kV, 20 mA, 10 min). A point-counting microscopical technique with computer-driven software (Optimas Corp., Bothell, Wash.) was employed to quantitate the total area of trabecular bone formed within each titanium cage, and the data were expressed in terms of percent trabecular bone volume.

Statistics

The experiments were designed with the recognition that there might be significant positional effects of grafts at the different spine levels. Nevertheless, our protocols produced too few numbers of grafts for any one to detect such effects. The data were expressed as the mean±standard error of the mean (SEM). The differences between the means were analyzed by Student's *t*-test when the variances were equal (ANOVA), or by a nonparametric two-tailed *t*-test, *F*-test, and Wilcoxon rank-order statistic when the variances were unequal. Differences between means at the 5% confidence level ($P<0.05$) were considered to be statistically significant. The statistical power at $\alpha=0.05$ ranged from 0.8 to 1.0 for the variables that showed statistical significance.

Results

At the time of sacrifice, 4 months postoperatively, host-derived trabecular bone had invested each of the control and experimental interbody cages (Fig. 1). Histomorphometry indicated that the different grafts and combinations of tissue types had produced volumes of new bone that were neither significantly different interalia, nor different from the outcome of the empty control implants (Fig. 2 A). This indicated that the postoperative recovery period was sufficiently long to model and remodel the original graft matrices. All bone present appeared microradiographically to be of uniform and equal density. Biomechanically, however, the behavior of the control fusion masses was inferior to that of the fusion masses formed under the influence of osteoconductive bony and apatitic substrates. An applied torque of ±2.5 N m (from –2.5 to +2.5 N m), which was insufficient to break the bony trabeculae, permitted a 1°–2° displacement in the experimental groups (Fig. 2B), versus 3°–4° displacement in the trabecular masses formed around the control cages. The POP grafts permitted, quantitatively, at least, the smallest angular displacement. The "pull-out" tensile test also affirmed that POP and most of the other osteoconductive experimental graft types, alone or in combination with autologous bone, performed optimally (Fig. 2C), and that their fusion masses were biomechanically superior to those formed around the control cages. The tensile failure load of the sheep demineralized osteoinductive bone was only equal to that of the control titanium cages that were implanted empty.

Discussion

This study was designed to determine whether POP could be used to promote interbody lumbar spinal fusions as effectively as autogenous iliac crest bone or a variety of other bone graft preparations. Therefore, comparisons were made to autografts, frozen allogeneic bone, demineralized sheep bone preparation (DBM), replamineform coralline skeleton (Interpore), and to admixtures of POP, DBM and Interpore. These materials were loaded into short (1.0× 1.5 cm) titanium mesh cages, inserted into lumbar disc spaces, and recovered for microradiographic-histomorphometric and biomechanical analysis after 4 months. The histomorphometric results suggested that the different graft types were equally effective at producing bone. The absence of obvious signs of aberrant bone formation (e.g., irregularities in trabecular thickness) indicated that the distributions of viable and dead bone were probably similar in each experimental group. Microradiography per se was incapable of making such distinctions. Moreover, biomechanical tests indicated that in terms of measures of torsional strain (Fig. 2B), tensile failure (Fig. 2C), and volume of bone formed within the titanium cages, the effects of POP and autogenous bone were as indistinguishable from each other as POP was to Interpore and 1:1 admixtures of those substrates with autogenous bone. Elkins and Jones also noted no difference in the degree of bone healing between autogenous cancellous bone, POP and a composite of POP and autogenous cancellous bone [13]. Despite contrary expectations, the osteoinductive demineralized sheep bone preparations proved the least effective of the different substrates in achieving a solid interbody fusion, even though tissue from other species prepared in an identical fashion [39] has proved to be osteoinductive [22, 40, 51]. The addition of autogenous bone did little to improve DBM performance. The advanced age of the donor animals could have been a factor in its poor performance, since production of bone morphogenetic proteins declines with increasing maturity [3]. Yet, it may be that mature sheep are poor BMP responders [15, 41]. This should be taken into consideration with further investigation.

The mechanism(s) responsible for the new bone formation that enveloped the titanium-carrier mesh is likely to involve vascular ingrowth from the marrow of the vertebral bodies, with the intercession of the vertebral periosteum and psoas muscle pericytes (osteoprogenitor cells). The probable involvement of these juxtavascular mesenchymal cells in psoas muscle was observed in sheep implanted with long (44×15-mm) tubular titanium cages to bridge an L4 osteotomy, where the chamber fully ossified within 6 months [20]. Because the most posterior annular tissue had not been completely removed, it is unlikely that

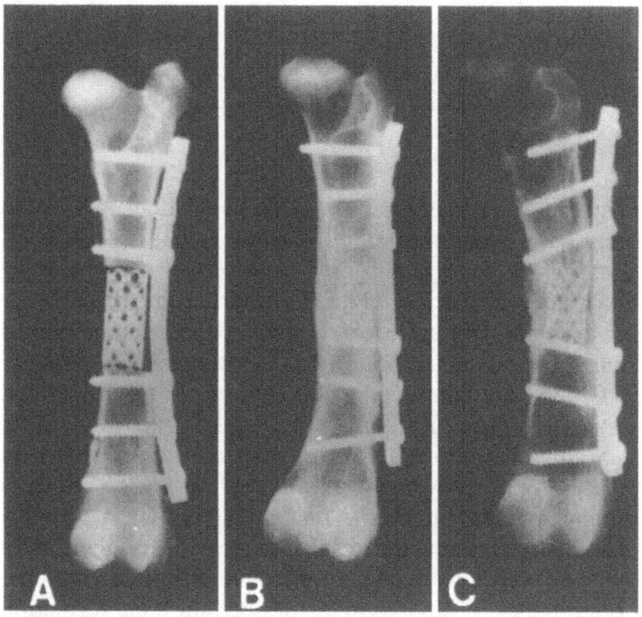

Fig. 3 Roentgenographs showing postoperative appearances of a femoral midshaft titanium cage implant in a sheep: immediately after surgery (**A**), 6 months after iliac crest autograft procedure (**B**), and 6 months after POP implant (**C**). All graft sites were stabilized by lateral eight-hole compression plate (with permission from Lippincott Williams & Wilkins)

the formation of the fusion masses was mediated in part by osteogenic potential of the dura. In addition, an important finding in this study was that the tissue formed within and around the titanium mesh implanted with POP and autogenous bone marrow had equal biomechanical competence in the bending and torsional modes.

In a previous publication we have reported that POP had an osteoconductivity equal to that of autogenous iliac crest marrow/bone (Fig. 3, Fig. 4) [20]. Our study corroborated the findings of Peltier and co-workers [35, 36], which showed that the most important property of POP as a "filler" was its apparent natural rate of absorption – one that was equal to the rate at which new bone grew into the defect. Peltier's findings were further reinforced by a previous observation by the present authors that equal volumes of bone were produced by POP and autogenous bone marrow preparations, and that the products were of equal biomechanical competence in bending and torsion testing modes [20].

Allergy to POP, although rare and related to minor additives, and inflammatory reactions should be considered when assessing the risk-benefit of using calcium sulphate as bone replacement material [38]. In a series of 15 implantations of calcium sulphate pellets (Osteoset, Wright Medical Technology) used for bone reconstruction after resection of bone tumors, three cases of inflammatory reactions were noted [38].

In one case, an allergic reaction provoked serious drainage and necessitated graft removal. In another case, inflammation resolved 2 months following implantation, whereas the third case was complicated by wound breakdown. However, other investigators have noted that POP is innocuous in terms of producing a local soft tissue chemical or pyogenic inflammatory reaction [20, 13, 35].

Fig. 4A–C Microradiographs showing the relative amount and structure of the bone formed external to (*top*) and within (*bottom*) the titanium cage midshaft femoral implants in sheep 6 months after surgery. **A** control/empty, **B** autogenous bone/marrow, **C** POP (with permission from Lippincott Williams and Wilkins)

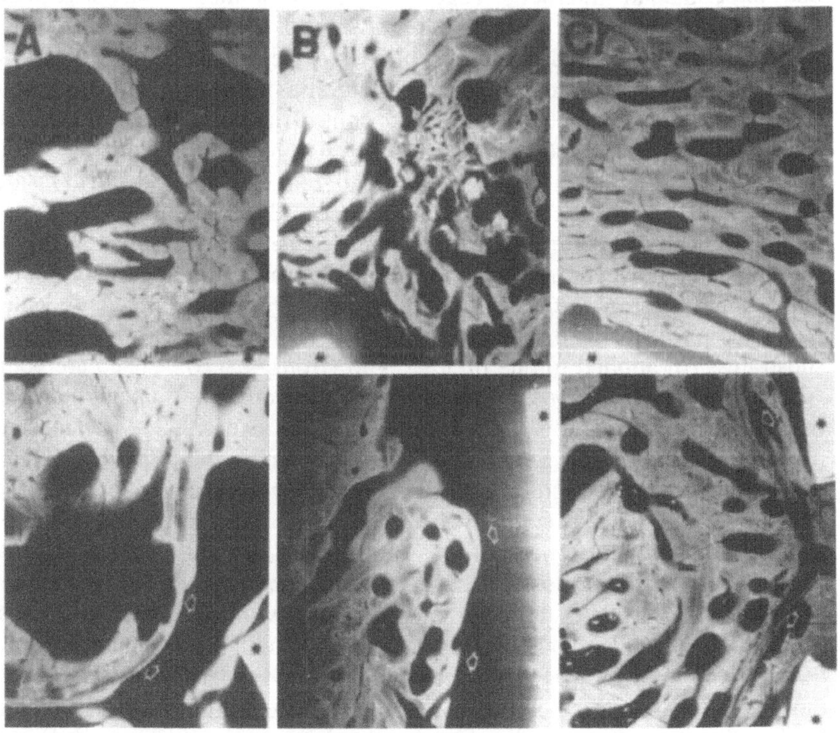

In a prospective clinical study of 50 patients using calcium sulphate pellets (Osteoset), no graft complication was encountered [50].

A recent clinical study of 50 patients showed that POP (an osteoconductive material) is very effective when used as a vehicle for a bioassayed demineralized bone matrix (an osteoinductive material), comparable to grafting with autograft [50]. These findings suggest that POP may be considered as a suitable vehicle through which osteoinductive material may express optimal osteoactivity.

POP may also be considered as an effective carrier for the local delivery of antibiotics. The elution of POP is 17% at 24 h; at 3 weeks trace amounts are still detected. This profile compares favorably to the more conventional carrier, polymethylmethacrylate, which releases 7% of its load by 24 h, with trace amounts detected at 14 days. Because POP remains effective for approximately 3 weeks, it offers a suitable means for long-term coverage of established osteomyelitis [31]. For acute contaminated open fractures, where brief antibiotic coverage is required, bone graft or demineralized bone matrix (DBM) may be used for local delivery, because they elute 70% and 45% of their antibiotic load by 24 h, respectively, and negligible amounts are detectable at 1 week [31].

We have not tested the effects of POP on common bone formation and resorption markers (e.g., alkaline phosphatase, osteocalcin, osteopontin). We are currently using histomorphometric studies to compare the rates of bone formation and resorption between normal bone and POP. In future studies, we intend to investigate the effects of POP in the proximity of neural elements such as dura and nerve roots.

In conclusion, the biomechanical histomorphometric outcomes of interpositional grafts of POP were equal to those of autogenous bone marrow grafts.

Acknowledgements The authors express their appreciation to Osteotech Inc. for the generous gift of the sheep demineralized bone preparation, and to Mr. Randal P. Morris (UTMB, Department of Orthopaedics and Rehabilitation) for technical assistance with the biomechanical testing. Also to the Department of Orthopaedic Surgery of UTMB for providing funds from Bixler's research grant.

References

1. Albee FH (1923) Fundamentals in bone transplantation: experience in three thousand bone graft operations. JAMA 81:1429–1432
2. Barth A (1893) Ueber histologische Befunde nach Knochenimplantationen. Arch Klin 46:409–417
3. Bessho K, Izuka T (1993) Changes in bone inducing activity of bone morphogenetic protein with aging. Ann Chir Gynaecol Suppl 207:49–53
4. Brown LT (1937) The mechanics of the lumbosacral and sacro-iliac joints. J Bone Joint Surg 19:770–775
5. Burwell RG (1985) The function of bone marrow in the incorporation of a bone graft. Clin Orthop Rel Res 200: 125–141
6. Challis JH, Lyttle JA, Stuart AE (1975) Strangulated lumbar hernia and volvulus following removal of iliac crest bone graft. Acta Orthop Scand 46:230–233
7. Cocking J (1971) Autologous bone grafting – complications at the donor site. J Bone Joint Surg Br 53:153
8. Cooper JW (1967) Cluneal nerve injury and chronic post surgical neuritis. J Bone Joint Surg 49:199
9. Drury BJ (1967) Clinical evaluation of back and leg pain due to irritation of the superior cluneal nerve. J Bone Joint Surg 49:199
10. Ducheyne P, Beight J, Cucler J, Evans B, Radin S (1990) Effect of calcium phosphate coating characteristics on early bone operative bone ingrowth. Biomaterials 11:531–540
11. Edberg E (1930) Some experiences of filling osseous cavities with plaster. Acta Chir Scand 67:313–319
12. Edwards JT, Diegmann MH, Scarborough NL (1998) Osteoinduction of human demineralized bone: characterization in a rat model. Clin Orthop 357: 219–228
13. Elkins AD, Jones LP (1988) The effects of plaster of Paris and autogenous cancellous bone on the healing of cortical defects in femur of dogs. Vet Surg 17:71–76
14. Escalas F, Dewald RL (1977) Combined traumatic arteriovenous fistula and ureteral injury: a complication of iliac bone grafting, a case report. J Bone Joint Surg 59:270–271
15. Fleet JC, Cashman K, Cox K, Rosen V (1996) The effects of aging on the bone inductive activity of recombinant human bone morphogenetic protein-2. Endocrinology 137:4606–4610
16. Friedlaender GE, Curting SL, Huo MH (1997) Bone grafts and bone graft substitutes. In: Frymoyer JW (ed) The adult spine: principles and practices, 2nd edn. Lippincott- Raven, Philadelphia, pp719–732
17. Froimson AI, Gummings AG Jr (1971) Iliac hernia following hip arthrodesis. Clin Orthop 30:89–91
18. Goshima J, Goldberg VM, Caplan AI (1991) The origin of bone formed in composite grafts of porous calcium phosphate ceramic loaded with marrow cells Clin Orthop 269:274–283
19. Hadjipavlou AG, Enker P, Dupuis P, Katzman S, Silver J (1996) The causes of failure of lumbar transpedicular spinal instrumentation and fusion: a prospective study. Int Orthop 20:35–42
20. Hadjipavlou AG, Simmons JW, Yang J, Nicodemus CL, Esch O, Simmons DJ (2000) Plaster of Paris as an osteoconductive material for interbody vertebral fusion in mature sheep. Spine 25:10–16
21. Heiple KG, Chase SW, Herndon CH (1963) A comparative study of the healing process following different types of bone transplantation. J Bone Joint Surg Am 45:1593–1612
22. Helm GA, Sheehan JM, Sheehan JP, et al (1997) Utilization of type I collagen gel, demineralized bone matrix and bone morphogenetic protein-2 to enhance autologous bone lumbar spinal fusion. J Neurosurg 86:93–100
23. Holms RE (1979) Bone regeneration within a coralline hydroxyapatite implant. Plast Reconstr Surg 63:626–633
24. Holms RE, Mooney V, Bucholz RW, Tencer AF (1984) A coralline replamineform hydroxyapatite implant for bone grafting. Clin Orthop 188: 282–292

25. Hong L, Hengshang X (1992) Tensile stength of the interface between hydroxyapatite and bone. J Biomed Mater Res 26:7–18
26. Hsu K, Zucherman JF, White AH (1987) Bone grafts and implants in spine surgery. In White AH, Rothman RH, Ray CD (eds) Lumbar spine surgery: techniques and complications. St. Louis, Mosby, pp 434–458
27. Kahn B (1979) Superior gluteal artery laceration: a complication of iliac bone graft surgery. Clin Orthop 149:204
28. Lexter E (1925) Joint transplantation and arthroplasty. Surg Gynecol Obstet 40:782–809
29. Lotem M, Maor P, Haimoff H. Woloch Y (1971) Lumbar hernia at an iliac bone graft donor site: a case report. Clin Orthop 80:130–132
30. Mackey D, Varlet A, Debeaumont D (1982) Antibiotic loaded Plaster of Paris pellets: an in vitro study of a possible method of local antibiotic therapy in bone infection. Clin Orthop 167: 263–268
31. Miclau T, Dahmers LE, Lindesey RW (1993) In vitro pharmacokinetics of antibiotic release from locally implantable materials. J Orthop Res 11:627–632
32. Muscher GF, Lane JM (1992) Clinical applications [of bone grafting] in orthopaedic surgery. In: Habal MB, Reddi AH (eds) Bone grafts and bone substitutes. W.B. Saunders, Philadelphia, pp 375–407
33. Nielsen A (1944) Filling of sterile and infected bone cavities by means of plaster of Paris. Acta Chir Scand 91: 17–27
34. Nystrom G (1928) Plugging of bone cavities with rivanol-plaster porridge. Acta Chir Scand 63:296
35. Peltier LF (1961) The use of plaster of Paris to fill defects in bone Clin Orthop 21:1–31
36. Peltier LR, Bickel EY, Lillo R, Thein MS (1957) The use of plaster of Paris to fill defects in bone. Ann Surg 146: 61–69
37. Phemister DB (1914) The fate of transplanted bone and regenerative power of its various constituents. Surg Gynecol Obstet 19:303–333
38. Robinson D, Alk D, Sandbank J, et al (1999) Inflammatory reactions associated with a calcium sulphate substitute. Ann Transpl 4:91–97
39. Russel J, Scarborough N, Chesmel K (1996) Ability of commercial demineralized freeze-dried bone allografts to induce new bone formation. J Periodontol 67:918–926
40. Sandhu HS, Kanim LE, Kabo JM, Toth JM, et al (1996) Effective doses of recombinant human bone morphogenetic protein-2 in experimental spinal fusion. Spine 21:2115–2122
41. Schwarz N, Dingers HP, Schiesser A, et al (1989) Dog bone less osteogenetic than rat bone: bone matrix transplants in nude rats. Acta Orthop Scand 60: 693–695
42. Seen N (1889) On the healing of aseptic bone cavities by implantation of antiseptic bone. Am J Med Sci 98:219–243
43. Shimazaki K, Mooney V (1985) Comparative study of porous hydroxyapatite and tricalcium phosphate as bone substitute. J Orthop Res 3:301–310
44. Simmons JW (1987) Bone banking. In: White AH, Rothman RH, Ray CD (eds) Lumbar spine surgery: techniques and complications. Mosby, St Louis, pp 459–470
45. Smith RT (1972) The mechanism of graft rejection. Clin Orthop 87:15–18
46. Tencer AF, Woodard PL, Swenson J, Brown KL (1987) Bone ingrowth into polymer coated synthetic coralline hydroxyapatite. J Orthop Res 5:275–282
47. Urist MR, Dawson E (1981) Intertransverse process fusion with the aid of chemosterilized autolyzed antigen-extracted allogenic (AAA) bone. Clin Orthop 165:97–113
48. Urist MR, Sato K, Brownell AG, et al (1983) Human bone morphogenetic protein (hBMP). Proc Soc Exper Biol Med 173:194–199
49. Vuono-Hawkins M, Zimermman MC, Lee CK, Carter FM, Parsons JR, Langrana NA (1994) Mechanical evaluation of canine intervertebral disk spacer. J Orthop Res 12:119–127
50. Wilkins RM, Kelly CM, Giusti DE (1999) Bioassayed demineralized bone matrix and calcium sulfate: use in bone-grafting procedures. Ann Chir Gynaecol 88:180–185
51. Yamaguchi A (1995) Regulation of differentiation pathway of skeletal mesenchymal cells in cell lines by transforming growth factor-beta superfamily. J Cell Biol 6:165–173
52. Younger EM, Chapman MW (1989) Morbidity at bone graft donor sites. J Orthop Trauma 3:192–195

Jeffrey M. Spivak
Amir Hasharoni

Use of hydroxyapatite in spine surgery

Abstract Hydroxyapatite- (HA-)based ceramics have been evaluated for a variety of applications in spinal surgery, utilizing in vivo animal models and human clinical series. In vivo animal studies have shown efficacy for these materials as a bone graft substitute in interbody fusions and as a bone graft extender or bioactive osteoinductive material carrier in posterolateral lumbar fusions. Clinically, HA ceramic has been shown to be effective as a bone graft extender in posterior spinal fusion surgery for childhood scoliosis, and as a structural bone graft substitute in anterior cervical spine fusions. As an osteoconductive material, it appears to function best as a bone graft extender or carrier for an osteoinductive bone growth factor rather than as a stand-alone bone graft substitute in nonstructural clinical applications. Injectable HA ceramics also hold promise as biocompatible and bioresorbable materials for use in spinal screw fixation strength augmentation and in minimally invasive vertebral body strength augmentation either following fracture or prophylactically in osteoporotic vertebrae.

Keywords Hydroxyapatite · Spinal fusion · Bone morphogenetic protein carrier · Vertebroplasty

J.M. Spivak (✉) · A. Hasharoni
New York University/
Hospital for Joint Diseases
Department of Orthopaedic Surgery,
and the Hospital
for Joint Diseases Spine Center,
301 East 17th St., Suite 400,
New York, NY 10003, USA
e-mail: jeffrey.spivak@med.nyu.edu

Introduction

Surgical techniques and instrumentation systems to provide segmental fixation, providing added stability and the ability to correct deformity, have become increasingly refined and available [3, 11]. This has been an important factor in the recent increase in popularity of spinal fusion surgery. For a spinal fusion (arthrodesis) to be successful, even in the presence of spinal instrumentation, living bone tissue must bridge adjacent vertebrae to provide long-term support. Failure of bony fusion (pseudoarthrosis) remains a significant problem in spine surgery. Basic indications for spinal fusion include spinal instability, correction and/or stabilization of spinal deformity, following complete discectomy (as in the anterior cervical spine) for decompression, and in certain cases of pain syndromes thought to be due to painful disc degeneration or focal spinal arthritis.

Bone grafting typically accompanies a spinal fusion. The grafted bone material spans the vertebral elements to be fused, providing a scaffold for ingrowth and replacement by a connected bridge of living host bone. Autologous bone graft from the iliac crest continues to be the gold standard material for use in achieving a successful spinal arthrodesis [9]. Even with the use of autologous bone graft, spinal fusions fail to heal and pseudoarthrosis develops in 5–35% of patients [5]. Mechanical enhancement of spinal fusion with rigid internal fixation has improved fusion rates in general, but it has not completely eliminated the occurrence of nonunion. As a result, osteogenic enhancement of spinal fusion is becoming increasingly sought after.

Problems certainly exist with the use of autologous bone grafting. Procurement of autologous bone adds to overall operative time and blood loss, and disrupts an otherwise normal structure of the body. Donor site complications reported include wound infection, hematoma, pelvic fracture, and cutaneous nerve neuromas [7, 38]. Significant complications with its use may occur in up to 10% of patients and minor complications may occur in as many as 25–30% of patients [4, 30]. Also, only a limited amount of autologous bone is available for grafting, and clinical scenarios exist where no autologous bone is available following multiple previous bone graft procedures. In addition, unpredictable bony incorporation and even resorption of autologous bone graft material is sometimes observed. These problems of donor site morbidity and pseudoarthrosis have fueled the search for a dependable bone graft substitute that possesses both osteoconductive and osteoinductive properties.

In addition to multiple local and systemic factors that influence bone formation, the selection of graft material will influence the outcome of a spinal fusion [9]. Graft materials placed into the spinal fusion bed participate in the fusion process in several ways, which depend on the properties of those materials. Osteogenic properties allow the grafts to directly produce bone, osteoinductive properties allow the grafts to stimulate osteoprogenitor mesenchymal cells to differentiate into bone producing cells, and osteoconductive properties allow the grafts to support bone growth and serve as a scaffold supporting neovascularization and ingrowth of osteoblasts and bone production. Bone graft substitutes that have a bone-like geometric construct, such as a porous hydroxyapatite ceramic, often have an osteoconductive property derived at least in part from its internal porous structure [3]. Porous ceramics in general are osteoconductive materials with the physical property of a graft material that allows the ingrowth of neovasculature and infiltration of osteogenic precursor cells during the bone growth process, known as creeping substitution. A graft material that is only osteoconductive transfers neither osteogenic cells nor inductive stimuli, but rather acts as a scaffold or trellis that supports the bone growth.

Ceramics

A number of osteoconductive ceramic bone graft substitutes have received attention as alternatives to autogenous bone. Calcium phosphate ($CaPO_4$) ceramics, which include hydroxyapatite (HA) and tricalcium phosphate (TCP), have been the most widely investigated and used in orthopedic surgery. Both are structured with pores that range from 100 to 200 μm in diameter. Their porosity enables mesenchymal cell migration, adhesion, proliferation and differentiation into osteoblasts within their pores. This unique structure constitutes their osteoconductive characteristics [3].

HA and TCP ceramics are both brittle materials with low fracture resistance. They can be varied in chemical and structural composition. Different preparative methods lead to either a compact or porous material with interconnective macropores that are the spatial and structural equivalent of cancellous bone. In a biologic system, more crystallization and higher material density result in greater mechanical strength and resistance to dissolution, and promote long-lasting stability. In contrast, an amorphous ultra-structure and greater porosity enhance interface activity and bone ingrowth, as well as early biodegradation of the material. Commercially available HA is resorbed very slowly, if at all, under normal physiologic conditions, whereas TCP generally is resorbed within 6 weeks after implantation. When used as a mixture, biodegradable HA/TCP graft material has the ability to dissolve, break down and allow new bone formation and remodeling required to attain optimal mechanical strength without interference. A fully non-resorbable graft material may hinder remodeling, prolong the strength deficiency of new bone and leave permanent stress risers in the fusion mass [4].

An alternative to synthetic calcium phosphate derivatives is natural coral, which has been used clinically to augment bone graft and in combination with platelet-derived growth factors. Composed of 97% calcium carbonate in the form of aragonite, coral is structurally similar to cancellous bone. It is extremely biocompatible and has yielded promising clinical results. The unique structural geometry of coral promotes rapid resorption and reossification without the risk of immunologic reaction or infectious disease transmission. An alternative formulation is coralline HA, which converts much of the calcium carbonate to HA [32].

Animal experimentation

The ability of calcium phosphate ceramics to act as bone graft substitutes for spinal fusion has been studied in many animal spinal fusion models with conflicting results [13, 21]. Part of the confusion may be due to the many different animal models utilized. The biology of healing of a spinal fusion differs depending on the anatomic structures surrounding the fusion region and the forces acting on the fusion bed. Also, the healing potential and amount of available bone surface area in the different anatomic fusion sites is variable. Interbody fusion models assess spinal fusion occurring within the disc space between two vertebral bodies. The structural grafts used in this type of fusion model are acted on by compressive mechanical loads and are within a bed of flat plates of vertebral endplate bone. Posterior and posterolateral fusion models assess spinal fusion of the adjacent posterior bony elements of the spine, including the lamina, facet joints, and transverse processes. Graft materials used in this location are generally not solid and structural, and heal under distraction or tension loads. The mass of morselized graft material is covered around the majority of its surface by muscle and other soft tissues, not bone. The concomitant use of spinal instrumentation with any fusion model affects the mechanical loading of the graft bed, generally limiting the amounts of load seen by the graft material. Instrumentation can also affect the type of load applied, such as allowing a facet joint fusion to occur under compression rather than tension. Differences in species used may also play a role. Taken together, these factors make direct comparisons of different studies impossible to interpret properly.

Emery et al. compared fusion rates of different osteoconductive commercially available ceramic materials in a canine thoracic anterior interbody fusion model [11]. They compared fusion rates of autogenous tricortical iliac crest graft to HA corraline, HA ceramic, HA/TCP (60/40%) ceramic composite, and a calcium carbonate ceramic. All fusions were performed using anterior spinal instrumentation. They found superior fusion rates for the autogenous iliac bone group as compared to all of the ceramic groups, both in histologic evaluation and biomechanical testing. Toth et al. assessed the effect of porosity of the ceramic composite in a goat anterior cervical spine fusion model [34]. Autograft was compared to 30%, 50%, and 70% porosity implants of 50/50 HA/TCP. The more porous implants were hypothesized to trade off some overall strength for improved bone ingrowth and union rate. Biomechanical and histologic evaluation of the fusion mass was done at 3 and 6 months after surgery. All of the tested ceramic implants performed equal to or better than autograft iliac crest bone. The more porous implants had a higher union rate early on, but also had a higher incidence of graft fracture. Overall fusion rates were 67% for the ceramic implants and 50% for autograft. The relatively low fusion rates in all groups were likely due to excessive neck motion in the goat; however, these low fusion rates put into question the ability of this model to be validly extrapolated to human anterior cervical fusions.

Delecrin et al. showed the influence of the fusion site micro environment on incorporation of ceramic and new bone formation in a canine posterior lumbar fusion model [9]. They evaluated bone growth into a macroporous ceramic implant in both an interlaminar fusion site and a posterolateral intertransverse fusion site, using block HA/TCP (60/40%) composite as a graft. The percentage of newly formed fusion bone was significantly higher at the laminar fusion site compared to the intertransverse site, where decorticated bone in the fusion bed was scarce. These results demonstrate a clear deficiency of osteoinduction properties of the graft, and a consequent reliance on bone growth induction, with the decorticated bleeding bone in the fusion bed serving as a source of stem cells and osteogenic factors.

Bozic et al. evaluated the effect of added direct-current electrical stimulation on the fusion rate of an osteoconductive coralline HA ceramic/bone marrow composite bone graft substitute in a rabbit intertransverse process (posterolateral) lumbar spinal fusion model [6]. The HA/bone marrow aspirate composite alone or combined with 40 mA or 100 mA direct-current electrical stimulation were compared to autograft bone. Fusion success was equivalent in the lower-current group and autograft group (50% vs 57%), but was significantly higher in the high-current test group (87%), demonstrating a dose-dependent effect of the direct-current stimulation. The fusion masses in the high-current group were also significantly stronger and stiffer biomechanically and showed a significantly larger fusion mass histologically. The ceramic/marrow aspirate alone test group had significantly fewer successful fusions (25%) than the autograft or current stimulation groups.

Zdeblick et al. analyzed the efficacy of porous HA graft as a substitute for autogenous or allogenic bone graft following anterior cervical discectomy in a goat cervical spine fusion model [39]. Results of single-level ACDF were satisfactory regardless of the graft material used. In multilevel fusions, the fusion rates drop dramatically and complications such as postoperative kyphosis and neural compression increase. Plate stabilization of the HA material led to graft incorporation rates comparable to the autogenous bone group and superior to the allograft bone results. Mechanically, however, while the HA and allograft groups were comparable, they were significantly inferior to the autogenous graft group, leading to early collapse of the fusion mass. Histological assessment revealed incomplete creeping substitution and failure of graft substitution in all three groups. Interestingly, following graft collapse in vivo, fusion rates were similar to unfractured grafts, but with residual severe postoperative kyphosis rendering its use impractical.

The efficacy of interconnected porous HA granules in achieving posterolateral lumbar fusion in sheep was examined by Baramki et al., who evaluated lumbar spinal fusion radiologically and mechanically in a sheep spine fusion model [2]. Bisegmental posterolateral intertransverse lumbar fusion with instrumentation was performed using either no graft material, autologous bone, HA alone, or a HA/autograft composite graft in a 1:1 ratio. The autologous bone group achieved a 100% fusion rate, compared with 72% fusion for the bone/HA composite group, 50% fusion for the HA alone group, and only 15% fusion for the sham operation without any graft material. Spinal arthrodesis using HA alone or mixed with bone as graft material promoted segmental fusions, but not reliably.

HA/TCP use as composite or as carrier systems in animal models

Ceramic composites, which consist of the osteoconductive ceramic combined with an osteoinductive agent such as demineralized bone matrix (DBM), bone marrow, extracted bone matrix proteins, or osteogenic growth factors such as recombinant bone morphogenetic protein (BMP), have been investigated extensively [12, 16, 19]. Walsh et al. sought to determine the effectiveness of HA/TCP/collagen composite composed of type I bovine dermal collagen, 65% HA, and 35% TCP ceramic as a bone graft substitute or expander for autologous bone graft in a posterolateral spine fusion model in sheep [36]. Dual-energy X-ray absorptiometry between the transverse processes revealed that the mineral densities formed by the collagen/HA/TCP composite was significantly higher than the autogenous bone graft group. Histologic analysis confirmed that the composite was highly compatible and was well incorporated into the fusion mass, and induced the formation of thick trabeculae and a mixture of lamellar and plexiform bone. The autogenous bone graft group had a smaller fusion complex, composed primarily of lamellar bone with thinner and fewer trabeculae. Both groups had similar mechanical properties. Another study, using a rabbit interbody fusion model, showed enhanced incorporation of porous HA blocks by the addition of DBM [27]. The animals implanted with the HA/DBM composite showed significant earlier fusion consolidation than the animals implanted with DBM alone, HA alone, or autograft. By 6 months, however, the results were comparable to those attained using autograft bone.

The efficacy of collagen/ceramic/autograft composite was also compared with that of autograft alone in a dog posterior spinal fusion model [40]. At 12 months, histologic quantification of bone ingrowth, as well as results from biomechanical testing, was similar in both groups. Muschler et al. compared posterior fusions in a dog segmental posterior spinal fusion model using autograft, collagen/ceramic composite, collagen/ceramic/autograft composite, and no graft material [22]. Autograft bone alone was the most effective graft material tested, and had a statistically superior union score. Results using the ceramic composites alone were no better than those without any graft materials. The addition of demineralized bone protein extract to the composite, however, significantly improved the union score, which was comparable to that obtained using composite plus autograft bone. Later, Muschler et al. evaluated the efficacy of collagen/ceramic (60% HA, 40% TCP) composite in inducing bone formation in comparison to autogenous iliac bone graft in a dog segmental posterior spinal fusion model. They found that such a composite was inferior to autogenous bone graft in inducing bone formation and fusion [23]. In addition, combining the collagen/ceramic composite with autogenous cancellous bone graft hindered bone formation, and reduced the rate of successful fusion. These results suggest that an autogenous cancellous bone graft carries both osteoconductive and osteoinductive potential, as compared to the lack of osteoinduction potential of the collagen/ceramic composite component of a mixed graft.

Growth factors are relatively short peptides that exert their mitogenic and differentiative effects on cells by binding to cell surface receptors and provoking a signal transduction cascade that results in cellular response. Takahashi et al. examined the efficacy of recombinant human bone morphogenetic protein-2 (rhBMP-2) in enhancing anterior cervical spine interbody fusion when added to a block HA graft in a goat cervical spine model with three-level anterior fusions [31]. Porous HA grafts that contained 0, 5, and 50 mg of rhBMP-2 were placed concurrently with anterior cervical spine fixation plates to achieve interbody fusion. The fusion rate, radiological findings, biomechanical stiffness, and histological appearance were evaluated at 1, 4 and 12 weeks postoperatively. At 12 weeks, manual testing showed a 100% fusion rate in the spines with HA grafts containing high-dose rhBMP-2; however, only a 50% fusion rate was shown in spines with grafts that contained no or low-dose rhBMP-2. On radiographic and histological studies, the biological process of fusion was seen to be more advanced with the larger concentration of rhBMP-2. Biomechanical testing demonstrated significantly higher stiffness values for grafts that contained high-dose rhBMP-2 than those without rhBMP-2 in flexion, extension, and lateral bending tests at 12 weeks. Histological analysis demonstrated that the rhBMP-2 increased the amount of bone apposition on the surface of the HA grafts and promoted bone formation in the porous structure without increasing the penetration distance.

Boden et al. used a non-human primate lumbar intertransverse process arthrodesis model to evaluate rhBMP-2 in a HA/TCP carrier as a complete bone graft substitute [4]. Twenty-one adult rhesus monkeys underwent a laminectomy and fusion with either autogenous iliac crest bone or 60/40 HA/TCP blocks saturated with a solution containing 0, 6, 9, or 12 mg of rhBMP-2. Fusion was not achieved in any of the monkeys treated with autogenous iliac crest bone graft. The monkeys treated with the HA/TCP blocks with rhBMP-2 achieved complete fusion. Histologic analysis showed some ingrowth of bone into the ends, but not through the ceramic block in the absence of rhBMP-2. When the ceramic blocks were loaded with rhBMP-2, there was a dose-dependent increase in the amount and quality of bone throughout the ceramic carrier based on qualitative assessment. The HA-TCP composite proved to be a suitable carrier for rhBMP-2 in this posterolateral spine fusion model in rhesus monkeys. Even in the presence of a laminectomy defect, there was no evidence of bone induction outside the confines of the ceramic carrier.

Osteogenin (BMP-3), an osteoinductive protein, was tested together with TCP acting as carrier by Breitbart and co-workers in a rabbit frontal bone model [7]. TCP alone was used as the control. At 1 month, there was minimal bone ingrowth and TCP resorption. At 3 months, both groups showed a modest amount of bone ingrowth. At 6 months, however, the osteogenin-treated group showed a significant increase in bone ingrowth and faster resorption of the TCP compared to the TCP treated group. They found that the addition of the bone inducer (osteogenin) to bone conductor (TCP) increased bone growth, and the bone was found to have differentiated more fully into lamellar bone in the presence of the bone growth and differentiation-inducing factor, as compared to woven bone on the TCP-only treated group.

Boden et al. compared efficacy of fusion using coralline HA with bone marrow, autogenous bone graft, or osteoinductive bone protein extract for single-level posterolateral lumbar spine fusions in a New Zealand White rabbit fusion model [5]. The animals received a coralline HA implant, either alone or in combination with bone marrow, autogenous iliac crest bone, or 500 ng bovine-derived osteoinductive bone protein extract. Coralline HA alone or with bone marrow produced no solid fusions. When combined with an equal amount of autogenous iliac crest bone, fusion appeared in 50%. When combined with the osteoinductive growth factor extract, the coralline HA resulted in solid fusion in 100%. The fusion masses in the growth factor group were significantly stronger and stiffer. This data indicated that coralline HA with bone marrow was not an acceptable bone graft substitute for posterolateral spine fusion in this model. When combined with autogenous iliac crest bone graft, coralline HA served as a graft extender, yielding results comparable to those obtained with autograft alone. Coralline HA served as an excellent carrier for the bovine osteoinductive bone protein extract, yielding superior results to those obtained with autograft or bone marrow.

One of the important characteristics of a delivery system based on HA/TCP composites is the pore size and overall implant porosity. Works by Itokazu et al. and Radin et al. concentrated on the applicability of HA/TCA to serve as chemotherapeutic, antibiotic and growth factors delivery systems [15, 26]. Urist and co-workers were the first to study the BMP delivery capabilities of TCP, and found that bone and cartilage formation were enhanced 12 fold by combining BMPs and TCP as a carrier [35]. It is not well understood to date, however, whether HA/TCP acts as a slow-release delivery system by directly or indirectly potentiating BMP activity, by protecting BMP from breakdown and digestion, or by serving to distribute BMP in a favorable three-dimensional pattern.

Human clinical studies

The clinical efficacy of ceramics as a graft material for spinal fusion has not been clearly established in animal studies. Better results in general were found with the ceramic composites and ceramic-as-a-carrier system studies. Human clinical series using ceramic alone or as a composite represent one step further in elucidating the safety and efficacy of these materials as an alternative to autologous bone graft [18].

A number of clinical series have been published reporting the benefit of ceramics in spinal fusions for patients with scoliosis. In a study of 12 patients with severe scoliosis by Passuti et al., internal fixation and blocks of HA/TCP (3/2) alone or mixed with autogenous cancellous bone were used to stabilize the spine and fuse the facet joints [24]. Clinical and radiographic assessments of the fusions were performed, and in two cases biopsies of the graft material were obtained. At an average follow-up of 15 months, all patients exhibited complete radiographic fusions. Histologic examination of the biopsy specimens revealed the formation of new bone, which was directly bounded to the ceramic implant surface and inside the macropores. Another study, done with natural coral acting as autograft substitute in 49 patients with idiopathic scoliosis, has shown that natural coral can be used successfully as a graft substitute [25].

In applying their results of animal studies to clinical practice, Delecrin et al., in a prospective randomized study, assessed the clinical and radiologic performances of a synthetic ceramic as a bone graft substitute in scoliosis surgery [10]. Fifty-eight patients with idiopathic scoliosis underwent posterior correction and arthrodesis by posterior spinal fusion using autogenous iliac bone grafts alone or in combination with porous biphasic calcium phosphate ceramic blocks comprised of HA/TCP. The mean postoperative observation time was 48 months. Patients in the ceramic group had a lower average blood loss than those in the iliac graft group and significantly less pain. Radiography demonstrated that successful incorporation of the ceramic blocks occurred within 12 months. Ransford et al. evaluated the use of synthetic porous ceramic as a substitute for autogenous bone graft in posterior spinal fusion for scoliosis in 341 patients undergoing surgery [28]. The 170 patients treated with 60/40% HA/TCP alone had the clear benefit of no donor site pain and morbidity. Overall fusion site morbidity and complication rate were comparable, regardless of the bone graft material used. These results justify the use of calcium phosphate ceramics as bone graft additives for instrumented posterior spinal fusion in some cases, such as when only a limited amount of autogenous bone graft exists.

The most human clinical experience with ceramic materials in spinal fusion exists for anterior interbody fusion of the cervical spine. Thalgott et al., in a nonrandomized, retrospective study of patients requiring anterior cervical discectomy and fusion, evaluated the pattern of incorporation, presence or absence of disc space collapse, maintenance of correction, and clinical outcomes in order to determine the efficacy of coralline HA as a bone replacement in anterior interbody fusions of the cervical spine used in conjunction with rigid plate fixation [32]. The incorporation rate of the HA block into vertebral bone was 100%, and the complication rate due to the graft material was extremely low.

Kim et al. have developed implants made of porous HA, used in more than 90 patients to achieve cervical interbody fusion [17]. Results were reported in 70 patients, whose surgical indications included cervical spondylosis, disc extrusion, ossification or hypertrophy of the posterior longitudinal ligament, and trauma. Flexion-extension radiographs and tomograms, obtained 6 and 12 months after surgery and every year thereafter, were obtained. Dislocation of the implant occurred in three patients. At 6–12 months after surgery, encasement of the implant and formation of union were observed in all patients. Normal lordosis, if present prior to surgery, was maintained post surgery. The authors found no neurological deterioration related to the site of fusion during the period of observation, and concluded that satisfactory interbody fusion can be achieved by using the HA implants. Similar good clinical results were reported by Hirabayashi and Kumano using HA ceramic spacers to maintain the laminar spread in open door cervical laminoplasty [14].

Other potential uses of HA ceramics in the spine

Injectable HA materials have been studied for use as "cements" to improve the strength of transpedicular vertebral screw fixation. Spivak and co-authors examined the improvement in posterior vertebral screw fixation strength in an unloaded in vivo canine model [29]. A crystalline-HA material was seen to significantly improve screw pull-out strength both initially and after 6 weeks in vivo in an over-drilled model, simulating a loose screw with poor initial fixation strength. Yerby et al. studied the use of an injectable ceramic in augmentation of revision pedicular instrumentation [37]. They examined the immediate effect of using an HA cement to augment revision pedicle screw insertion after failure of the primary pedicle screw fixation in human cadaveric spines by mechanical testing. The pull-out strength of the HA cement-augmented screws was 325% greater than control screws reinserted without HA augmentation. The major potential clinical advantages of an injectable HA "cement" for this application would be a more biocompatible alternative to the polymethylmethacrylate (PMMA) currently used, and the elimination of potential thermal injury due to the exothermic curing reaction of PMMA. These results suggest that HA cements may be a mechanically viable alternative to PMMA for augmenting the strength of primary and revision pedicular instrumentation, and should be considered for future experimental, animal, and clinical testing [33].

Injectable HA materials have also been studied experimentally for use in augmenting the strength of fractured vertebral bodies. Mermelstein et al. conducted a biomechanical study on the stabilization of human cadaveric thoracolumbar burst fractures in order to demonstrate that the addition of a calcium phosphate cement into the fractured vertebral body through a transpedicular approach is a feasible technique [20]. Transpedicular vertebral body reconstruction with HA cement reduced pedicle screw-bending moments by 59% in flexion and 38% in extension and mean initial stiffness in the flexion-extension plane was increased by 40%.

Cunin et al. used osteoporotic human cadaveric thoracic vertebral bodies and in situ vertebral bodies from living mature sheep as model systems to assess coral resorption and new bone formation after injection of coral granules [8]. The distribution of coral granules injected into human cadaveric thoracic vertebral bodies was homogeneous as assayed radiographically. In order to evaluate the use of natural coral as an osteoconductive material, cavities were drilled into vertebral bodies of ten mature ewes and were either left empty or filled with coral. Quantitative evaluation of coral resorption and new bone formation was made 2 months and 4 months after implantation. Osteogenesis was increased in cavities filled with coral in comparison with cavities left empty at both 2 months and 4 months. These results demonstrate the osteoconductivity of coral in granular form for vertebral filling. Interestingly, interconnectivity between adjacent bone trabeculae and newly formed bone was restored.

Bai et al. conducted a biomechanical study comparing two materials for augmentation of osteoporotic vertebral bodies and vertebral bodies after compression fracture in order to compare an injected, biodegradable calcium phosphate bone substitute with injected PMMA bone cement for strengthening osteoporotic vertebral bodies and improving the integrity of vertebral compression fractures in 40 fresh osteoporotic thoracolumbar vertebrae [1]. Osteoporotic vertebrae were injected either with calcium phosphate or PMMA and there was a non-injected control group. Each specimen was then loaded in anterior compression until failure. The second part of the study involved injection of calcium phosphate or PMMA into postfractured vertebrae. The fracture strength and stiffness in the calcium phosphate bone substitute group and those in the PMMA group were similar and significantly higher than those in the intact control group. Anterior vertebral height was increased significantly compared to initial postfracture vertebral body height, with no difference between calcium phosphate and PMMA injections. This study demonstrated that the injection of a biodegradable calcium phosphate bone substitute to strengthen osteoporotic vertebral bodies or improve vertebral compression fractures may provide an alternative to the use of PMMA.

Summary

HA ceramics seem to hold promise for use as an extender of autologous iliac crest bone grafting in spinal fusions. Used alone, they have not been proven to be as efficacious as autograft. In many animal models, the usage of HA/TCP resulted in less than desired fusion results. However, the reported results of spinal fusion using ceramic materials are conflicting both in animal and human clinical studies. These discrepancies are in part due to inherent differences in the healing process and healing potential of the various types of spinal fusions performed clinically and in animal experimentation. Data from a number of animal studies suggest a potential use for ceramic composites as a bone graft replacement or augmentation material for interbody spinal fusion surgery. The HA/TCP ceramic composite, either with or without added collagen, can serve as a scaffold onto which mesenchymal cells grow and differentiate into bone-producing osteoblasts, form creeping cones of bone in the scaffold, replace and finally degrade the scaffold, forming a solid fusion mass. Combining an osteoconductive ceramic material such as an HA composite with an osteoinductive agent such as rhBMP-2, OP-1, DBM, extracted bone matrix proteins, AGF, osteogenin, or others seems to be the most promising combination for achieving a reliably successful spinal fusion without the use of autogenous bone graft. The use of HA ceramics in augmentation of spinal fixation strength and in augmentation of vertebral body strength holds much promise for future clinical applications.

References

1. Bai B, Jazrawi LM, Kummer FJ, Spivak JM (1999) The use of an injectable, biodegradable calcium phosphate bone substitute for the prophylactic augmentation of osteoporotic vertebrae and the management of vertebral compression fractures. Spine 24:1521–1526
2. Baramki HG, Steffen T, Lander P, Chang M, Marchesi D (2000) The efficacy of interconnected porous HA in achieving posterolateral lumbar fusion in sheep. Spine 25:1053–1060
3. Boden SD, Schimandle JH (1995) Biologic enhancement of spinal fusion. Spine 20:113S–123S
4. Boden SD, Martin GJ Jr, Morone MA, Ugbo JL, Moskovitz PA (1999) Posterolateral lumbar intertransverse process spine arthrodesis with recombinant human bone morphogenetic protein 2/HA-TCP after laminectomy in the nonhuman primate. Spine 24:1179–1185
5. Boden SD, Martin GJ Jr, Morone M, Ugbo JL, Titus L, Hutton WC (1999) The use of coralline HA with bone marrow, autogenous bone graft, or osteoinductive bone protein extract for posterolateral lumbar spine fusion. Spine 24:320–327
6. Bozic KJ, Glazer PA, Zurakowski D, Simon BJ, Lipson SJ, Hayes WC (1999) In vivo evaluation of coralline HA and direct current electrical stimulation in lumbar spinal fusion. Spine 24:2127–2133
7. Breitbart AS, Staffenberg DA, Thorne Ch, et al (1995) Tricalcium phosphate and osteogenin: a bioactive onlay bone graft substitute. Plast Recons Surg 96: 699–708
8. Cunin G, Boissonnet H, Petite H, et al (2000) Experimental vertebroplasty using osteoconductive granular material. Spine 25:1070-1076
9. Delecrin J, Aguado E, Guyen JM, et al (1997) Influence of local environment on incorporation of ceramic for lumbar fusion. Spine 22:1683–1689
10. Delecrin J, Takahashi S, Gouin F, Passuti N (2000) A synthetic porous ceramic as a bone graft substitute in the surgical management of scoliosis: a prospective, randomized study. Spine 25:563–569
11. Emery SE, Fuller DA, Stevenson S (1996) Ceramic anterior spinal fusion. Spine 21:2713–2719
12. Gao T, Lindholm TS, Marttinen A, Urist MR (1996) Composites of bone morphogenetic protein and type 4 collagen, coral derived coral HA, and tricalcium phosphate ceramics. Int Orthop 20:321–325
13. Guigui P, Plais PY, Flautre B, et al (1994) Experimental model of posterolateral spinal arthrodesis in sheep. Spine 19:2798–2803
14. Hirabayashi S, Kumano K (1999) Contact of hydroxyapatite spacers with split spinous processes in double-door laminoplasty for cervical myelopathy. J Orthop Sci 4:264–268
15. Itokazu M, Sugiyama T, Ohno T, Wada E, Katagiri Y (1997) Development of porous apatite ceramic for local delivery of chemotherapeutic agents. Cancer 536–538
16. Kawamura M, Iwata H, Sato K, Miura T (1987) Chondroosteogenic response to crude bone matrix proteins bound to hydroxyapatite. Clin Orthop 217:281–292
17. Kim P, Wakai S, Matsuo S, Moriyama T, Kirino T (1998) Bisegmental cervical interbody fusion using hydroxyapatite implants: surgical results and long-term observation in 70 cases. J Neurosurg 88:21–27
18. Le Huec JC, Lesprit E, Delavigne C, Clement D, Chauveaux D, Le Rebeller A (1997) Tricalcium phosphate ceramics and allografts as bone substitutes for spinal fusion in idiopathic scoliosis. Acta Orthop Belg 63:202–210
19. Lowery GL, Kulkarni S, Pennisi AE (1999) Use of autologous growth factors in lumbar spinal fusion. Bone 25 [2 Suppl]:47S–50S
20. Mermelstein LE, McLain RF, Yerby SA (1998) Reinforcement of thoracolumbar burst fractures with calcium phosphate cement. A biomechanical study. Spine 23:664-670; discussion 670,671
21. Mooney V, Massie JB, Lind BI, Rah JH, Negri S, Holmes RE (1998) Comparison of hydroxyapatite granules to autogenous bone graft in fusion cages in a goat model. Surg Neurol 49:628–633; discussion 633,634
22. Muschler GF, Huber B, Ullman T, Barth R, Easley K, Otis JO,Lane JM (1993) Evaluation of bone-grafting materials in a new canine segmental spinal fusion model. J Orthop Res 11:514-524
23. Muschler GF, Negami S, Hyodo A, et al (1996) Evaluation of collagen ceramic composite graft materials in a spinal fusion model. Clin Orthop 328: 250-260
24. Passuti N, Daculsi G, Rogez JM,et al (1989) Macroporous calcium phosphate ceramic performance in human spine fusion. Clin Orthop 248:169–174
25. Pouliquen JC, Noat M, Verneret C, Guillemin G, Patat JL (1989) Coral substituted for bone grafting in posterior vertebral arthrodesis in children. Initial results. Rev Chir Orthop Reparatrice Appar Mot 75:360-369
26. Radin S, Campbell JT, Ducheyne P, Cuckler JM (1993) Calcium phosphate ceramic coatings as carriers of vancomycin. Biomaterials 18:777–782
27. Ragni P, Ala-Mononen P, Lindholm TS (1993) Spinal fusion induced by porous hydroxyapatite blocks (HA). Experimental comparative study with HA, demineralized bone matrix and autogenous bone marrow. Ital J Orthop Traumatol 19:133-144
28. Ransford AO, Morley T, Edgar MA, et al (1998) Synthetic porous ceramic compared with autograft in scoliosis surgery. J Bone Joint Surg Br 80: 13–18

29. Spivak JM, Neuwirth MG, Labiak JJ, Kummer FJ, Ricci JL (1994) Hydroxyapatite enhancement of posterior spinal instrumentation fixation. Spine 19:955–964
30. Summers BN, Eisenstein SM (1989) donor site pain from the ilium: a complication of lumbar spine fusion. J Bone Joint Surg Br 71:667–680
31. Takahashi T, Tominaga T, Watabe N, Yokobori AT Jr, Sasada H, Yoshimoto T (1999) Use of porous hydroxyapatite graft containing recombinant human bone morphogenetic protein-2 for cervical fusion in a caprine model. J Neurosurg 90 [4 Suppl]:224
32. Thalgott JS, Fritts K, Giuffre JM, Timlin M (1999) Anterior interbody fusion of the cervical spine with coralline hydroxyapatite. Spine 24:1295–1299
33. Timura J, Kitsugi T, Lida H, et al (1997) Bone bonding ability of bioactive bone cements. Clinical Orthop 343:183–191
34. Toth JM, An HS, Lim TH, et al (1995) Evaluation of porous biphasic calcium phosphate ceramics for anterior cervical interbody fusion in a caprine model. Spine 20:2203–2210
35. Urist M, Lietze A, Dawson E (1986) (β-tricalcium phosphate delivery system for bone morphogenetic protein. Clin Orthop 187:277–280
36. Walsh WR, Harrison J, Loefler A, et al (2000) Mechanical and histologic evaluation of Collagraft in an ovine lumbar fusion model. Clin Orthop 375:258–266
37. Yerby SA, Toh E, McLain RF (1998) Revision of failed pedicle screws using hydroxyapatite cement. A biomechanical analysis. Spine 23:1657–1661
38. Younger EM, Chapman MW (1989) Morbidity of bone graft donor sites. J Orthop Trauma 3:192–195
39. Zdeblick TA, Cooke ME, Kunz DN, et al (1994) Anterior cervical discectomy and fusion using a porous hydroxyapatite bone graft substitute. Spine 19: 348–2357
40. Zerwekh JE, Kourosh S, Scheinberg R, et al (1992) Fibrillar collagen-biphasic calcium phosphate composite as a bone graft substitute for spinal fusion. J Orthop Res 10:562-572

P. F. Heini
U. Berlemann

Bone substitutes in vertebroplasty

P.F. Heini (✉) · U. Berlemann
Department of Orthopaedic Surgery,
Spine Service, Inselspital,
University of Bern,
Freiburgstrasse, 3010 Bern, Switzerland
e-mail: paul.heini@insel.ch,
Tel.: +41-31-6322111,
Fax: +41-31-6323600

Abstract Vertebroplasty – percutaneous cement augmentation of vertebral bodies – is an efficient procedure for the treatment of painful vertebral fractures in osteoporosis. At the present time, polymethylmethacrylate (PMMA) is the only available cement with reports of clinical application and experience. The material is easy to handle, the radiopacity can be adapted by adding contrast dye, and it is mechanically efficient. Composite cements (acrylic cements in conjunction with ceramics) are bioactive, highly radiopaque, and feature excellent mechanical properties. One such cement, Cortoss, is currently undergoing clinical trials for vertebroplasty and has so far been shown to be a potentially valuable alternative to PMMA. Several in vitro studies with injectable calcium phosphate (CaP) cements show their feasibility and mechanical effectiveness. Animal studies confirm their biocompatibility and osteoconductivity. However, handling problems and the limited radiopacity of these cements currently preclude their clinical use.

Keywords Vertebroplasty · Polymethylmethacrylate · Osteoporosis · Bone cement · Calcium phosphate · Bone substitutes

Introduction

Galibert and Deramond first introduced the technique of percutaneous vertebroplasty with polymethylmethacrylate (PMMA) as a reinforcement procedure for the treatment of vertebral angiomas in 1987 [26]. Following encouraging early clinical results, particularly with respect to pain relief, indications for PMMA augmentation were extended. At present, osteoporotic compression fractures of the spine represent the most important indication for vertebroplasty, followed by metastatic bone diseases. Clinical series of vertebroplasty almost exclusively report the use of PMMA; however, several disadvantages have been recognized and described [16, 18, 25, 31, 32, 36, 53]. PMMA cures with a strongly exothermic reaction, potentially damaging adjacent soft tissue structures, particularly in the event of cement extrusion. In addition, with maximal PMMA filling, adjacent vertebral overload has been reported, possibly provoking fractures [6] (Fig. 1a,b). For the purpose of vertebral augmentation, PMMA seems to be a successful, but not an optimal material. Researchers and clinicians therefore have to consider and evaluate alternative substances for use in vertebroplasty.

Bone substitutes have always been an important issue in orthopedics, especially in spine surgery. The use of (solid) autogenous bone grafts (iliac crest, ribs, fibulae) is associated with considerable morbidity and mechanical limitations [3, 14, 23] (Fig. 2a–c). PMMA was and still is the material of choice for defect reconstruction, especially in palliative treatment of spinal metastasis [33]. Allografts have a long history as a bone substitute, but their value remains controversial [11, 13, 56]. Bone growth factors show an enormous potential with encouraging experimental and initial clinical results [8, 9, 10, 49].

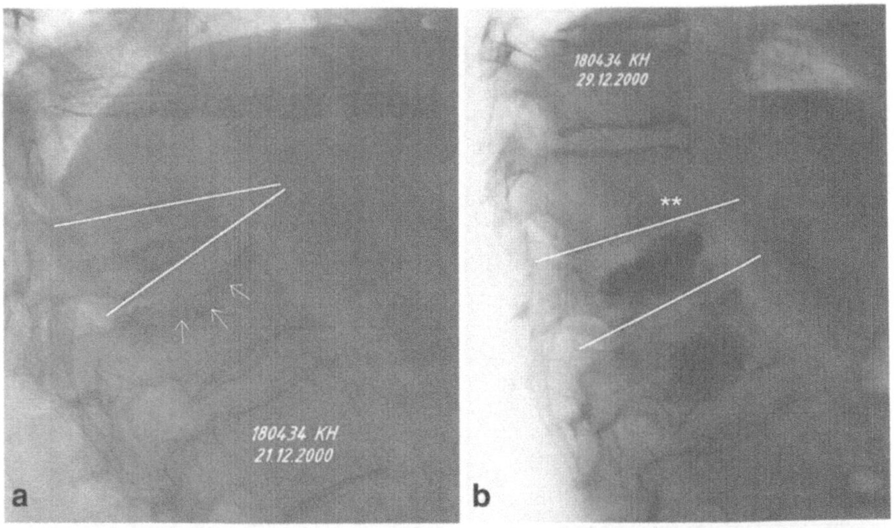

Fig. 1 **a** Osteoporotic collapse of T12 and endplate fracture of L1 (*arrows*) in a 66-year-old man due to long-term steroid medication. **b** After reduction of T12 with correction of kyphosis by 18° (kyphoplasty) and vertebroplasty at L1, the first standing X-ray shows immediate impression of the endplate adjacent to the augmentation (*asterisk*)

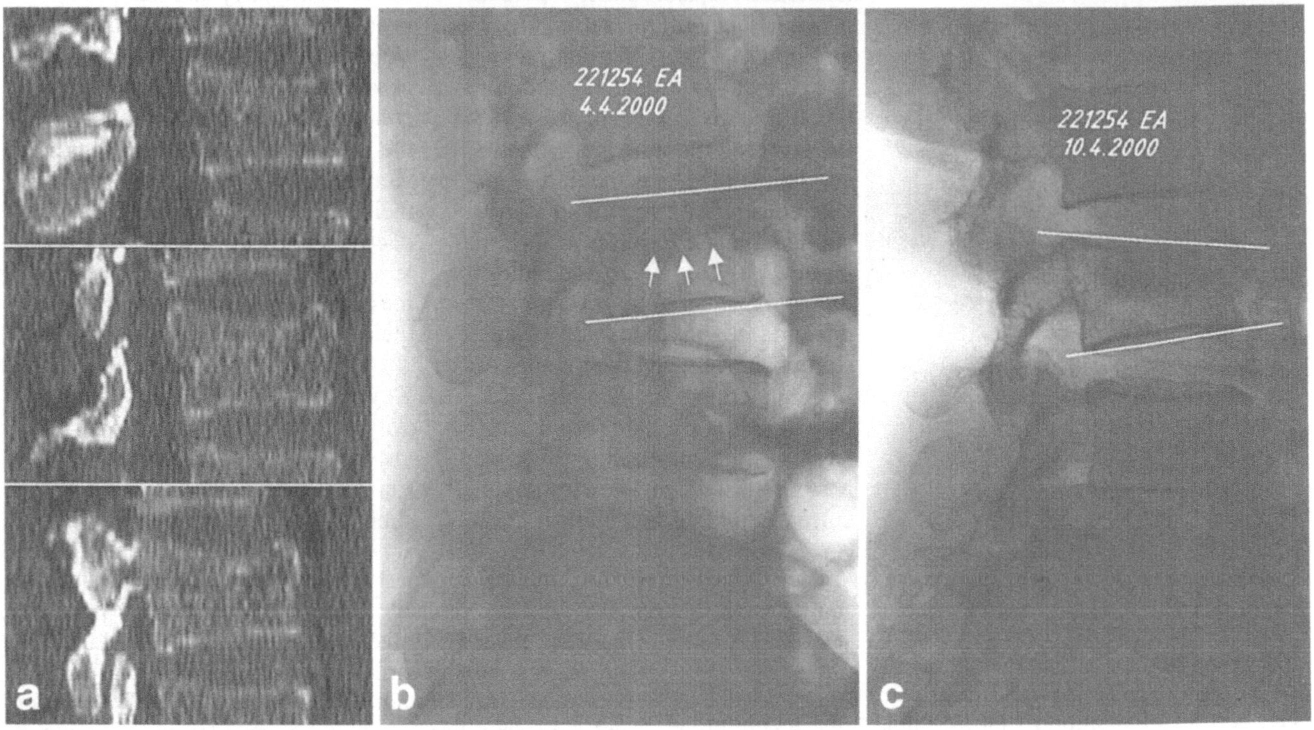

Fig. 2 **a** L3 compression fracture, AO type A 1.2.1 in a 45-year-old woman. **b** Percutaneous anatomical reduction of the endplate using a bone tamp technique (kyphoplasty) and filling of the defect with autologous bone (*arrows*). **c** Loss of reduction to preoperative status after mobilization

Contemporary bone substitutes

Several bone substitutes are in clinical use, mainly as bone graft expanders for spinal fusion [8, 22, 28, 29, 34, 43, 45, 46, 57]. Biomaterials (materials intended to interface with biological systems to evaluate, treat, augment, or replace any tissue, organ, or function of the body [54]) can be divided into three different classes:

1. Metals
   a) Titanium
   b) Stainless steel
   c) Tantalum (e.g., Hedrocel)
2. Polymers (large group of materials of heterogenous origin)
   a) Polymethyl methacrylate
   b) Polyhydroxyethyl methacrylate
   c) Polyethylene
   d) Polyglycolide, polylactide
   e) Polyether-ether-ketone (PEEK)

Table 1 Calcium phosphates (CaP) and calcium salts used in CaP cements

Name	Abbreviation	Formula
Dicalcium phosphate dihydrate	DCPD	$CaHPO_4 \bullet 2H_2O$
Dicalcium phosphate, anhydrous	DCPA	$CaHPO_4$
Tetracalcium phosphate	TTCP	$Ca_4(PO_4)_2O$
Dicalcium phosphate	DCP	$CaHPO_4$
α-Tricalcium phosphate	αTCP	$Ca_3(PO_4)_2$
β-Tricalcium phosphate	βTCP	$Ca_3(PO_4)_2$
Calcium-deficient hydroxyapatite	CDHA	$Ca_9H(PO_4)_5OH$
Monocalcium phosphate monohydrate	MCPM	$Ca(H_2PO_4)_2 \bullet H_2O$
Calcium pyrophosphate	CPP	$Ca_2P_2O_7$
Hydroxyapatite	HA	$Ca_5(PO_4)_3OH$
Hydroxyapatite, precipitated	PHA	$Ca_{10-x}(HPO_4)_x(PO_4)_{6-x}(OH)_{2-x}$
Calciumsulfate, dihydrated	CSD	$CaSO4 \bullet 2H_2O$
Calcium sulfate, hemihydrated	CSH	$CaSO_4 \bullet 0.5H_2O$

3. Ceramics (crystalline metallic oxides, carbides, nitrides, and borides fused by sintering)
   a) Bioactive glasses (e.g., Bioglass): high resorption rate
   b) Calcium ceramics
   c) Calcium sulfate: not osteoconductive, fast degradation
   d) Calcium phosphate: tricalcium phosphate, hydroxyapatite (osteoconductive)
   e) Calcium carbonate: fast degradation (osteoconductive)

For the clinician, it is extremely difficult to approach this topic and survey the numerous products on the market. We have therefore tried to list the most common bone substitutes available in Europe and United States and focused on injectable bone cements (Tables 1, 2). The information on the products were obtained from the literature and from the Internet. However, we cannot guarantee that it is comprehensive. The same cement material is sometimes marketed by different distributors under different brand names (i.e., α-BSM is produced by Etex and sold in Europe by Merck as Biobon and in the United States by Lorenz Surgical as embarc). Furthermore, basic knowledge about bone cements is required in order to understand important details of different substances. Several articles concerning this issue help to close an existing gap in this field.

Bone substitutes for vertebroplasty

Requirements for an ideal augmentation material

A bone substitute for vertebroplasty needs to have the following properties:

- Injectability
- Ease of handling
- High radiopacity
- Adapted viscosity (not too low)
- Lasting, constant viscosity (5–10 min)
- Long setting time (≈15 min)
- Low curing temperature
- Adapted, lasting mechanical properties
- Biocompatibility
- Bioactivity
- Low price
- Slow biodegradation

An optimal bone substitute for vertebroplasty must be easy to apply, i.e., the components are easy to handle, the mixing procedure is simple, and the material can be applied percutaneously through cannulas into the vertebral body. This requires a low initial viscosity of the material, which has to be balanced against potential extravasation if the material is too liquid. Sufficient radiopacity is of utmost importance in order to be able to follow the cement flow. The setting time should be about 10 min, and viscosity of the cement should remain constant during this period to allow controlled application. The curing temperature must be as low as possible.

The optimal mechanical properties (i.e., compressive strength/stiffness) have not yet been defined. Following the operative procedure, the material should provide immediate reinforcement of the vertebral body and allow early ambulation of the patients. Stiffness and yield strength should resemble values of natural bone. Excessively high stress differences in comparison to nonaugmented areas should be avoided. Finally, reinforcement should not deteriorate over time.

The material must not cause adverse reactions in the surrounding tissue. A bioactive cement seems to be advantageous; however, whether or not a biodegradable cement is important is an open question.

Finally, the material should be reasonably priced in order to allow wide-spread application from the point of view of cost-effectiveness and economic restrains.

At present, different compositions of injectable bone substitutes are available (Table 3); several of these are still under laboratory development and not yet ready for clinical application.

Table 2 Overview of bone substitutes

Name	Substance	Producer
Calcium phosphates		
Calciresorb	βTCP	Ceraver Osteal
chronOS	βTCP	Mathys
Vitoss	βTCP	Orthovita
Biosorb	βTCP	SBM France
Bio Base	αTCP	Bio Vision
Vitoss	βTCP	Orthovita
Biologic HA		
Interpore Pro Osteon 500/200 HA/CC®	Coral calcium carbonate → HA	Interpore International
Endobon	Bovine HA	Merck KGaA
Pyrost	Bovine HA	Osteo/Stryker Howmedica
Synthetic HA		
Synatite	HA	SBM France
Cerapatite	HA	Ceraver Osteal
permaOS	HA	Mathys
Biphasic ceramics		
Triosite	60% HA, 40% TCP	Zimmer
BCP	60% HA, 40% TCP	Bioland biomateriaux/Sofamor Danek
Ceraform	65% HA, 35% TCP	Teknimed
Biocer-Biogel 2 (Phocalcite, Biogreffe)	75% HA, 25% TCP	Bioland biomateriaux/DePuy
Calciresorb 35–Cerapatite 65	35% β-TCP, 65% HA	Ceraver Osteal
Calcium phosphate cements		
Bone Source	TTCP, DCP	Orthofix/Howmedica
Norian SRS	α-TCP, $CaCO_3$, MCPM	Norian
α BSM = Biobon = embarc	ACP, DCPD	Etex/Merck/Biomet/ Lorenz Surgical
Mimix	TCP, TTCP, citric acid	Lorenz Surgical
Biocement D	α-TCP, DCP, $CaCO_3$, PHA	Merck/Biomet
Cementek	α-TCP, TTCP, $Ca(OH)_2$, H_3PO_4	Teknimed
Fracture Grout	TTCP, $CaCO_3$, H_3PO_4	Norian
Biopex	α-TCP, TTCP, DCPD	Mitsubishi
Allografts		
Tutoplast	Collagen, HA	Tuogen
Xenografts		
Surgibone	Bovine HA-like, 20–29% collagen	Unilab Surgibone
Bio Oss/Orthoss	Bovine HA-like	Geistlich
Collagraft	Hydroxyapatite, bovine collagen	Zimmer
Healos	Bovine HA, collagen	Orquest/Sulzer
Others		
Osteoset	Calcium sulfate	Wright Medical Technologies
Stimulan	Calcium sulfate	Encore Orthopaedics
Biocoral	Coralline calcium carbonate	Inoteb
Bioglass	Silicate hydroxyapatite	US Biomaterials
Collapat	HA collagen	Osteo
Grafton	Demineralized bone matrix (allograft)	Osteotech
Dynagraft	Demineralized allograft	GenSci/DePuy

DCP, dicalcium phosphate; DCPD, dicalcium phosphate dihydrate; HA, hydroxyapatite; PHA, precipitated hydroxyapatite; TCP, tricalcium phosphate; TTCP, tetracalcium phosphate.

Polymethylmethacrylyate

At present, PMMA is the only material that can be used for vertebroplasty with which there is extensive in vitro and in vivo experience. PMMA cements most commonly used are Simplex P, Cranioplastic, and Palacos LV 40 [20, 32, 36, 53] Due to the insufficient radiopacity of the material, contrast dye needs to be added. This seems to work

Table 3 Overview of bone substitutes for vertebroplasty

Substance	Chemistry	Applicability	Biomechanics	Biology	Remarks
PMMA, e.g.,. Simplex, Palacos LV40[a]	*Monomer:* methylmethacrylate/ dimethyl-*p*-toluidin (liquid); *polymer:* methylmethacrylate/ methylacrylate; benzoylperoxide (solid)	Low viscosity, easy to handle, easy to inject, setting time 6–8 min, high curing temperature	In vitro tests on vertebroplasty model very efficient [1, 4,31], toxic monomers may get into circulation [18], in vitro compressive strength 70–100 MPa, PMMA = gold standard	No testing on in vivo vertebroplasty model, vast clinically experience, long-term experience for bone defects in tumors and total joint replacement [7,47]	Cheap, radiopacity needs to be enhanced by contrast dye [32], curing temperature probably not important for vertebroplasty [31], a special, experimental formula of Simplex with increased radiopacity shows good mechanical setting time 5 min properties [1]
Composite cements					
Cortoss (Orthovita)	*bis*-GMA/*bis*-EMA/ TEGDMA	Low-viscosity paste, setting time 5–8 min, curing temperature 63°C, long phase of applicability, easy to handle	In vitro tests on vertebroplasty model in axial compression very efficient, in vitro compressive strength 211 MPa [1, 4,40]	Rabbit femur model shows bone apposition at the surface, sheep femur no interference with bone healing [19]	Bioactive glass ceramic reinforced composite, designed as bone void filler, high radiopacity, some osteoconductive potential – chemical bone bonding to the surface, currently being clinically tested for vertebroplasty
Hydroxyapatite composite resin (CAP) (Kuraray)	Hydroxyapatite acrylic monomer: (*bis*-phenol-A glycidyl methacrylate 2.2-*bis*-(4-methacryloylethoxyphenyl) propane/ TEGDMA)	Paste, injectable in vitro, limited penetration into cancellous bone, setting time 4.9 min, curing temperature 46°C	In vitro tests on reinforcement of pedicle screw fixation, no tests regarding vertebroplasty, in vitro testing of cement: compressive strength 259 MPa [52]	Rabbit femur model, histological investigation up to 36 weeks: bone ingrowth at the surface [48]	No references/information on clinical use
CaP cements					
Bone Source (Howmedica)	Tetracalcium phosphate + dicalcium dihydrate hydroxyapatite, setting time 7 s (in sodium monophosphate), 25 s in water	Designed for repair of cranial defects, injectable in vitro by 12-G needle, compressive strength 50 MPa	In vitro tests in axial compression vertebroplasty model showed no significant increase of yield strength compared to the intact verte-bral body [5,44]		
Norian	Carbonated apatite cement, calcium carbonate, α-tricalcium phosphate and calcium phosphate monohydrate	Injectable in vitro with an irrigation/suction technique in a vertebroplasty model [51], not currently applicable in vivo	In vitro tests on axial compression model, no change in stiffness, energy absorption higher in reinforced vertebrae only after collapse of more than 25% of vertebral height, in vitro compressive strength 50 MPa [51]	Rabbit femoral defect model, canine metaphyseal defect model [15], not assessed on vertebroplasty	Clinical use as bone void filler in metaphyseal defects [15]
Biopex (Mitsubishi)	75% α-TCP, 18% TTCP, 5% DCPD, 2% HA, setting time 7 min	Easy to handle and inject, two formulas depending on the water to powder ratio	No tests on vertebroplasty model, augmentation of screw fixation in femoral neck fractures [50], compressive strength determined in body fluid shows slow increase to maximum strength (80 MPa) within 7 days [41]	Rabbit mandibula model shows slow remodeling of Biopex [41]	No information/experience on vertebroplasty

Table 3 (continued)

Substance	Chemistry	Applicability	Biomechanics	Biology	Remarks
Biobon = α-BSM (Etex/Biomet Merck)	Apatitic CaP	Injectable with a 11-G needle, setting time 20 s	Vertebroplasty model with significant increase of stability like PMMA [2]	Sheep tibia fracture model, rabbit tibia defect model [39], no data on in vivo vertebroplasty model	Used in dentistry, fast resorption
Cementek	α-TCP, TTCP, $Ca(OH)_2$, H_3PO_4	Compressive strength 20 MPa	No information on vertebroplasty	Rabbit mandibula defect model [27, 42]	
HAC (Howmedica)	No information	Injectable in vitro	In vitro test of a T11 fracture in a cadaver spine model, cementing with HAC and PMMA restores stability after destabilization due to a fracture [21]	No in vivo vertebroplasty model	Probably a variation of Bone Source
Mimix	TCP, TTCP, citric acid	No information	Designed and approved for craniofacial indications		
EBS (experimental brushite cement)	β-TCP, MCPM	Injectable formula, compressive strength 20–60 MPa, setting time 5 min	Axial compression model shows significant increase of yield strength and stiffness, less pronounced than PMMA [31]	Metaphyseal rabbit defect model osteoconductive [35]	Experimental formula, not suitable for clinical use
Collagraft (Zimmer)	65% HA, 35% TCP + type I bovine collagen	Paste	No information on mechanical properties available	Multiple animal and clinical studies show its efficiency regarding osteoconductivity (long bones, spinal fusion) [10, 12, 57]	Not designed for vertebroplasty, no experimental data regarding vertebroplasty
Biocement D	α-TCP, DCP, $CaCO_3$, PHA		No information on vertebroplasty [37,38]		

PMMA, polymethylmethacrylate; GMA, phenol glycidyl dimethacrylate; EMA, phenol ethoxydimethacrylate; TEGDMA, triethyleneglycol dimethacrylate; CaP, calcium phosphate; TCP, tricalcium phosphate; TTCP, tetracalcium phosphate; DCPD, dicalcium phosphate dibasic; HA, hydroxyapatite, MCPM, monocalcium phosphate monohydrate; PHA, hydroxyapatite, precipitated.
[a]Minimal requirements: compressive strength, 70 N/mm^2; maximum curing temperature, 90°C (ISO 5833).

reliably, but there are no data available regarding the mechanical and biological effects of adding dye to the cement. Furthermore, PMMA is not bioactive and generates high polymerization temperatures. Belkoff reported about a modified PMMA with increased $BaSO_4$ content(Simplex). In vitro tests have confirmed its feasibility and mechanical effect. Clinical experience, however, has not been reported [5].

Composite cements

Composite cements (acrylic cements in conjunction with ceramics) are bioactive but behave basically like PMMA. Orthovita is promoting a PMMA-like material (Cortoss) which is bioactive and easy to handle. In vitro studies and animal studies have confirmed its efficacy and biocompatibility [1, 4, 19, 24, 55]. This material seems to be advantageous compared with PMMA as it features an optimal and constant viscosity (the components are mixed in the extrusion cannula) and a high radiopacity. Furthermore, the curing temperature is lower than that of regular PMMA. These properties, together with a good penetration into the cancellous bone, reduce the risk if extravasation. Clinical trials on vertebroplasty with this cement are currently being performed.

The remaining materials presented in this article are not ready for clinical use for vertebroplasty at this time. Most of these cements were designed for dentistry and craniofacial surgery and have proven to be biologically suitable. The need for appropriate bone substitutes in spine surgery, especially in vertebroplasty, has lead to these products being evaluated and adapted for these new applications. All the information on injectable bone cements has been summarized here, with a special focus on materials that have been tested in vitro for vertebroplasty or screw fixation in the spine.

Kuraray is producing a composite cement of hydroxyapatite (HA) and an acrylic monomer (CAP) that seems to be easy to handle. It shows some bioactivity and a high mechanical performance [48]. In vitro tests on pedicle screw fixation have been performed, but not on vertebroplasty [52].

Calcium phosphate cements

Bone Source is an injectable cement primarily designed to repair cranial defects. Lim et al. tested PMMA and Bone Source in vertebral bodies in an axial compression model and achieved a significant increase of yield strength for intact reinforced vertebrae in comparison to the native state. This was more pronounced for PMMA, whereas the increase of a fractured vertebrae was only significant with PMMA but not with calcium phosphate (CaP) [44]. Belkoff compared the use of Bone Source and PMMA in isolated vertebral bodies in an axial compression model and again found a significant increase of the peak load for PMMA; however, CaP cement did not improve the mechanical properties [5].

Schildhauer published a report on the use of Norian for reinforcement of vertebral bodies. Filling could only be achieved by using an irrigation/suction/injection technique. The amount of cement injected is not reported. An increase in energy absorption was able to be achieved, but only the vertebral body height had been reduced by 50%. The change in yield strength and stiffness is not reported [51]. Heini used Norian for in vitro reinforcement of vertebral bodies; however, its material properties precluded application through a cannula, as it separated under pressure to the liquid and solid phase [30]. However, its usefulness as a bone substitute in other applications was able to be demonstrated [15].

Biopex is a bone cement with remarkable mechanical properties. Experimental data are available on its use for screw fixation in femoral neck fractures [50]. No further tests have been performed. Personal in vitro handling tests show that the cement can be injected very easily over a long period. Its biological behavior was assessed in a rabbit mandibula model [41].

Biobon (or α-BSM or embarc) is a CaP cement that was originally designed for dentistry and craniofacial surgery. Its mechanical efficacy in a vertebroplasty model was assessed and compared with PMMA and shows a significant effect [2, 39]. Whether its radiopacity and handling will allow clinical application is not clear.

Mimix is a cement designed and approved for craniofacial surgery. No test results or information is available for vertebroplasty.

Cementek is a cement paste with suitable mechanical properties. No experience in clinical use has been reported for any application. Its biological behavior was assessed in a rabbit mandibula defect model [27, 42].

EBS (end product: experimental brushite cement) shows good mechanical properties and biological behavior. A biomechanical study on a vertebroplasty model showed a significant increase in the yield strength and stifness [31, 35]. There are no clinical data available yet.

Collagraft is a paste consisting of CaP cement and bovine collagen. This bone substitute has already been in clinical use for a long time and has proved to be useful for long bone defects and spinal fusion [10, 12, 57]. No information on its mechanical properties or experimental data on vertebroplasty is available.

Biocement D is a calcium-deficient HA cement containing dicalcium phosphate (DCP) and collagen in order to improve the injectability [37, 38]. No further information is available regarding mechanical or biological properties.

Drake et al. compared the stability of a thoracic spine specimen (T7–L1) in a T11 fracture model intact or reinforced with PMMA or HA cement (Howmedica). The three-dimensional load displacement behavior showed significant restoration of stability for both materials following destabilization. There are no further specifications regarding the cement [21].

Conclusion

An optimized cement formula is definitely required for vertebroplasty. The disadvantages of PMMA are its high curing temperature and the potential adverse biological effects. Vertebroplasty has become an important treatment option and has a great potential. There are some promising cements under development, and several of these products will likely soon be available.

Optimal viscosity and sufficient radiopacity are the most important parameters to be addressed. The optimal mechanical properties and filling patterns required for optimal reinforcement need to be evaluated further. It seems that PMMA augmentation leads to a significant increase in vertebral body stiffness, thereby increasing the risk of fractures at adjacent vertebral bodies [6]. On the other hand, it does not seem reasonable to reinforce vertebrae in such manner that their mechanical properties only improve after a considerable collapse has already occurred [51]. Biodegradation is an open question: When treating osteoporotic vertebral fractures by cement augmentation, fast cement resorption without new bone formation will have a contrary effect, as the induced resorption may weaken the vertebral body and promote further collapse. It would be useful to assess the biological behavior and dynamics of biodegradation in a standardized animal model (i.e., osteoporotic sheep).

The material most appropriate for our patients will eventually be a bioactive/slowly resorbable cement with mechanical properties comparable to a healthy vertebral body (not equal to cancellous bone) with an adapted viscosity and high radiopacity, available at a reasonable price.

References

1. Ahrens J, Fuller M, Burton D, Regan J (2001) In vitro comparison of two different filler materials for vertebroplasty. Transactions of the 47th annual meeting of the Orthopaedic Research Society, San Francisco, 25–28 February 2001
2. Bai B, Jazrawi LM, Kummer FJ, Spivak JM (1999) The use of an injectable, biodegradabel Calcium Phosphate Bone Substitute for the prophylactic augmentation of osteoporotic vertebrae and the management of vertebral compression fractures. Spine 25(15):1521–1526
3. Bauwart C, Asher M, Hassanein R (1995) Iliac crest bone graft harvest donor site morbidity: a statistical evaluation. Spine 13:566–569
4. Belkoff SM, Mathis JM, Erbe EM, Fenton DC (2000) Biomechanical evaluation of a new bone cement for use in vertebroplasty. Spine 25(9):1061–1064
5. Belkoff S, Mathis J, Deramond H, Jasper L (2001) An ex vivo biomechanical evaluation of a hydroxyapatite cement for use in vertebroplasty. Transactions of the 47th annual meeting of the Orthopaedic Research Society, San Francisco, 25–28 February 2001
6. Berlemann U, Ferguson SJ, Nolte LP, Heini PF (2000) Adjacent vertebral failure following vertebroplasty: a biomechanical evaluation. J Bone Joint Surg [Br] (accepted for publication)
7. Bini SA, Gill K, Johnston JO (1995) Giant cell tumor of bone. Curettage and cement reconstruction. Clin Orthop 321:245–250
8. Boden S, Martin G, Morone M, Ugbo J, Moskovitz P (1999) Posterolateral lumbar intertransverse process spine arthrodesis with recombinant human bone morphogenetic protein-2/hydroxyapatite- tricalcium phosphate after laminectomy in the nonhuman primate. Spine 24:1179–1185
9. Boden S, Zdeblick T, Sandhu H, Heim S (2000) The use of rhBMP-2 in interbody fusion cages: definitive evidence of osteoinduction in humans: a preliminary report. Spine 25:376–380
10. Boden SD, Schimandle JH (1995) Biologic enhancement of spinal fusion. Spine 20(24S):113S–123S
11. Brown M, Malinin T, Davis P (1976) A roentgenographic evaluation of frozen allografts versus autografts in anterior cervical spine fusion. Clin Orthop 119:231–236
12. Chapman MW, Bucholz R, Cornell C (1997) Treatment of acute fractures with a collagen-calcium phosphate graft material. A randomized clinical trial. J Bone Joint Surg [Am] 79(4): 495–502
13. Cloward R (1980) Gas-sterilized cadaver bone grafts for spinal fusion operations. A simplified bone bank. Spine 5(1):4–10
14. Cockin J (1971) Autologous bone grafting complications at the donor-site. J Bone Joint Surg Br 53:253
15. Constantz BR, Ison IC, Fulmer MT, Poser RD, Smith ST, VanWagoner M, Ross J, Goldstein SA, Jupiter JB, Rosenthal DI (1995) Skeletal repair by in situ formation of the mineral phase of bone. Science 267(5205):1796–1799
16. Cotten A, Boutry N, Cortet B, Assaker R, Demondin X, Leblond D, Chastanet P, Duquesnoy B, Deramond H (1998) Percutaneous vertebroplasty: state of the art. Radiographics 18:311–320
17. Daculsi G, LeGeros R, Nery E, Lynch K, Kerebel B (1989) Transformation of biphasic calcium phosphate ceramics in vivo: ultrastructural and physicochemical characterization. J Biomed Mater Res 23:883–894
18. Dahl OE, Garvik LJ, Lyberg T (1994) Toxic effects of methylmethacrylate monomer on leukocytes and endothelial cells in vitro. Acta Orthop Scand 65(2):147–153
19. Dallap B, Gadaleta SJ, Prabhu V et al (1998) Histological, radiological and mechanical comparison of polymethylmethacrylate (PMMA) and a novel cement in an ovine model. Transactions of the 45th annual meeting of the Orthopaedic Research Society, New Orleans, 16–19 March 1998
20. Deramond H, Depriester C, Galibert P, Le Gras D (1998) Percutaneous vertebroplasty with polymethylmetacrylate. Technique, indications, and results. Radiol Clin North Am 36:533–546
21. Drake J, Rogge T, Taggard D, Goel V, Hitchon P (2001) Stability assessment of two vertebroplasty materials. Transactions of the 47th annual meeting of the Orthopaedic Research Society, San Francisco, 25–28 February 2001
22. Emery S, Fuller D, Stevenson S (1996) Ceramic anterior spinal fusion: biologic and biomechanical comparison in a canine model. Spine 21:2713–2719
23. Fernyhough J, Schimandle J, Weigel M, Edwards C, Levine A (1992) Chronic donor-site pain complicating bone graft harvesting from the posterior iliac crest for spinal fusion. Spine 17:1474–1480
24. Fujita H, Ido K, Matsuda Y et al (2000) Evaluation of bioactive bone cement in canine total hip arthroplasty. J Biomed Mater Res 49:273–288
25. Galibert P, Deramond H (1990) La vertébroplastie acrylique percutanée comme traitement des angiomes vertébraux et des affections dolorigènes et fragilisantes du rachis. Chirurgie 116:326–335
26. Galibert P, Deramond H, Rosat P, Le Gars D (1987) Note préliminaire sur le traitement des angiomes vertébraux par vertébroplastie percutanée. Neurochirurgie 33:166–168
27. Garbarsky A, Mejdoubi E, Caratero C, Lacout JL (1995) Hydraulic phosphate cement for orthopaedic and dental applications. Bull Inst Oceanogr Monaco 14(3):35–41
28. Guigui P, Plais P, Flautre B (1994) Experimental model of posterolateral spinal arthrodesis in sheep. 1. Experimental procedures and results with autologous bone graft. Spine 19:2791–2797
29. Guigui P, Plais P, Flautre B (1994) Experimental model of posterolateral spinal arthrodesis in sheep. 2. Application of the model: evaluation of vertebral fusion obtained with coral (Porites) or with a biphasic ceramic (Triosite). Spine 19:2798–2803
30. Heini PF, Kaufmann M, Angst M (1998) Effect of bone cement augmentation on the mechanical properties of human cadaveric vertebrae. Abstract presented at the Eurospine '98, Second Combined Meeting of the Leading European Spine Societies, Innsbruck, 24–27 June 1998
31. Heini PF, Berlemann U, Kaufmann M, Lippuner K, Fankhauser Ch, van Landuyt P (2001) Augmentation of mechanical properties in osteoporotic vertebral bones – a biomechanical investigation of vertebroplasty efficacy with different bone cements. Eur Spine J 10(2):164–171

32. Heini PF, Walchli B, Berlemann U (2000) Percutaneous transpedicular vertebroplasty with PMMA: operative technique and early results. A prospective study for the treatment of osteoporotic compression fractures. Eur Spine J 9(5):445–450
33. Heini PF (1998) Orthopedic aspects of vertebral metastases. Ther Umsch 55(7):418–22
34. Heise U, Osborn J, Duwe F (1990) Hydroxyapatite ceramic as a bone substitute. Int Orthop 14:329–338
35. Ikenaga M, Hardouin P, Lemaître J, Andrianjatovo H, Flautre B (1998) Biomechanical characterization of a biodegradable calcium phosphate hydraulic cement: a comparison with porous biphasic calcium phosphate ceramics. J Biomed Mater Res 40:139–144
36. Jensen ME, Evans AJ, Mathis JM, Kallmes DF, Cloft HJ, Dion J (1997) Percutaneous polymethylmethacrylate vertebroplasty in the treatment of osteoporotic vertebral body compression fractures: technical aspects. Am J Neuroradiol 18:1897–1904
37. Khairoun I, Boltong MG, Driessens FCM, Planell (1997) Effect of calcium carboanate on clinical compliance of apatitic calcium phosphate bone cement. J Biomed Mater Res 38(4): 356–360
38. Khairoun I, Driessens FCM, Boltong MG, Planell JA, Wenz R (1999) Addition of cohesion promotors to calcium phosphate cements. Biomaterials 20: 393
39. Knaack D, Goad ME, Aiolova M, Rey C, Tofighi A, Chakravarthy P, Lee DD (1998) Resorbable calcium phosphate bone substitute. J Biomed Mater Res 43(4):399–409
40. Krause WR, Park SH, Straup RA (1989) Mechanical properties of BIS-GMA resin short glass fiber composites. J Biomed Mater Res 23(10):1195–1211
41. Kurashina K, Kurita H, Hirano M, Kotani A, Klein CPAT, de Groot K (1997) In vivo study of calcium phosphate cements: implantation of an atricalcium phosphate/dicalcium phosphate dibasic/tetracalcium phosphate monoxide cement paste. Biomaterials 18:539–543
42. Lacout JL, Mejdoubi E, Hamad M (1996) Crystallization mechanism of calcium phosphate cements for biologic uses. J Materials Sci Materials Med 7:371–374
43. Le Henc J, Lesprit E, Delavigne C et al (1997) Tricalcium phosphate ceramics and allografts as bone substitutes for spinal fusion in idiopathic scoliosis: comparative clinical results at four years. Acta Orthop Belg 63:202–211
44. Lim T, Brebach GT, Renner SM, Kim WJ, Kim JG, An HS (2001) Effect of a new calcium phosphate cement on the compression strength of vertebroplasty. Transactions of the 47th annual meeting of the Orthopaedic Research Society, San Francisco, 25–28 February 2001
45. Moore D, Chapman M, Manske D (1987) The evaluation of a biphasic calcium phosphate ceramic for use in grafting long-bone diaphyseal defect. J Orthop Res 5:356–365
46. Passati N, Daculsi G, Rogez J, Martin S, Bainvel J (1989) Macroporous calcium phosphate ceramic performance in human spine fusion. Clin Orthop 248:169–176
47. Persson BM, Ekelund L, Lovdahl R, Gunterberg B (1984) Favourable results of acrylic cementation for giant cell tumors. Acta Orthop Scand 55(2):209–214
48. Saito M, Maruoka A, Mori T, Sugano N, Hino K (1994) Experimental studies on a new bioactive bone cement: hydroxyapatite composite resin. Biomaterials 15(2):156–160
49. Sandhu H, Kanim L, Toth J et al (1997) Experimental spinal fusions with recombinant human bone morphogenetic protein-2 without decortication of osseous elements. Spine 22:1171–1176
50. Sato T, Bourgeault C, Kyle R (2001) Calcium phosphate augmentation of screw fixation in femoral neck fracture. Transactions of the 47th annual meeting of the Orthopaedic Research Society, San Francisco, 25–28 February 2001
51. Schildhauer TA, Bennett AP, Wright TM, Lane JM, O'Leary PF (1999) Intravertebral body reconstruction with an injectable in situ-setting carbonated apatite: biomechanical evaluation of a minimally invasive technique. J Orthop Res 17:67–72
52. Turner A, Gillies R, Svehla M, Saito M, Walsh W (2001) Augmentation of pedicle screw fixation with a bioactive cement. Transactions of the 47th annual meeting of the Orthopaedic Research Society, San Francisco, 25–28 February 2001
53. Weill A, Chiras J, Simon JM, Rose M (1996) Spinal metastases: indications for and results of percutaneous injection of acrylic surgical cement. Radiology 199:241–247
54. Williams D (1996) Editorial. Biomaterials 17(1):1–2
55. Yamamuro T, Nakamura T, Ilida H (1998) Development of bioactive bone cement and its clincal applications. Biomaterials 19:1479–1482
56. Zdeblick T, Ducker T (1991) The use of freezedried allograft bone for anterior cervical fusions. Spine 16:726–732
57. Zerwekh J, Kourosh S, Scheinberg R (1992) Fibrillar collagen-biphasic calcium phosphate composite as a bone graft substitute for spinal fusion. J Orthop Res 10:562–572

GPSR Compliance

The European Union's (EU) General Product Safety Regulation (GPSR) is a set of rules that requires consumer products to be safe and our obligations to ensure this.

If you have any concerns about our products, you can contact us on ProductSafety@springernature.com

In case Publisher is established outside the EU, the EU authorized representative is:

Springer Nature Customer Service Center GmbH
Europaplatz 3
69115 Heidelberg, Germany

Batch number: 10684220

Printed by Printforce, the Netherlands